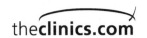

SURGICAL CLINICS
OF NORTH AMERICA

Perioperative Issues for Surgeons:
Improving Patient
Safety and Outcomes

GUEST EDITOR
Lena M. Napolitano, MD

CONSULTING EDITOR
Ronald F. Martin, MD

December 2005 • Volume 85 • Number 6

SAUNDERS

An Imprint of Elsevier, Inc.
PHILADELPHIA   LONDON   TORONTO   MONTREAL   SYDNEY   TOKYO

W.B. SAUNDERS COMPANY
A Division of Elsevier Inc.

1600 John F. Kennedy Blvd., Suite 1800, Philadelphia, PA 19103-2899

http://www.theclinics.com

SURGICAL CLINICS OF NORTH AMERICA
December 2005
Editor: Catherine Bewick

Volume 85, Number 6
ISSN 0039–6109
ISBN 1-4160-2795-5

Reprints. For copies of 100 or more of articles in this publication, please contact the commercial Reprints Department Elsevier Inc., 360 Park Avenue South, New York, New York 10010-1710. Tel. (212) 633-3813, Fax: (212) 462-1935, email: reprints@elsevier.com

The ideas and opinions expressed in *The Surgical Clinics of North America* do not necessarily reflect those of the Publisher. The Publisher does not assume any responsibility for any injury and/or damage to persons or property arising out of or related to any use of the material contained in this periodical. The reader is advised to check the appropriate medical literature and the product information currently provided by the manufacturer of each drug to be administered to verify the dosage, the method and duration of administration, or contraindications. It is the responsibility of the treating physician or other health care professional, relying on independent experience and knowledge of the patient, to determine drug dosages and the best treatment for the patient. Mention of any product in this issue should not be construed as endorsement by the contributors, editors, or the Publisher of the product or manufacturers' claims.

Surgical Clinics of North America (ISSN 0039–6109) is published bimonthly by Elsevier; Corporate and editorial Offices: 1600 John F. Kennedy Blvd., Suite 1800, Philadelphia, PA 19103-2899. Accounting and circulation offices: 6277 Sea Harbor Drive, Orlando, FL 32887-4800. Periodicals postage paid at Orlando, FL 32862, and additional mailing offices. Subscription prices are $200.00 per year for US individuals, $315.00 per year for US institutions, $100.00 per year for US students and residents, $245.00 per year for Canadian individuals, $385.00 per year for Canadian institutions, $260.00 for international individuals, $385.00 for international institutions and $130.00 per year for Canadian and foreign students/residents. To receive student/resident rate, orders must be accompanied by name of affiliated institution, date of term, and the *signature* of program/residency coordinator on institution letterhead. Orders will be billed at individual rate until proof of status is received. Foreign air speed delivery is included in all *Clinics* subscription prices. All prices are subject to change without notice. POSTMASTER: Send address changes to *The Surgical Clinics of North America*, W.B. Saunders Company, Periodicals Fulfillment, Orlando, FL 32887-4800. **Customer Service: 1-800-654-2452 (US). From outside of the US, call 1-407-345-1000.**

The Surgical Clinics of North America is also published in Spanish by McGraw-Hill Interamericana Editores S.A., P.O. Box 5-237 06500 Mexico D.F. Mexico; and in Portuguese by Interlivros Edicoes Ltda., Rua Comandante Coelho 1085, CEP 21250, Rio de Janeiro, Brazil; and in Greek by Paschalidis Medical Publications, Athens Greece.

The Surgical Clinics of North America is covered in *Index Medicus, EMBASE/Excerpta Medica, Current Contents/Clinical Medicine, Current Contents/Life Sciences, Science Citation Index*, and *ISI/BIOMED*.

Printed in the United States of America.

CONSULTING EDITOR

RONALD F. MARTIN, MD, Staff Surgeon, Department of Surgery, Marshfield Clinic, Marshfield, Wisconsin; Clinical Associate Professor of Surgery, University of Vermont, Burlington, Vermont; Lieutenant Colonel, Medical Corps, United States Army Reserve

GUEST EDITOR

LENA M. NAPOLITANO, MD, FACS, FCCP, FCCM, Professor of Surgery, Chief, Surgical Critical Care, Associate Chair of Surgery for Critical Care, Department of Surgery, University of Michigan Health System, University Hospital, Ann Arbor, Michigan

CONTRIBUTORS

MARIA D. ALLO, MD, FACS, FCCM, Chairperson, Department of Surgery, Santa Clara Valley Medical Center, San Jose California; Chief, Division of General Surgery, and Clinical Professor of Surgery, Stanford University, Stanford, California

DANIEL A. ANAYA, MD, Resident in General Surgery, Department of Surgery, University of Washington, Seattle, Washington

PHILIP S. BARIE, MD, MBA, FCCM, FACS, Professor of Surgery and Public Health, Division of Critical Care and Trauma, Weill Medical College of Cornell University, New York, New York

BARBARA L. BASS, MD, FACS, Carolyn and John F. Bookout, Distinguished Endowed Chair, Department of Surgery, The Methodist Hospital, Houston, Texas; Professor of Surgery, Weill Medical College, Cornell University, Ithaca, New York

MIKE BELKIN, MD, Associate Professor of Surgery and Chief, Division of Vascular Surgery, Brigham and Women's Hospital, Harvard Medical School, Boston, Massachusetts

RAMON BERGUER, MD, Clinical Professor of Surgery, University of California Davis, Sacramento, California; Chief of Surgery, Contra Costa Regional Medical Center, Martinez, California

BRENNAN J. CARMODY, MD, FACS, Clinical Instructor in Surgery, General Surgery Division, Virginia Commonwealth University, Richmond, Virginia

MIRJAM CHRIST-CRAIN, MD, Senior Registrar, Clinic of Endocrinology, Diabetes and Clinical Nutrition, University Hospital Basel, Basel, Switzerland

MITCHELL JAY COHEN, MD, Clinical Instructor, Department of Surgery, University of California San Francisco, San Francisco General Hospital, San Francisco, California

T. FORCHT DAGI, MD, MPH, FACS, FCCM, Division of Health Sciences and Technology, The Harvard-MIT Program in Health Sciences and Technology; Department of Surgery, The Uniformed Services University of the Health Sciences, Newton Center, Massachusetts

ERIC J. DeMARIA, MD, FACS, Professor of Surgery and Chairman, General Surgery Division, Virginia Commonwealth University, Richmond, Virginia

DEV M. DESAI, MD, PhD, Assistant Professor of Surgery, Division of General and Transplant Surgery, Department of Surgery, Duke University School of Medicine, Durham, North Carolina

SOUMITRA R. EACHEMPATI, MD, FACS, Associate Professor of Surgery, Division of Critical Care and Trauma, Weill Medical College of Cornell University, New York, New York

BRENDA G. FAHY, MD, Professor of Anesthesiology, Director of Critical Care, University of Kentucky Chandler Medical Center, Lexington, Kentucky

VERNA C. GIBBS, MD, Professor of Clinical Surgery, Department of Surgery QI Program, University of California at San Francisco, San Francisco; Attending Surgeon, San Francisco Veterans Affairs Medical Center, San Francisco, California

ZAKI-UDIN HASSAN, MD, Assistant Professor of Anesthesiology, University of Kentucky Chandler Medical Center, Lexington, Kentucky

TRACI L. HEDRICK, MD, Resident Physician, Department of Surgery, University of Virginia Health System, Charlottesville, Virginia

KATHLEEN M. HEINTZ, DO, Assistant Professor of Medicine, Division of Cardiology and Critical Care Medicine, Cooper University Hospital, Robert Wood Johnson Medical School, Camden, New Jersey

PAUL J. HELLER, MD, Veterans Administration Connecticut Healthcare System, Anesthesia Service, West Haven, Connecticut

STEVEN M. HOLLENBERG, MD, Professor of Medicine, Division of Cardiology and Critical Care Medicine, Cooper University Hospital, Robert Wood Johnson Medical School, Camden, New Jersey

BRANNON R. HYDE, MD, Department of Surgery, The University of Texas Medical Branch, Galveston, Texas

RAYMOND J. JOEHL, MD, FACS, Professor of Surgery, Loyola University Medical Center, Maywood, Illinois; Chief, Surgical Service, and Manager, Surgery Service Line, Edward Hines, Jr. Veterans Administration Hospital, Hines, Illinois

PAUL C. KUO, MD, MBA, Professor and Chief, Division of General and Transplant Surgery, Vice-Chair for Research, Department of Surgery, Duke University School of Medicine, Durham, North Carolina

DAVID B. LORAN, MD, Department of Surgery, The University of Texas Medical Branch, Galveston, Texas

PAUL M. MAGGIO, MD, Assistant Professor of Surgery, Division of Trauma Burn/Critical Care, Department of Surgery, University of Michigan Health System, University Hospital, Ann Arbor, Michigan

LENA M. NAPOLITANO, MD, FACS, FCCP, FCCM, Professor of Surgery, Chief, Surgical Critical Care, Associate Chair of Surgery for Critical Care, Department of Surgery, University of Michigan Health System, University Hospital, Ann Arbor, Michigan

AVERY B. NATHENS, MD, MPH, Associate Professor, Department of Surgery, University of Washington; Division of General and Trauma Surgery, Harborview Medical Center, Seattle, Washington

CHRISTOPHER D. OWENS, MD, Vascular Surgery Fellow, Brigham and Women's Hospital, Harvard Medical School, Boston, Massachusetts

HIRAM C. POLK, Jr, MD, Professor of Surgery, Department of Surgery, University of Louisville School of Medicine, Louisville, Kentucky

H. DAVID REINES, MD, FACS, Vice Chairman, Department of Surgery, Inova Fairfax Hospital, Falls Church, Virginia; Professor of Surgery, Virginia Commonwealth University, Falls Church, Virginia

ROBERT G. SAWYER, MD, Associate Professor, Departments of Surgery and Health Evaluation Sciences, University of Virginia Health System, Charlottesville, Virginia

WILLIAM P. SCHECTER, MD, FACS, Professor and Vice-Chair, University of California San Francisco; Chief of Surgery, San Francisco General Hospital, San Francisco, California

PATRICIA C. SEIFERT, RN, MSN, FAAN, Cardiac Care Coordinator, Cardiovascular Operating Room, Inova Heart and Vascular Institute, Falls Church, Virginia

PAUL A. TAHERI, MD, Associate Professor of Surgery, Chief, Division of Trauma Burn/Critical Care, Department of Surgery, University of Michigan Health System, University Hospital, Ann Arbor, Michigan

MAUREEN TEDESCO, MD, Resident in Surgery, Stanford University, Stanford, California

MATTHIAS TURINA, MD, Ferguson Research Fellow, Price Institute of Surgical Research, Department of Surgery, University of Louisville School of Medicine, Louisville, Kentucky

KAREN STANLEY WILLIAMS, MD, Associate Professor of Anesthesiology, Department of Anesthesiology and Critical Care, George Washington University Medical Center, Washington, District of Columbia

JOSEPH B. ZWISCHENBERGER, MD, Professor of Surgery, Medicine and Radiology, Director General of Thoracic Surgery, Department of Surgery, The University of Texas Medical Branch, Galveston, Texas

CONTENTS

This article reviews evidence supporting the exercise of risk assessment and demonstrates how it assists in determining which patients should undergo a planned invasive procedure. The article focuses on the preoperative functional assessment of three major organ systems—cardiac, pulmonary, and renal–and reviews guidelines for determining which patients need additional testing of organ system function. The article also discusses how to improve the condition of selected patients so that the surgeon can achieve the best possible result and outcome.

Advances in technology and pharmacology continue to change techniques for anesthesia. So-called "fast-track" anesthesia has led to the development of new anesthetic agents and changes in anesthetic practice, including the increased use of regional anesthesia, techniques involving continuous plexus catheters to improve postoperative analgesia, and total intravenous anesthesia. Technological advances now provide additional options for airway management when a difficult airway is encountered. Advances have also produced additional intraoperative monitoring through the use of depth-of-anesthesia monitors and transesophageal echocardiography. Future areas of development are likely to include target-controlled infusion pumps as well as techniques and medications that improve fast-track anesthesia safely.

Perioperative Issues: Myocardial Ischemia and Protection – Beta-Blockade

Paul M. Maggio and Paul A. Taheri

Approximately one third of patients undergoing noncardiac surgery have coronary artery disease, and cardiovascular complications are an important cause of perioperative morbidity and mortality. Several algorithms are available to assess the risk for perioperative cardiac events. Although preoperative risk assessment is useful in identifying patients at greatest risk for cardiac complications, recent investigations have provided additional guidance in choosing interventions to improve perioperative outcomes. These investigations show that perioperative beta-blockers significantly reduce morbidity and mortality in noncardiac surgery and appear to offer the greatest benefit to high-risk patients. Because of the lower complication rate in intermediate- and low-risk patients and the absence of large randomized controlled trials, the role of beta-blockers in this population is less well-defined.

Perioperative Cardiac Issues: Postoperative Arrhythmias

Kathleen M. Heintz and Steven M. Hollenberg

This article reviews current concepts about the diagnosis and acute management of postoperative arrhythmias. A systematic approach to diagnosis of arrhythmias and evaluation of predisposing factors is presented, followed by consideration of common bradyarrhythmias and tachyarrhythmias in the postoperative setting. Postoperative arrhythmias are common and represent a major source of morbidity after surgical procedures, both cardiac and noncardiac. Postoperative dysrhythmias are most likely to occur in patients with structural heart disease. The initiating factor for an arrhythmia following surgery is usually a transient insult such as hypoxemia, cardiac ischemia, catecholamine excess, or electrolyte abnormality. Management includes correction of these imbalances and, if clinically indicated, medical therapy directed at the arrhythmia itself.

Surgical Site Infections

Philip S. Barie and Soumitra R. Eachempati

This article examines the epidemiology and risk factors for the development of surgical site infections (SSIs), the importance of appropriate administration of prophylactic antibiotics, nonpharmacologic strategies, and the role of new "active" devices in reducing SSIs. A review of the pertinent English-language literature shows that many factors contribute to the risk of a patient developing an SSI. These include the patient's health status, preparation of the patient before surgery, and the use of appropriate antibiotic prophylaxis. Careful preparation of the patient and care after surgery is especially important. The use of new "active" antibacterial devices may reduce risk further. Surgeons can minimize the risk to the patient of the development of SSI through strict adherence to established surgical guidelines for perioperative care.

Health-Care–Associated Infections and Prevention
Traci L. Hedrick and Robert G. Sawyer

Health-care-associated infections (HAIs) are an important cause of perioperative morbidity and mortality. Currently, one out of every 10 surgical patients develops an HAI. Causes of HAIs vary, but include the transient immunodeficiency associated with surgery, immobility, and the presence of indwelling devices. With rates of antimicrobial resistance increasing, prevention remains the best solution. The investigators review the most frequently encountered health-care–associated infections with an emphasis on preventative strategies. The article addresses issues related to the diagnosis, treatment, and prevention of health-care–related pneumonia, health-care–associated urinary tract infections, and intravascular-catheter–related infections. The article also discusses the utility of hand hygiene policies.

Impact of Diabetes Mellitus and Metabolic Disorders
Matthias Turina, Mirjam Christ-Crain, and Hiram C. Polk, Jr

Metabolic and endocrine disorders are common in the perioperative surgical patient. During surgical stress and critical illness, each hormonal system reveals characteristic changes that can be of diagnostic and prognostic significance. A number of endocrinopathies, electrolyte problems, or metabolic derangements may either preexist or develop during the course of surgical treatment. Early correction and tight control of blood glucose levels was shown to improve outcome in critically ill surgical patients. However, many other pharmacological interventions to correct endocrine alterations in critical illness have proven unsuccessful, most likely because of the many overlapping actions between the endocrine and immune systems, and are not standard of care in surgical patients.

Thrombosis and Coagulation: Deep Vein Thrombosis and Pulmonary Embolism Prophylaxis
Daniel A. Anaya and Avery B. Nathens

Venous thromboembolism (deep venous thrombosis and pulmonary embolism, VTE) is a common complication in surgical patients and is the primary cause of preventable deaths in hospitalized patients. Despite well-known risk factors, VTE prophylaxis is frequently not practiced according to recommended guidelines. Patients can readily be stratified according to their risk of perioperative VTE, and mechanical and pharmacologic prophylactic regimens can be tailored to their individual risk. Pharmacologic VTE prophylaxis should be the standard of care in most clinical settings given its ease of administration, low risk, and cost-effectiveness.

The surgical management of the anticoagulated patient requires an understanding of the fundamentals of blood thrombosis, the mechanisms that enable anticoagulants to work, and the indications for anticoagulation. As percutaneous cardiac and peripheral procedures become increasingly sophisticated, we can expect to encounter more patients on aspirin and clopidogrel. Management strategies will require continued appraisal of available literature for evidence-based surgical practice. This article summarizes how coagulation takes place and explains the role of certain agents that alter coagulation, such as aspirin, clopidogrel, warfarin, heparin and low-molecular-weight heparin. The article also discusses thrombosis risks involving patients with nonvalvular atrial fibrillation, patients with mechanical heart valves and patients with a history of deep vein thrombosis.

This article addresses the management of postoperative bleeding. The problem is called postoperative bleeding rather than postoperative hemorrhage to emphasize the fact that perfect postoperative hemostasis rather than acceptable postoperative blood loss is the ideal. Postoperative bleeding is a risk of all surgical procedures. The best way to reduce the risk of hemorrhage is to identify and correct potential causes of coagulopathy both pre- and post-operatively.

Perioperative anemia is common and is associated with increased need for blood transfusion in the perioperative period. Perioperative anemia has also been linked to increased morbidity and mortality in surgical patients. Anemia may impede a patient's ability to recover fully and participate in postoperative rehabilitation. Preoperative treatment of anemia is associated with a reduction in the need for blood transfusion in the perioperative period. Additional advances in surgical technology that reduce blood loss intraoperatively are associated with a reduction in postoperative anemia and should be used whenever possible. All strategies to prevent anemia in the perioperative period should be considered in an effort to minimize exposure of surgical patients to blood transfusion.

pharmacologic therapies. The toxicity profile of these therapies can strongly influence the decision algorithms for delivering care in the perioperative period. In this manuscript, the investigators describe the potential effects of drugs commonly used for treatment of patients with cancer, HIV, or transplanted organs, and the impact of these drugs on the care of these patients in the perioperative setting. The article addresses such topics as cardiotoxicity, pulmonary toxicity, hepatotoxicity, genitourinary toxicity, neurotoxicity, myelosuppression, cutaneous toxicity, mitochondrial toxicity, lipodystrophy, hypersensitivity, and liver dysfunction. The article also describes the use of corticosteroids, calcineurin inhibitors, sirolimus, and antimetabolites.

Surgeons and hospitals must be aware of the special considerations for treating obese patients. Obesity involves increased incidence of several comorbidities, such as coronary heart disease and hypertension, which increase perioperative risk. Obesity has been identified as an independent risk factor for surgical site infection and the obese population has a higher than normal incidence of perioperative deep venous thrombosis and pulmonary embolism. For these and other reasons, medical professionals must make thorough evaluations to properly identify and address medical comorbidities and other issues associated with obese patients. Medical professionals must, for example, use invasive arterial monitoring for severely obese patients and ensure that operating room tables can accommodate obese patients.

An operating room's condition is rarely directly implicated in disease transmission. Even so, to prevent such rare transmissions, hospitals must be thoughtful in designing operating rooms as important adjuncts to infection control. Proper ventilation in and near the operating room is the single most important component in establishing an environment that stops the spread of infection. Other considerations include attention to traffic control, equipment maintenance and storage, and construction materials that enhance the ability to maintain clean rooms. Hospitals can avert potential infectious problems through preventive maintenance and the use of infection control risk assessments (ICRAs) for pre-emptive consideration of infectious risks before renovations, repairs and new construction. Guidelines should be consulted and incorporated into each operating room's policies and procedures.

FORTHCOMING ISSUES

RECENT ISSUES

The Clinics are now available online!

www.theclinics.com

SURGICAL
CLINICS OF
NORTH AMERICA

Surg Clin N Am 85 (2005) xvii–xviii

Foreword

Perioperative Issues for Surgeons: Improving Patient Safety and Outcomes

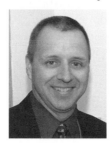

Ronald F. Martin, MD
Consulting Editor

This issue of the *Surgical Clinics of North America* deals with the perioperative concerns of our patients. It covers a wide range of topics from hospital systems issues to specific medical concerns of varying subsets of patients. This issue once again underscores the importance of the surgeon understanding the system in which he or she works. The complexity of the patients we care for is increasing and will likely continue to do so for the balance of our careers.

The days when surgeons could (at least according to lore) control everything about their working environment are gone. In fact, many surgeons faced with increasing responsibilities for increased "productivity," decreasing reimbursement, and an increasing desire for shorter hours have opted to delegate many of the responsibilities that used to be ours. Preoperative "clearance" is something one gets from a medical colleague; total parenteral nutrition is managed by the Metabolic Support Service; operative instruments and supplies are purchased in consolidated contracts. Although it is not necessarily the best use of a surgeon's time to personally tend to every detail of a patient's hospitalization or care, we still are responsible for the end result. For better or worse, patients tend to give us more credit than we deserve when things go well and place most of the blame on us when they do not. Ironically, many surgeons are fine with the former and indignant at the latter.

doi:10.1016/j.suc.2005.10.001

There is a fine line between delegation of responsibility and abdication of responsibility. A similar fine line exists between being a rugged individualist and a prima donna who is incapable of being a "team player." With so many competing needs evolving in hospital systems, it is incumbent upon us to know how we fit into the overall system. Because many of these matters have the potential to become confrontational, it is always of value to understand the needs of potential "competitors" for resources and to speak their language. There are few things that will quell the ire of a surgeon whose requests are denied by administration as much as making that surgeon part of the administration and saying, "Show us how."

On the medical side of perioperative patient issues, it remains an imperative that we discuss our plans with our colleagues as directly as possible. As the complexity and types of procedures and operations we perform increases, it becomes more clear how little nonsurgeons really understand what we can and cannot do. It is only through continued education of ourselves and others that we will keep the system working smoothly.

Despite the fact that we are greatly pressed for time, I would urge us all to participate in those matters that contribute to running effective hospital and prehospital systems as much as we can. We may not get paid for it, but we will certainly be rewarded—and so will our patients. This issue that Dr. Napolitano and her colleagues have contributed will serve as an excellent source of information for us to help our patients and one another.

Ronald F. Martin, MD
Department of Surgery
Marshfield Clinic
1000 North Oak Avenue
Marshfield, WI 54449, USA

E-mail address: martin.ronald@marshfieldclinic.org

ELSEVIER
SAUNDERS

SURGICAL
CLINICS OF
NORTH AMERICA

Surg Clin N Am 85 (2005) xix–xx

Preface

Perioperative Issues for Surgeons: Improving Patient Safety and Outcomes

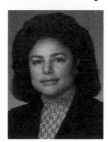

Lena M. Napolitano, MD
Guest Editor

Optimal perioperative (pre- and postoperative) care of the patient undergoing surgery is ultimately linked to optimal patient outcome.

Millions of patients undergo surgery each year. Approximately 300,000 patients in the United States and 500,000 patients worldwide undergo coronary artery bypass surgeries (the most common cardiac surgical procedure) annually. Similarly, approximately 400,000 total knee replacements and over 300,000 hip replacements are performed each year in the United States. The number of patients who undergo bariatric surgery more than quadrupled between 1998 and 2002 (from 13,386 to 71,733), with part of the increase driven by a 900% increase in operations on older patients between the ages of 55 and 64.

Surgical procedures are commonly performed in older patients with significant comorbidities. By the year 2030, it is estimated that 20% of Americans will be older than 65, while one out of four elderly individuals will be older than 85 years of age. According to recent estimates, 50% of those over age 65 will undergo surgery as compared with only 12% of those aged 45 to 60 years. Despite the higher numbers of elderly patients having surgery, mortality and morbidity rates have been on the decline, in part due to significant advances in perioperative care.

Recent studies have also shown a decline in the perioperative mortality rates in all age groups. Advances in surgical and anesthetic techniques combined with sophisticated perioperative monitoring and critical care

doi:10.1016/j.suc.2005.10.002   *surgical.theclinics.com*

management are factors that have contributed to improved perioperative patient outcomes. An evidence-based approach to achieve optimal perioperative care can therefore ultimately impact on improved outcome in millions of patients undergoing surgery annually in the United States.

In this issue of the *Surgical Clinics of North America*, the fundamental strategies for optimal perioperative care are reviewed. The preoperative assessment of the surgical patient should begin well in advance of the anticipated surgical date. A preoperative assessment is useful to identify factors associated with increased risks of specific complications and initiation of a management plan that minimizes these risks. Appropriate prophylaxis strategies (including deep venous thrombosis prophylaxis and strategies for prevention of surgical site infection) are necessary in almost all patients. Optimal intraoperative care includes several safety initiatives that are discussed in detail. Postoperative care strategies (including pain control, prevention and treatment of nausea and vomiting, clinical pathways) are essential. Prevention of postoperative complications (cardiac, infectious) can be achieved with multidisciplinary efforts. Finally, research to more critically examine risk-adjusted surgical patient outcomes is underway.

I would like to thank the authors for generously contributing their time and expertise in the preparation of this issue. I would also like to acknowledge Catherine Bewick of Elsevier for her tireless support and assistance in bringing this issue to completion. I hope that this issue serves as a timely and current reference to assist in the provision of evidence-based perioperative care to surgical patients in an effort to ultimately improve patient outcomes.

Lena M. Napolitano, MD
Department of Surgery
University of Michigan Medical Center
1500 E. Medical Center Drive
1C340 University Hospital, Box 0033
Ann Arbor, MI 48109-0033, USA

E-mail address: lenan@umich.edu

ELSEVIER
SAUNDERS

SURGICAL
CLINICS OF
NORTH AMERICA

Surg Clin N Am 85 (2005) 1061–1073

Preoperative Evaluation: Pulmonary, Cardiac, Renal Dysfunction and Comorbidities

Raymond J. Joehl, MD[a,b,*]

[a]Loyola University Medical Center, 2160 South First Avenue, Maywood, IL 60153, USA
[b]Edward Hines, Jr. VA Hospital, Fifth Avenue and Roosevelt Road,
P.O. Box 5000, Hines, IL 60141, USA

As physicians and surgeons, we are interested in improving our patients' general well-being. When we recommend a surgical procedure, we expect a good outcome. Stated differently, we recommend invasive procedures and operations to our patients when we have a reasonable expectation that, by excising a tumor, removing the source of inflammation or infection, or by performing a reconstructive procedure to improve organ-system function or the patient's functional status, we will improve the patient's overall condition. We also recommend surgery when we know that the benefits of the operation or intervention far outweigh the associated risk of the procedure. Additionally, to ensure the best possible result and outcome, we are interested in minimizing complications that are known to occur with a given procedure.

Our knowledge and experience help us select those patients who are best suited for an operation or who will likely have the best result and outcome. The process of selecting the best candidates for an operation has many facets, including an initial patient assessment and identification of patient characteristics that affect outcome. This selection process is an exercise in risk assessment. Often, by optimizing the patient's condition, surgeons can achieve the best possible result and outcome. Furthermore, surgeons may find after this risk assessment that the risks of the procedure outweigh the benefits. Surgeons thus may not recommend an invasive procedure, especially if it is unusually complex and risky.

* Surgical Service (112), Edward Hines, Jr. Hospital (VA Hines Hospital), Fifth Avenue and Roosevelt Road, P.O. Box 5000 Hines, IL 60141.
 E-mail address: raymond.joehl@med.va.gov

0039-6109/05/$ - see front matter. Published by Elsevier Inc.
doi:10.1016/j.suc.2005.09.015
surgical.theclinics.com

In this article, the author reviews evidence supporting this exercise of risk assessment and demonstrates how it assists in the selection of patients who should undergo the planned invasive procedure. The author focuses on the preoperative functional assessment of three major organ systems—cardiac, pulmonary, and renal—and reviews guidelines for determining which patients need additional testing of organ system function. As for which additional tests would further clarify or complete the risk assessment, the author leaves these determinations to the medical and cardiology consultants who evaluate specific patients.

Preoperative cardiac risk assessment

In approaching preoperative cardiac risk assessment, four facts must be recognized:

1. As many as one third of surgical patients have significant coronary artery disease.
2. Patients with known peripheral vascular disease and those over age 60 years have increased risk of perioperative cardiac events.
3. operations associated with major extra-cellular fluid shifts or prolonged operating times have increased cardiac risk.
4. Vascular, thoracic, upper abdominal, and major orthopedic open procedures are associated with the highest cardiac risk.

In the Department of Veterans Affairs surgical database of more than 80,000 veterans reported in 1995, cardiac complications were prevalent in this older population. The overall 30-day mortality rate was 3.1% and cardiac complications occurred in 4.5%, with myocardial infarction occurring in 0.7%, cardiopulmonary resuscitation required in 1.5%, and 2.3% experiencing pulmonary edema [1]. Thus, estimation of perioperative cardiac risk and efforts to minimize that risk may eliminate postoperative cardiac complications.

Preoperative cardiac evaluations clearly provide benefits resulting in improved morbidity and mortality. Information learned from a cardiac risk assessment helps in providing informed consent to patients, may assist in improving a patient's condition to lower the risk of perioperative morbidity and mortality, and assists the surgeon in selecting the best candidates for an operation. On the other hand, additional testing associated with cardiac risk assessment may be unnecessary, ineffective or harmful, or may delay surgical treatment, which may lead to a decline of a patient's physical or emotional condition. However, clinical cardiac risk screening via a thoughtful history of exercise tolerance and level of daily physical activity can stratify patients into low- and high-risk categories, making it possible to accurately identify those patients in the intermediate- or high-risk categories who might benefit from noninvasive or invasive cardiac testing [2].

The challenge to surgeons and their medical colleagues is to identify those patients who need perioperative cardiac risk assessment. Many patients do not require cardiac evaluation. For example, evidence does not support an in-depth cardiac evaluation for patients who are having minor surgery under local anesthesia and who have no pre-existing medical problems, or who have had recent normal cardiac studies and no new symptoms [3]. Certainly, however, other noncardiac problems (eg, pulmonary, renal, neurological problems) may need to be addressed before surgery in these patients.

The process of cardiac risk assessment begins with a thorough history and physical examination. Specific items to include in the history are listed in Box 1.

Significant abnormalities on baseline diagnostic tests include ECG abnormalities, signs of pulmonary edema on chest radiograph, abnormal blood tests, and abnormal blood. Table 1 shows a modified cardiac risk index, which stratifies patients into low-, intermediate- and high-risk categories [4].

The American College of Cardiology and the American Heart Association (ACC/AHA) recently published an update to the Guideline for Perioperative Cardiovascular Evaluation for Noncardiac Surgery [5]. Clinical predictors of increased perioperative cardiovascular risk compiled in the guideline are listed in Box 2. Implementation of the ACC/AHA guidelines

---

Box 1. Information for patient's history in assessing cardiac risk

- the patient's age
- history of myocardial infarction
- previous coronary revascularization
- episodes of congestive heart failure
- cerebrovascular disease
- hypertension
- heart murmur
- diabetes
- lung disease
- type of surgery indicated (emergency or not)
- anesthesia type
- previous problems with surgery or anesthesia

Physical findings of significance include:
- abnormal heart rate and rhythm
- abnormal blood pressure
- jugular venous distension
- presence of an S3 heart sound
- heart murmur
- signs of obstructive pulmonary disease
- presence of peripheral vascular disease

Table 1
Modified cardiac risk index

Assessment	Variable	Points
History	Emergency surgery	10
	Age>70 years	5
	MI<6 months ago	20
	MI>6 months ago	10
	Angina class[a]	
	Class III	10
	Class IV	20
Physical examination	Suspected critical aortic stenosis	20
History and laboratory	Poor general medical status, defined as any of:	
	pO_2<60 mmHg, pCO_2>50 mmHg, K^+<3 mmol/L	5
	BUN>50 mmol/L, creatinine>2 mg/dL, bedridden	5
Electrocardiogram	Arrhythmias	
	rhythm other than sinus or sinus plus atrial premature beats	5
	>5 premature ventricular contractions	5
Chest radiograph	Alveolar pulmonary edema	
	Within 1 week	10
	Ever	5
Total: add points		

Class I, 0–15 points represent low-to-intermediate risk; class II, 16–30 points; class III, >30 points. Classes II and III represent high-risk categories.

Abbreviations: BUN, blood urea nitrogen; MI, myocardial infarction; pCO_2, partial pressure of carbon dioxide; pO_2, partial pressure of oxygen.

[a] Canadian Cardiovascular Society classification of angina: 0, asymptomatic; I, angina with strenuous exercise; II, angina with moderate exertion; III, angina with walking one-to-two blocks or climbing one flight of stairs or less at a normal pace; IV, inability to perform any physical activity without developing angina.

Adapted from Detsky AS, Abrams HB, McLaughlin JR, et al. Predicting cardiac complications in patients undergoing non-cardiac surgery. J Gen Intern Med 1986;1:211–9; with permission.

for cardiac risk assessment before noncardiac surgery in an internal medicine preoperative assessment clinic led to a more appropriate use of preoperative stress testing and beta-blocker therapy while preserving a low rate of cardiac complications [6].

Once a patient's risk is determined, then decisions regarding further diagnostic testing can be made. For example, patients with intermediate risk might need further clarification of risk and additional testing, depending on the type of planned operation. For example, total hip arthroplasty, a high-risk procedure, might call for further clarification of risk, while a cataract extraction, a low-risk procedure, would not. The classification of cardiac risk stratification for noncardiac surgical procedures is listed in Box 3. Patients at high risk, such as a patient with a murmur of aortic stenosis, which carries great risk, will definitely need additional testing, such as echocardiography [7], dipyridamole myocardial stress perfusion imaging [8], traditional exercise stress testing [9], or coronary angiography [10].

Box 2. Clinical predictors of increased perioperative cardiovascular risk leading to myocardial infarction, heart failure, or death

Major
1. Unstable coronary syndromes
   - Acute or recent myocardial infarction with evidence of important ischemic risk by clinical symptoms or noninvasive study
   - Unstable or severe angina (Canadian class III or IV)
2. Decompensated heart failure
3. Significant arrhythmias
   - High-grade atrioventricular block
   - Symptomatic ventricular arrhythmias in the presence of underlying heart disease
   - Supraventricular arrhythmias with uncontrolled ventricular rate
4. Severe valvular disease

Intermediate
1. Mild angina pectoris (Canadian class I or II)
2. Previous myocardial infarction by history or pathological evidence
3. Q waves
4. Compensated or prior heart failure
5. Diabetes mellitus (particularly insulin-dependent)
6. Renal insufficiency

Minor
1. Advanced age
2. Abnormal ECG (eg, left ventricular hypertrophy, left bundle branch block, ST-T abnormalities)
3. Rhythm other than sinus (eg, atrial fibrillation)
4. Low functional capacity (eg, inability to climb one flight of stairs with a bag of groceries)
5. History of stroke
6. Uncontrolled systemic hypertension

Data from Eagle KA, Berger PB, Calkins, et al. ACC/AHA guideline update for perioperative cardiovascular evaluation for noncardiac surgery—executive summary. A report of the American Heart Association Task Force on Practice Guidelines (Committee to Update the 1966 Guidelines on Perioperative Cardiovascular Evaluation for Noncardiac Surgery). Anesth Analg 2002;94:1052–64.

Box 3. Cardiac risk[a] stratification for noncardiac surgical procedures

High (reported cardiac risk often >5%)
- Emergent major operations, particularly in the elderly
- Aortic and other major vascular surgery
- Peripheral vascular surgery
- Anticipated prolonged surgical procedures associated with large fluid shifts and blood loss

Intermediate (reported cardiac risk generally <5%)
- Carotid endarterectomy
- Head and neck surgery
- Intraperitoneal and intrathoracic surgery
- Orthopedic surgery
- Prostate surgery

Low (reported cardiac risk generally <1%)
- Endoscopic procedures
- Superficial procedure
- Cataract surgery
- Breast surgery

---

[a] Combined incidence of cardiac death and nonfatal myocardial infarction.

Data from Eagle KA, Berger PB, Calkins, et al. ACC/AHA guideline update for perioperative cardiovascular evaluation for noncardiac surgery—executive summary. A report of the American Heart Association Task Force on Practice Guidelines (Committee to Update the 1966 Guidelines on Perioperative Cardiovascular Evaluation for Noncardiac Surgery). Anesth Analg 2002;94: 1052–64.

Interventions to decrease high perioperative cardiac risk are especially necessary in patients for whom the high cardiac risk poses a greater threat to the patient's livelihood than that posed by the noncardiac surgical problem. Stated differently, treating the cardiac condition is more urgent than treating the noncardiac surgical condition. Ultimately, the decision to undergo a cardiac intervention (eg, angioplasty, stenting) or coronary revascularization should be based on the same clinical grounds that determine the need for these interventions in the nonoperative setting.

Consideration for other interventions to optimize cardiac function should also be given to the patient at high risk for cardiac complications. Beta-blocker therapy will reduce mortality and other nonfatal cardiac events in patients at risk or who have known coronary artery disease, or those patients who are older than 65 years of age and who have hypertension, diabetes, or elevated cholesterol [11]. Use of perioperative pulmonary artery catheterization to monitor hemodynamic status is helpful to improve cardiac function and reduce complications in patients who have history of congestive heart failure, who will sustain significant blood loss during the procedure (eg, hip arthroplasty), or who will sustain significant fluid shifts because of prolonged operating time (eg, Whipple procedure) [12]. Perioperative epidural anesthesia in patients with hip fractures reduces cardiac events and complications significantly [13]. Maintaining normal body temperature perioperatively in elderly patients undergoing major surgery reduces postoperative morbid cardiac events [14].

Preoperative pulmonary risk assessment

Pulmonary complications are as likely as cardiac complications to cause perioperative mortality and to prolong hospital confinement [15]. In a case-control study of patients having elective abdominal aortic surgery, pulmonary complications were 2.6 times more common than cardiac complications. Also, pulmonary complications were more likely to be severe, and mortality was equally likely to be from pulmonary as from cardiac complications. Also, in another study of patients age 70 years or older with pulmonary complications, only pulmonary and renal complications predicted long-term mortality during 2 years of follow-up [16]. Therefore, surgeons must determine the risk of postoperative pulmonary complications as part of routine preoperative evaluation. By doing so, surgeons identify patients who may benefit from strategies to reduce risk of clinically significant pulmonary complications, including pneumonia, atelectasis, bronchospasm, prolonged mechanical ventilation, and an exacerbation of pre-existing chronic lung disease.

In general, surgeons determine the risk of postoperative pulmonary complications by performing a thorough history and physical examination, and in certain circumstances, surgeons also perform spirometry and additional laboratory testing. Determination of a patient's general health status using the American Society of Anesthesiologists (ASA) Physical Status [17] is an excellent predictor of perioperative mortality and is a useful tool to determine pulmonary risk (Table 2). Patients with an ASA class greater than II have a 1.5- to 3.2-fold increased risk of pulmonary complications [18].

Other specific factors to consider are detailed. The age of a male patient was shown to be a minor predictor of pulmonary risk in the Department of Veterans Affairs National Surgical Quality Improvement Program (NSQIP) [19]. The presence of chronic obstructive pulmonary disease (COPD) is the most important patient-related risk factor for developing pulmonary complications postoperatively. A patient with COPD has a 6% to 28% risk of developing pulmonary complications, depending on the severity of airflow obstruction [18], which cannot be stratified more precisely than "high," "moderate" or "low." Smoking is a significant risk factor. Smokers have

Table 2
American Society of Anesthesiologists (ASA) physical status classification

ASA Class	Description of Patient Characteristics
I	A normal healthy patient
II	A patient with mild systemic disease
III	A patient with severe systemic disease that is not incapacitating
IV	A patient with an incapacitating systemic disease that is a constant threat to life
V	A moribund patient who is not expected to survive 24 hours with or without an operation
E	Suffix to indicate an emergency operation for any ASA class of patient

a 1.4- to 4.3-fold greater risk of pulmonary complications than do patients who have never smoked [18]. In patients with asthma and other reversible airways obstruction, risk is increased only if the patient is actively wheezing or if the peak airway flow is <80% of personal best or predicted [20]. Inquiring about exercise capacity is an important part of pulmonary risk assessment. In a questionnaire study of 600 patients having noncardiac surgery, patients who admitted they could not walk four blocks were 9.0% more likely to have pulmonary complications than those able to walk four blocks. Meanwhile, patients who admitted that they could not climb two flights of stairs were 6.3 percent more likely to have pulmonary complications than were patients who could [21]. The increased likelihood of pulmonary complications for these patients was modest but statistically insignificant. Direct observation of patients, however, yielded more significant results. Those who could climb four flights of stairs had an 11% pulmonary complication rate while those who could climb only three or fewer flights had a 52% complication rate [22].

Generally, obesity should not be considered a major risk factor for postoperative pulmonary complications [18] after gastric bypass surgery [23], laparoscopic cholecystectomy [24], or cardiac surgery [25]. Likewise, obstructive sleep apnea is a minor risk factor, primarily related to the period of highest risk, typically during intubation. The patient with obstructive sleep apnea may require fiber-optic intubation. Thus, expertise in such intubation should be readily available. Sleep apnea also may be associated with unplanned or prolonged ICU stays [26].

Certain noncardiac and nonpulmonary surgical procedures are associated with increased risk of postoperative pulmonary complications. These complications are rare following procedures not related to the chest and abdomen. Risk of postoperative pulmonary complications increases as the incision approximates the diaphragm [18]. Upper-abdominal procedures have higher risk than lower-abdominal procedures [18] and laparoscopic procedures [27]. The duration of an operation is important in determining risk of postoperative pulmonary complications, which increases significantly in procedures lasting more than 3 hours [18].

Surgeons should consider performing preoperative spirometry (also known as pulmonary function tests) only in patients with a history of smoking or COPD, or those with unexplained symptoms that may stem from undiagnosed pulmonary disease. Spirometry includes measurement of forced expiratory volume in one second (FEV_1) and forced vital capacity (FVC). Alternatively, surgeons should not routinely perform spirometry before surgery, even in patients having a high-risk procedure, unless there is a specific indication as defined previously. In a study among smokers having abdominal surgery, those smokers with an FEV_1 of <40% have a higher incidence of bronchospasm, but no increased risk of prolonged mechanical ventilation, ICU stay, or death [28]. While no evidence supports this practice, surgeons should consider withholding preoperative spirometry in patients with known COPD or asthma except when clinical evaluation cannot establish whether a patient is in optimal condition or if information suggests deterioration of a condition since a previous spirometry.

Preoperative arterial blood gas is useful to evaluate for preexisting hypoxia or hypercarbia. If significant hypercarbia exists preoperatively, then high FiO_2 concentrations should be avoided in the perioperative period. Unusual preoperative blood gas levels should not be a reason to deny surgery. A study of high-risk patients having lung resection found that $PaCO_2$ did not predict postoperative pulmonary complications [29]. Other metabolic factors, such as renal function (measured by blood urea nitrogen (BUN)) and nutritional status (measured by serum albumin), have been shown to influence the risk of postoperative pulmonary complications. Levels of BUN >30gm/dL and serum albumin <3.0 gm/dL were moderate predictors of pulmonary risk, with odds ratios for respiratory complications of 2.29 and 2.53, respectively [19].

Several non-drug interventions are known to decrease risk of postoperative pulmonary complications. Patients who stop smoking at least 8 weeks before an elective operation have a significantly lower risk of postoperative pulmonary complications than those who continue to smoke or who stop smoking fewer than 8 weeks before surgery. The risk of pulmonary complications is greater among recent quitters (<8 weeks) and current smokers [30]. Other ways to reduce risk include modification of the surgical approach to limit the procedure to less than 3 hours [16], the use laparoscopic techniques if possible [27], and the use of less ambitious surgical procedures in patients at high risk. Lung expansion maneuvers have been shown to reduce risk of postoperative pulmonary complications, especially if patients are instructed in the use of these maneuvers before surgery [31].

In patients with asthma or COPD, surgeons should reduce and optimize treatment for airflow obstruction. Patients who are not at their personal best baseline or whose peak flow is <80% of predicted should be treated with bronchodilators or a short course of steroids [20]. Also, surgeons should consider for preoperative chest physical therapy patients who have a) an ineffective cough and copious upper airway secretions, b) persistent sputum production despite other therapies, and c) poor functional capacity because of exertional dyspnea. Indications for preoperative treatment of bacterial bronchitis or pneumonia with antibiotics are identical to those for patients who have asthma or COPD and are not preparing for an operation [18].

Surgeons often assume during daily visits to hospitalized patients that treatment is adequate for addressing postoperative pain to reduce postoperative pulmonary complications. However, sometimes surgeons find that patients, fearing significant pain and or muscle spasm in or around the surgical wound, are splinting the chest, abdomen or diaphragm to avoid stretching an abdominal or chest incision. This splinting impairs deep breathing and contributes to reduced lung expansion. Several measures, in addition to systemic narcotic or nonsteroidal analgesic medications, are useful to relieve postoperative pain. These measures include epidural analgesia or intercostal nerve blocks in high-risk patients undergoing thoracic, abdominal, or aortic operations [32]. Additionally, providing patients with information and advice before an operation is valuable and important. Educating the patient on what to expect and how to respond after the operation relieves anxiety. The patient who is prepared well for a major operation and who has practiced various maneuvers to increase lung expansion should be better able to perform these maneuvers after the operation. Close monitoring of patients at high risk of postoperative pulmonary complications either in an ICU or in another specialized hospital unit capable of readily and expeditiously assisting these patients helps prevent pulmonary complications and improve results and outcomes.

Preoperative assessment of renal and hepatic dysfunction and other comorbidities

Surgeons must perform focused reviews of systems to expand on known comorbid conditions and detect other undiagnosed medical conditions that predict perioperative morbidity and mortality. Renal dysfunction is often asymptomatic and is a significant predictor of perioperative cardiac morbidity [33] and pulmonary complications [19]. As a result, routine testing of renal function in patients who are over 50 years old and who are having major surgery is reasonable and worthwhile. Hepatic dysfunction related to alcoholic liver disease, cirrhosis, or nutritional deficits is an important predictor of poor outcome after major surgery. Several older observational studies show that surgery during acute hepatitis is associated with >10% mortality rate. Many studies have shown that the presence and severity of cirrhosis, usually alcohol-related, predicts poor perioperative outcome in abdominal and other types of surgery [34].

Malnutrition, as manifested by decreased serum albumin levels, is a powerful predictor of perioperative morbidity. In a study of the Department of Veterans Affairs NSQIP database of 50,000 veterans undergoing surgery, evidence of hypoalbuminemia was the largest predictor of perioperative morbidity after adjusting for other factors predicting poor outcome [35]. Other Department of Veterans Affairs studies using the NSQIP database have shown that preoperative serum albumin and ASA Physical Status (see Table 2) were the preoperative variables most consistently predictive of 30-day operative morbidity and mortality in all eight individual surgical specialties studied, including general surgery, orthopedic surgery, urology, vascular surgery, neurosurgery, otolaryngology, noncardiac thoracic surgery and plastic surgery, and in all eight surgical specialties as a whole [36,37].

Uncontrolled diabetes mellitus can lead to volume depletion and hyperosmolar states and contribute to poor wound healing. In 100 diabetic patients undergoing abdominal or cardiac surgery, a single serum glucose level >220 mg/dL on the first postoperative day was predictive of subsequent infection [38]. In a randomized trial conducted in ICU patients, of which two thirds had cardiac surgery, those patients randomly receiving intensive insulin therapy for glucose levels >110 mg/dL had 46% fewer episodes of multiorgan failure from sepsis. Also, the mortality rate decreased from 10.9% to 7.2% [39].

Tobacco use increases risk of perioperative pulmonary complications. Smoking increased the rate of pulmonary complications fivefold in a prospective study of 400 patients having elective surgery [40]. Risk of pulmonary complications reaches its lowest level after 8 weeks of tobacco abstinence, as shown in a study of 200 patients having coronary bypass surgery [30].

References

[1] Khuri SF, Daley J, Henderson W, et al. The National Veterans Administration surgical risk study: risk adjustment for the comparative assessment of the quality of surgical care. J Am Coll Surg 1995;180:519–31.

[2] Vanzetto G, Machecourt J, Blendea D, et al. Additive value of thallium single-photon emission computed tomography myocardial imaging for prediction of perioperative events in clinically selected high cardiac risk patients having abdominal aortic surgery. Am J Cardiol 1996;77:143–8.

[3] Schein OD, Katz J, Bass EB, et al. The value of routine preoperative medical testing before cataract surgery. Study of medical testing for cataract surgery. N Engl J Med 2000;342: 168–75.

[4] Detsky AS, Abrams HB, McLaughlin JR, et al. Predicting cardiac complications in patients undergoing non-cardiac surgery. J Gen Intern Med 1986;1:211–9.

[5] Eagle KA, Berger PB, Calkins H, et al. ACC/AHA guideline update for perioperative cardiovascular evaluations for noncardiac surgery—executive summary. A report of the American College of Cardiology/American Heart Association Task Force on Practice Guidelines (Committee to Update the 1996 Guidelines on Perioperative Cardiovascular Evaluation for Noncardiac Surgery). Anesth Analg 2002;94:1052–64.

[6] Almanaseer Y, Mukherjee D, Kline-Rogers EM, et al. Implementation of the ACC/AHA guidelines for preoperative cardiac risk assessment in a general medicine preoperative clinic: improving efficiency and preserving outcomes. Cardiology 2005;103(1):24–9.

[7] Rohde LE, Polanczyk CA, Goldman L, et al. Usefulness of transthoracic echocardiography as a tool for risk stratification of patients undergoing major noncardiac surgery. Am J Cardiol 2001;87:505–9.

[8] Etchells E, Meade M, Tomlinson G, et al. Semiquantitative dipyridamole myocardial stress perfusion imaging for cardiac risk assessment before noncardiac vascular surgery: a meta-analysis. J Vasc Surg 2002;36:534–40.

[9] Gauss A, Rohm HJ, Schauffelen A, et al. Electrocardiographic exercise stress testing for cardiac risk assessment in patients undergoing noncardiac surgery. Anesthesiology 2001;94: 38–46.

[10] Mason JJ, Owens DK, Harris RA, et al. The role of coronary angiography and coronary revascularization before noncardiac vascular surgery. JAMA 1995;273:1919–25.

[11] Mangano DT, Layug EL, Wallace A, et al. Effect of atenololon mortality and cardiovascular morbidity after noncardiac surgery. Multicenter Study of Perioperative Ischemia Research Group. N Engl J Med 1996;335:1713–20.

[12] Practice guidelines for pulmonary artery catheterization. A report by the American Society of Anesthesiologists Task Force on Pulmonary Artery Catheterization. Anesthesiology 1993;78:380–94.

[13] Matot I, Oppenheim-Eden A, Ratrot R, et al. Preoperative cardiac events in elderly patients with hip fracture randomized to epidural or conventional analgesia. Anesthesiology 2003;98: 156–63.

[14] Frank SM, Fleisher LA, Breslow MJ, et al. Perioperative maintenance of normothermia reduces the incidence of morbid cardiac events. A randomized trial. JAMA 1997;277:1127–34.

[15] Lawrence VA, Hilsenbeck SG, Mulrow CD, et al. Incidence and hospital stay for cardiac and pulmonary complications after abdominal surgery. J Gen Intern Med 1995;10:671–8.

[16] Manku K, Bacchetti P, Leung JM. Prognostic significance of postoperative in-hospital complications in elderly patients. I. Long-term survival. Anesth Analg 2003;96:583–9.

[17] Owens WD, Felts JA, Spitznagel EL Jr. ASA physical status classifications: a study of consistency ratings. Anesthesiology 1978;49:239–43.

[18] Smetana GW. Preoperative pulmonary evaluation. N Engl J Med 1999;340:937–44.

[19] Arozullah AM, Daley J, Henderson WG, et al. Multifactorial risk index for predicting postoperative respiratory failure in men after major noncardiac surgery. The National VA Surgical Quality Improvement Program. Ann Surg 2000;232:242–53.

[20] Guidelines for the diagnosis and management of asthma. National Heart, Lung, and Blood Institute. National Asthma Education Program. Expert Panel Report. J Allergy Clin Immunol 1991;88:425–534.

[21] Reilly DF, McNeely MJ, Doerner D, et al. Self-reported exercise tolerance and the risk of serious perioperative complications. Arch Intern Med 1999;159:2185–92.

[22] Girish M, Trayner E Jr, Dammann O, et al. Symptom-limited stair climbing as a predictor of postoperative cardiopulmonary complications after high-risk surgery. Chest 2001;120: 1147–51.

[23] Pasulka PS, Bistrian BR, Benotti PN, et al. The risks of surgery in obese patients. Ann Intern Med 1986;104:540–6.

[24] Angrisani L, Lorenzo M, DePalma G, et al. Laparoscopic cholecystectomy in obese patients compared with non-obese patients. Surg Laparosc Endosc 1995;5:197–201.

[25] Moulton MJ, Creswell LL, Mackey ME, et al. Obesity is not a risk factor for significant adverse outcomes after cardiac surgery. Circulation 1996;94:1187–92.

[26] Rennotte MT, Baele P, Aubert G, et al. Nasal continuous positive airway pressure in the perioperative management of patients with obstructive sleep apnea submitted to surgery. Chest 1995;107:367–74.

[27] A prospective analysis of 1518 laparoscopic cholecystectomies. The Southern Surgeons Club. N Engl J Med 1991;324:1073–8.

[28] Warner DO, Warner MA, Offord KP, et al. Airway obstruction and perioperative complications in smokers undergoing abdominal surgery. Anesthesiology 1999;90:372–9.

[29] Kearney DJ, Lee TH, Reilly JJ, et al. Assessment of operative risk in patients undergoing lung resection. Importance of predicted pulmonary function. Chest 1994;105:753–9.

[30] Bluman LG, Mosca L, Newman N, et al. Preoperative smoking habits and postoperative pulmonary complications. Chest 1998;113:883–9.

[31] Castillo R, Haas A. Chest physical therapy: comparative efficacy of preoperative and postoperative in the elderly. Arch Phys Med Rehabil 1985;66:376–9.

[32] Ballantyne JC, Carr DB, deFerranti S, et al. The comparative effects of postoperative analgesic therapies on pulmonary outcome: cumulative meta-analyses of randomized, controlled trials. Anesth Analg 1998;86:598–612.

[33] Lee TH, Marcantonio ER, Mangione CM, et al. Derivation and prospective validation of a simple index for prediction of cardiac risk of major noncardiac surgery. Circulation 1999;100:1043–9.

[34] Rizvon MK, Chou CL. Surgery in the patient with liver disease. Med Clin North Amer 2003; 87:211–27.

[35] Gibbs J, Cull W, Henderson W, et al. Preoperative serum albumin level as a predictor of operative mortality and morbidity: results of the National VA Surgical Risk Study. Arch Surg 1999;134:36–42.

[36] Khuri SF, Daley J, Henderson W, et al. Risk adjustment of the postoperative mortality rate for the comparative assessment of the quality of surgical care: results of National Veterans Affairs Surgical Risk Study. J Am Coll Surg 1997;185:325–38.

[37] Daley J, Khuri SF, Henderson W, et al. Risk adjustment of the postoperative morbidity rate for the comparative assessment of the quality of surgical care: results of National Veterans Affairs Surgical Risk Study. J Am Coll Surg 1997;185:339–52.

[38] Pomposelli JJ, Baxter JK III, Babineau TJ, et al. Early postoperative glucose control predicts nosocomial infection rate in diabetic patients. JPEN J Parenter Enteral Nutr 1998;22:77–81.

[39] van den Berghe G, Wouters P, Weekers F, et al. Intensive insulin therapy in the critically ill patients. N Engl J Med 2001;345:1359–67.

[40] Brooks-Brunn JA. Predictors of postoperative pulmonary complications following abdominal surgery. Chest 1997;111:564–71.

ELSEVIER
SAUNDERS

SURGICAL
CLINICS OF
NORTH AMERICA

Surg Clin N Am 85 (2005) 1075–1089

Anesthetic Choices in Surgery

Zaki-Udin Hassan, MD, Brenda G. Fahy, MD*

*University of Kentucky Chandler Medical Center, 800 Rose Street,
Room N-204, Lexington, KY 40536*

The type and location of surgical procedure may limit anesthetic techniques and choice of anesthetic agents. Available techniques depend on several factors (Box 1) presenting three basic anesthetic options: regional anesthesia, including subarachnoid block, epidural anesthesia, and peripheral nerve block; monitored anesthesia care (MAC); and general anesthesia. Regional anesthesia (eg, an epidural) may be combined with general anesthesia. Following preoperative evaluation (See article by Joehl elsewhere in this issue.), which should include an assessment of potential problems in airway management, sufficient information should be available to permit the selection of the most suitable anesthetic technique. Whole textbooks have been written concerning anesthetic techniques. Because of space limitations, this chapter will briefly discuss anesthetic techniques available for the surgical patient with comments on some of the latest techniques, including peripheral nerve blocks, airway adjuncts, so-called "fast-track" anesthetics, and advances in technology.

Anesthetic techniques

Regional anesthesia

Among the options for regional anesthesia (Table 1), subarachnoid block and epidural anesthesia are most effective for abdominal, perineal, and lower-extremity surgery. Commonly aggregated under the heading "neuraxial anesthesia," subarachnoid block and epidural anesthesia may be administered as either single-shot or continuous techniques and may include opioids as well as local anesthetics. Patients who are anticoagulated, including those

---

* Corresponding author.
E-mail address: bgfahy2@email.uky.edu (B.G. Fahy).

0039-6109/05/$ - see front matter © 2005 Elsevier Inc. All rights reserved.
doi:10.1016/j.suc.2005.09.017

surgical.theclinics.com

Box 1. Anesthetic choices in surgery

1) Factors in selection
   a) Requirements of surgery (including type and location)
   b) Anesthesiologist's experience and expertise
   c) Patient preference
   d) Surgeon preference
2) Anesthetic choices
   a) Regional anesthesia
      • Surgical procedure in appropriate location (eg, extremities, lower abdomen, perineum, urinary tract)
      • Subarachnoid, epidural or peripheral nerve blocks
   b) Monitored anesthesia care
      • Particular patient or procedure requires higher doses of sedative medications
      • Coexistent diseases require close monitoring, which may include hemodynamic or ventilator support
   c) General anesthesia
      • Required because of location of surgical procedure (eg, upper abdominal thoracic procedures, spine, head and neck)

---

taking low-molecular heparins and antiplatelet drugs, have a contraindication for neuraxial anesthesia because of epidural hematoma risk.

Blockade of the brachial plexus, lumbar plexus, and specific peripheral nerves offers certain advantages over other techniques. Those advantages include postoperative analgesia and fewer systemic physiologic changes. Carotid endarterectomy may be done with peripheral nerve blocks using superficial and deep cervical plexus blocks, thus permitting awake neurological assessment. Upper- and lower-extremity procedures may require regional blocks, which provide anesthesia for the specific nerve or nerves involved. These blocks can be used alone or in combination with other peripheral nerve blocks to provide surgical anesthesia.

Increasingly favored over injections of local anesthetic, the use of these techniques involving regional anesthesia continues to increase, as advances in nerve stimulators [1] and ultrasound guidance [2,3] devices aid in making blocks more successful while reducing the likelihood of complications (Table 2). New technologies are also permitting continuous catheter techniques [4,5] that prolong surgical anesthesia and postoperative analgesia. However, the performance of these peripheral nerve blocks requires an anesthesiologist skilled in these techniques as well as a cooperative patient and surgeon.

Table 1
Common regional anesthetic techniques by surgical site

Surgical site		Appropriate nerve block
Upper extremity	Upper Arm including shoulder	Interscalene brachial plexus nerve block,
	Arm, elbow, forearm	Infraclavicular or supraclavicular brachial plexus nerve block or Bier block
	Lower forearm, wrist, hand	Axillary nerve block, elbow block, Bier block
	Hand, metacarpal	Axillary block, wrist block, elbow block
	Digits	Wrist block, digital block
Lower extremity	Entire extremity including hip	Subarachnoid block, lumbar epidural
	Hip, anterior thigh	Femoral, obturator and lateral femoral cutaneous nerve (3 in 1) block
	Knee, lower leg, foot	Sciatic and 3-in-1 nerve block
	Lower leg, ankle and foot	Common peroneal and tibial nerve block, saphenous nerve and ankle block, bier block
	Digits	Metatarsal block, digital block
Abdomen	Lower abdomen, pelvic viscera	Subarachnoid block, lumbar epidural block
	Inguinal region	Ilioinguinal and iliohypogastric nerve blocks, subarachnoid block, lumbar epidural block
	Perineum and urinary tract	Pudendal nerve block, paracervical nerve block, penile block, subarachnoid block, lumbar epidural block
Head and neck	Midface, upper and lower jaw discrete surgical procedures	Maxillary and mandibular nerve blocks
	Cervical plexus (C2 to C4) (eg carotid endarterectomy)	Superficial and deep cervical plexus blocks

Monitored anesthesia care

MAC involves patient monitoring with the surgeon providing local anesthesia and the anesthesia personnel providing supplemental sedation as required. Anesthesia personnel are usually required to provide MAC when a particular patient or procedure requires higher doses of sedative medication or when coexistent diseases require closer monitoring. A propofol infusion in sedative doses is now often used for MAC, but must be administered cautiously because its effects are additive with other agents and may result in deeper levels of sedation with potential general anesthetic induction in higher doses. In contrast to MAC, conscious sedation occurs when nonanesthesia personnel provide moderate sedation while the patient receives a local anesthetic injection at the site of the procedure. Conscious

Table 2
Complications of upper extremity blocks[a]

Block	Potential complications
Interscalene block	Respiratory compromise
	Pneumothorax
	Epidural or intrathecal injection
Supraclavicular block	Respiratory compromise
	Pneumothorax
	Horner's syndrome neuropathy
Infraclavicular	Pneumothorax
Axillary	No risk of pneumothorax
Bier block (Intravenous regional block)	Accidental early tourniquet deflation
	Local anesthetic
	Phlebitis
	Compartment syndrome
	Loss of limb

[a] Nerve damage or neuritis, although uncommon, can occur with any peripheral nerve block. This complication is usually self-limited. Local anesthetic toxicity as a result of infraclavicular injection may occur.

sedation requires patient responsiveness to stimulation (verbal or tactile), maintaining a patent airway without assistance, and cardiovascular stability.

Because sedation is a continuum, one cannot always predict how an individual will respond to certain medications, especially propofol. Even when administered for moderate or light sedation, propofol can rapidly cause profound changes in depth of sedation, resulting in deep sedation or general anesthesia with no specific antagonist medication available. For this reason, nonanesthesia personnel administering propofol should be proficient in airway management and advanced life support to rescue a patient from a level of sedation that is deeper than intended. A recent package insert for Diprivan-brand propofol carried the following warning:

> For general anesthesia or monitored anesthesia care sedation, DIPRIVAN Injectable Emulsion should be administered only by persons trained in the administration of general anesthesia not involved in the conduct of the surgical/diagnostic procedure. Patients should be continuously monitored, and facilities for maintenance of a patent airway, artificial ventilation, and oxygen enrichment and circulation resuscitation must be immediately available.

General anesthesia

With advances in minimally invasive surgical techniques and a rising number of office-based procedures, more ambulatory surgeries are taking place. This trend has been one of the most important factors in altering anesthetic practices. Increasingly, anesthetic practices must accommodate surgical conditions that call for a rapid recovery phase, including early emergence from anesthesia and faster patient return to normal function. Fast-tracking after ambulatory surgery entails taking the patient directly from the operating room to the surgery day unit, thus bypassing the postanesthesia care unit (PACU). Fast-tracking may also call for simply discharging the patient from the PACU to home [6,7]. This concept of fast-tracking spans the spectrum of anesthesia as it applies to procedures requiring postoperative hospitalization (eg, cardiac surgery), allowing earlier discharge [8]. The trend toward fast-tracking has led to the development of anesthetic agents that enable shorter recovery phases. Such agents include the inhalation agents sevoflurane and desflurane, and shorter-acting induction agents, such as propofol. Two of the limiting factors in fast-tracking are postoperative pain, nausea, and vomiting. For information in greater detail see the article about postoperative pain by Cohen and Schechter and the article about postoperative nausea and vomiting by Williams elsewhere in this issue.

Isoflurane, sevoflurane, and desflurane [9] are common inhalation agents for general anesthesia. Halothane and enflurane are used less commonly because halothane is associated with side effects affecting the heart and liver, and enflurane is associated with renal dysfunction. Isoflurane has a slower uptake and elimination than sevoflurane or desflurane and is frequently used in longer cases in part because shorter-acting inhalation agents cost more. Compared with isoflurane, sevoflurane is associated with a faster emergence and is more suitable for inhalation induction. Sevoflurane has been associated with emergence delirium, which appears to be inversely related to age and is most frequent in children 5 years old or younger. Desflurane has the fastest recovery of inhalation agents but is associated with tachycardia and hypertension. Also, its pungent odor makes it undesirable for use in inhalation induction.

Propofol is commonly used not only because its short-duration characteristics dovetail with fast-tracking [9], but also because of its antiemetic properties. Propofol is often used when administering total intravenous anesthesia (TIVA), during which inhalation agents are avoided. Postoperative high-dose infusions can lead to propofol infusion [10] syndrome, which causes severe and potentially life-threatening metabolic acidosis. First reported in children, this complication is more common in critically ill children. However, it does also occur in critically ill adults [11]. Although two cases of lactic acidosis attributed to intraoperative propofol have recently appeared in the literature [12], speculation has been raised as to whether propofol was causative [13].

Although TIVA may include propofol, many different combinations of other intravenous agents, including benzodiazepines and opioids [14], are also available. Indications for TIVA include a history of malignant hyperthermia, a disorder specific to anesthesia. TIVA is useful in such cases because it avoids potential triggering inhalation agents and succinylcholine.

Because TIVA is more costly to administer than anesthesia using inhalation agents, TIVA is often limited to specific indications or short cases.

One of the latest intravenous sedatives, dexmedetomidine, is a highly selective alpha-2 adrenergic agonist that has been described as an adjunct to reduce other anesthetic requirements during anesthesia [15]. So far, the Food and Drug Administration has approved the sedative only for brief periods (<24 hours) of postoperative sedation. Although dexmedetomidine has excellent sedative properties, high incidence of bradycardia associated with its administration limits its usefulness [16,17].

Airway adjuncts

Airway management is a crucial skill in anesthetic management, requiring facility with a variety of techniques to establish an airway. The American Society of Anesthesiologists has developed a difficult-airway algorithm [18] for cases where a difficult intubation is anticipated and for cases where such difficulties are unexpected (Box 2; Fig. 1). Although all of the various airway

---

Box 2. Guideline for managing difficult airways

1. Assess the likelihood and clinical impact of basic management problems.
   a. Difficult ventilation
   b. Difficult intubation
   c. Difficulty with patient cooperation or consent
   d. Difficult tracheostomy
2. Pursue opportunities to deliver supplemental oxygen throughout the process of difficult airway management.
3. Consider the relative merits and feasibility of basic management choices.
   a. Awake intubation versus intubation attempts after induction of general anesthesia
   b. Noninvasive techniques for initial approach to intubation versus invasive technique for initial approach to intubation
   c. Presentation of spontaneous ventilation versus ablation of spontaneous ventilation
4. Develop primary and alternative strategies.

From American Society of Anesthesiologists Task Force on Management of the Difficult Airway. Practice guidelines for management of the difficult airway: an updated report by the American Society of Anesthesiologists Task Force on Management of the Difficult Airway. Anesthesiology 2003;98(5):1269–77; with permission.

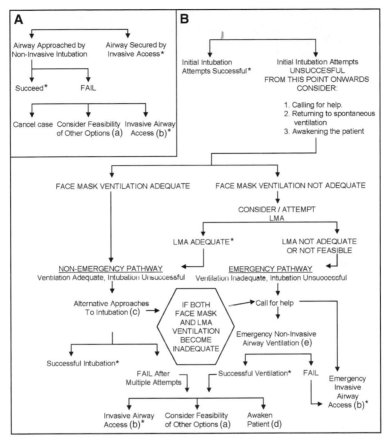

A

Airway Approached by   Airway Secured by
Non-Invasive Intubation   Invasive Access*

Succeed*   FAIL

Cancel case   Consider Feasibility   Invasive Airway
              of Other Options (a)   Access (b)*

B

Initial Intubation   Initial Intubation Attempts
Attempts Successful*   UNSUCCESFUL
                              FROM THIS POINT ONWARDS
                              CONSIDER:

1. Calling for help.
2. Returning to spontaneous
   ventilation
3. Awakening the patient

FACE MASK VENTILATION ADEQUATE   FACE MASK VENTILATION NOT ADEQUATE

CONSIDER / ATTEMPT
LMA

LMA ADEQUATE*   LMA NOT ADEQUATE
                       OR NOT FEASIBLE

NON-EMERGENCY PATHWAY   EMERGENCY PATHWAY
Ventilation Adequate, Intubation Unsuccessful   Ventilation Inadequate, Intubation Unsuccessful

Alternative Approaches   IF BOTH   Call for help
To Intubation (c)   FACE MASK
                              AND LMA
                              VENTILATION   Emergency Non-Invasive
                              BECOME   Airway Ventilation (e)
                              INADEQUATE

Successful Intubation*   FAIL   Emergency
                                                                        Invasive
          FAIL After   Successful Ventilation*   Airway
          Multiple Attempts   Access (b)*

Invasive Airway   Consider Feasibility   Awaken
Access (b)*   of Other Options (a)   Patient (d)

★ Confirm Tracheal Intubation or LMA Placement with Exhaled C02
LMA = Laryngeal Mask Airway

Fig. 1. (A) Algorithm for awake intubation. (B) Algorithm for intubation after induction of general anesthesia. (a) Other options include surgery using face mask or laryngeal mask airway anesthesia, local anesthesia infiltration, or regional nerve blockade. The choice of any of these options usually implies that mask ventilation will not be problematic. Therefore, these options may be of limited value if this step in the algorithm has been reached via the emergency pathway. (b) Invasive airway includes surgical or percutaneous tracheostomy or cricothyrotomy. (c) Alternative noninvasive approaches to difficult intubation include the use of different laryngoscope blades, a laryngeal mask airway device as an intubation conduit (with or without fiberoptic guidance), fiber-optic intubation, an intubating stylet or tube changer, a light wand, retrograde intubation, and blind oral or nasal intubation. (d) Consider re-preparing the patient for awake intubation or canceling surgery. (e) Options for emergency noninvasive airway ventilation include the use of a rigid bronchoscope, esophageal-tracheal Combitube ventilation, or transtracheal jet ventilation. (*From* American Society of Anesthesiologists Task Force on Management of the Difficult Airway. Practice guidelines for management of the difficult airway: an updated report by the American Society of Anesthesiologists Task Force on Management of the Difficult Airway. Anesthesiology 2003;98(5):1269–77; with permission.)

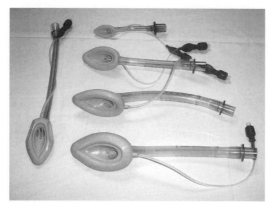

Fig. 2. LMAs™ are available in different sizes for use in pediatric and adult populations.

adjuncts are beyond the scope of this chapter, some of the newer airway adjuncts are discussed, including the laryngeal mask airway (LMA) device (Fig. 2), the esophageal-tracheal Combitube, and the intubating lighted stylet or light wand.

One of the most important recent advances in airway management is the LMA (Fig. 3) because placement does not require direct visualization of the vocal cords (Fig. 4). When correctly placed, an LMA can allow ventilation. LMAs, which do not protect against aspiration, come in different sizes for pediatric and adult use. Modifications of the LMA have led to the development of an intubating LMA (Fig. 5), through which a specialized endotracheal tube is passed without direct visualization (Figs. 6 and 7) or with the

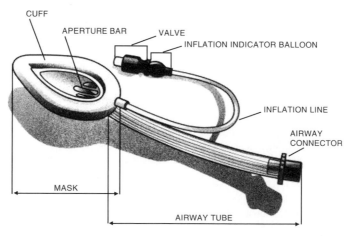

Fig. 3. Components of an LMA™. (Courtesy of LMA™ North America, Inc., San Diego, CA; with permission.)

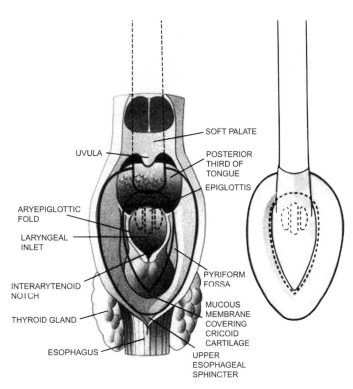

Fig. 4. Dorsal view of an LMA™ showing correct pharyngeal position. (Courtesy of LMA™ North America, Inc., San Diego, CA; with permission.)

aid of a fiber-optic bronchoscope. In a patient who cannot be ventilated by mask or LMA, nor be endotracheally intubated, a surgical airway made via a cricothyroidotomy or tracheostomy may be required to save the patient's life.

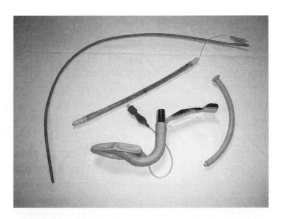

Fig. 5. Components of an intubating LMA™.

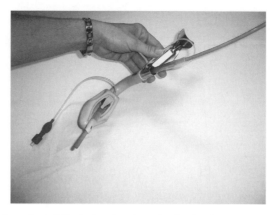

Fig. 6. Insertion of specially designed endotracheal tube through intubating LMA™.

A Combitube® (Fig. 8), placed without vocal-cord visualization, is a double-lumen airway with two inflatable balloons. One lumen contains ventilating side holes at the pharynx level and is closed at the distal end, while the other lumen is patent with a cuff similar to an endotracheal tube (Fig. 9). If the tube is placed into the trachea (Fig. 10), the smaller cuff is inflated. If the tube is placed in the esophagus (see Fig. 9), the second larger pharyngeal

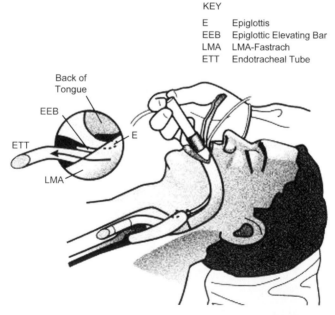

Fig. 7. Insertion technique for intubating LMA™ with passage of specially designed endotracheal tube. E, epiglottis; EEB, epiglottic elevating bar; ETT, endotracheal tube. (Courtesy of LMA™ North America Inc., San Diego, CA; with permission.)

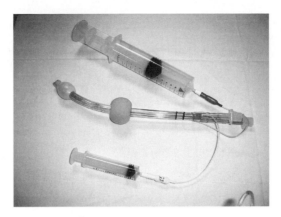

Fig. 8. Combitube® with oropharyngeal and distal cuffs inflated.

balloon is inflated, which isolates the oropharynx from the hypopharynx, permitting ventilation.

The lighted stylet or light wand [19] (Fig. 11) is positioned within an endotracheal tube and then placed in the posterior pharynx. Tracheal entry is confirmed by visualization of a red translucency in the neck. Once this red translucency is apparent, the endotracheal tube is advanced and the stylet is removed. Endotracheal tube placement is then confirmed with standard methods. Because visualization of the tracheal transillumination requires a darkened room, this technique may not always be practical.

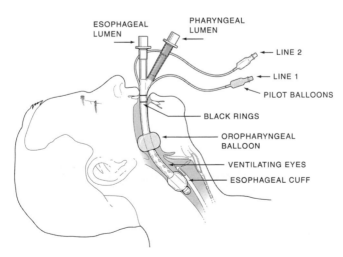

Fig. 9. Combitube® in esophageal position that occurs most commonly with placement. (Courtesy of Mallinckrodt Incorporated, Pleasanton, CA; with permission. Combitube® is a registered trademark of Tyco Healthcare Group LP.)

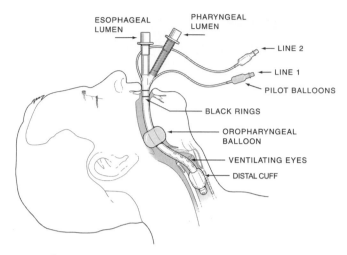

Fig. 10. Combitube® in tracheal position. (Courtesy of Mallinckrodt Incorporated, Pleasanton, CA; with permission. Combitube® is a registered trademark of Tyco Healthcare Group LP.)

Anesthetic technology and monitoring developments

In addition to continuous developments concerning catheters with peripheral nerve blocks, other developments related to anesthetic technology include improvements in infusion devices, such as target-controlled infusion pumps, and intraoperative anesthetic monitoring advances, as represented by depth-of-anesthesia monitors and the expanded use of transesophageal echocardiography (TEE). Target-controlled infusion pumps for propofol are commercially available in most parts of the world, but, at the time of publication, not North America. These infusion systems enable anesthesia personnel to select the target blood concentration for a particular effect and then control depth of anesthesia by adjusting the requested target blood concentration to account for such variables as patient response and type of surgery. This system, based on pharmacokinetic models, delivers an intravenous infusion with the goal of maintaining a constant level of anesthetic drug [20]. Further developments in the area of target-controlled infusions continue.

Anesthesiologists have always been concerned about patient awareness with recall of intraoperative events. This concern has prompted numerous attempts to develop a reliable monitor for depth of anesthesia. Currently under development are monitors that that record and process the electroencephalographic or auditory evoked potentials. Other monitors in development are designed to detect changes in autonomic function. All currently available depth-of-anesthesia monitors have some limitations and have not proven effective for all populations. The bispectral index (BIS) is one of the more commonly used commercially available depth-of-anesthesia monitors. The BIS is a derived index from electroencephalographic

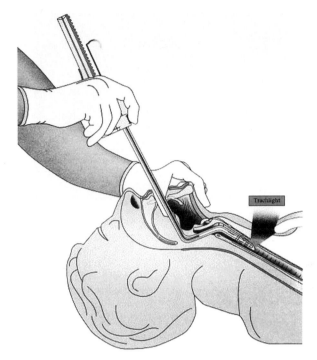

Fig. 11. Light-guide intubation involves transillumination of the neck's soft tissues. A bright, well-defined, circumscribed glow is seen anteriorly when the endotracheal tube with the light wand enters the glottic opening. If the glow is not well circumscribed or not seen, the light wand has entered the esophagus. (Courtesy of Laerdal Medical Corporation Wappingers Falls, NY; with permission. © 2005 Laerdal Medical Corporation.)

parameters. The index generates a linear dimensionless number ranging from 0 to 100 with values between 40 and 60 recommended by its manufacturer as indicators of adequate depth of anesthesia. Questions surround the reliability of the BIS, which may vary with the anesthetic agents [21,22], and its cost-effectiveness [23]. These issues are beyond the scope of this article.

Intraoperative TEE is more sensitive than electrocardiography for detecting myocardial ischemia and has category I indications for evaluating a hemodynamically unstable patient. Because of this higher sensitivity, intraoperative TEE can differentiate between myocardial ischemia, ventricular failure, valvular dysfunction, hypovolemia, low systemic vascular resistance, and cardiac tamponade. Originally used with cardiothoracic anesthesia, TEE has taken on a role in noncardiac surgery as well. TEE interpretation requires specialized training and TEE limitations include contraindication to esophageal probe insertion (esophageal varices) and anatomic difficulties. TEE technology now includes three-dimensional image construction (Fig. 12), providing additional real-time information about volume status, myocardial ischemia, regional wall abnormalities and valvular dysfunction.

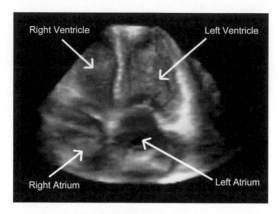

Fig. 12. Three-dimensional transesophageal echocardiography image.

Summary

Advances in technology and pharmacology continue to change techniques for anesthesia. Fast-track anesthesia has led to the development of newer anesthetic agents and changes in anesthetic practice, including the increased use of regional anesthesia, techniques involving continuous plexus catheters to improve postoperative analgesia, and TIVA. Technological advances now provide additional options for airway management when a difficult airway is encountered and additional intraoperative monitoring with depth-of-anesthesia monitors and transesophageal echocardiography. Future areas of development are anticipated to include target-controlled infusion pumps and techniques and medications that improve fast-track anesthesia safely.

References

[1] Hadzic A, Vloka J, Hadzic N, et al. Nerve stimulators used for peripheral nerve blocks vary in their electrical characteristics. Anesthesiology 2003;98(4):969–74.
[2] Greher M, Kapral S. Is regional anesthesia simply an exercise in applied sonoanatomy? Aiming at higher frequencies of ultrasonographic imaging. Anesthesiology 2003;99(2):250–1.
[3] McGoldrick KE. Ultrasound guidance in regional anaesthesia. Survey of Anesthesiology 2005;49(2):108–9.
[4] Capdevilla X, Macaire P, Dadure C, et al. Continuous psoas compartment block for postoperative analgesia after total hip arthroplasty: new landmarks, technical guidelines, and clinical evaluation. Anesth Analg 2000;94:1606.
[5] Liu SS. Continuous plexus and peripheral nerve blocks for postoperative analgesia. Anesth Analg 2003;96(1):263–72.
[6] Coloma M, Zhou T, White PF, et al. Fast-tracking after outpatient laparoscopy: reasons for failure after propofol, sevoflurane, and desflurane anesthesia. Anesth Analg 2001;93(1):112–5.
[7] Chan VW, Peng PW, Kaszas Z, et al. A comparative study of general anesthesia, intravenous regional anesthesia, and axillary block for outpatient hand surgery: clinical outcome and cost analysis. Anesth Analg 2001;93(5):1181–4.

[8] Cheng DCH, Wall C, Djaiani G, et al. Randomized assessment of resource use in fast-track cardiac surgery 1-year after hospital discharge. Anesthesiology 2003;98(3):651–7.

[9] Gupta A, Stierer T, Zuckerman R, et al. Comparison of recovery profile after ambulatory anesthesia with propofol, isoflurane, sevoflurane and desflurane: a systematic review. Anesth Analg 2004;98(3):632–41.

[10] Cray SH, Robinson BH, Cox PN. Lactic academia and bradyarrhythmia in a child sedated with propofol. Crit Care Med 1998;26(12):2087–92.

[11] Cremer OL, Moons KG, Bouman EA, et al. Long-term propofol infusion and cardiac failure in adult head-injured patients. Lancet 2001;357(9250):117–8.

[12] Burow BK. Metabolic acidosis associated with propofol in the absence of other causative factors. Anesthesiology 2004;101(1):239–41.

[13] Funston JS. Two reports of propofol anesthesia associated with metabolic acidosis in adults. Anesthesiology 2004;101(1):6–8.

[14] Tesniere A, Servin F. Intravenous techniques in ambulatory anesthesia. Anesthesiol Clin North America 2003;21(2):273–88.

[15] Aho M, Lehtinen AM, Scheinin M, et al. Dexmedetomidine, an alpha 2 adrenoceptor agonist, reduces anesthetic requirements for patients undergoing minor gynecologic surgery. Anesthesiology 1990;73:230–5.

[16] Venn RM, Grounds RM. Comparison between dexmedetomidine and propofol for sedation in the intensive care unit: patient and clinician perceptions. Br J Anaesth 2001;87:684–90.

[17] Triltsch AE, Welte M, von Homeyer P, et al. Bispectral index-guided sedation with dexmedetomidine in intensive care: a prospective, randomized, double blind, placebo-controlled phase II study. Crit Care Med 2002;30:1007–14.

[18] Caplan RA, Benumof JL, Berry FA, et al. Practice guidelines for management of the difficult airway: an updated report by the American Society of Anesthesiologists Task Force on Management of the Difficult Airway. Anesthesiology 2003;98(5):1269–77.

[19] Wong S, Coskunfirat ND, Hee H, et al. Factors influencing time of intubation with a light-wand device in patients without known airway abnormality. J Clin Anes 2004;16(5):326–31.

[20] van den Nieuwenhuyzen MC, Engbers FH, Vuyk J, et al. Target-controlled infusion systems: role in anaesthesia and analgesia. Clin Pharmacokinet 2000;38(2):181–90.

[21] Barr G, Jakobsson JG, Owall A, et al. Nitrous oxide does not alter bispectral index: study with nitrous oxide as sole agent and as an adjuvant to IV anaesthesia. Br J Anaesth 1999;82:827–30.

[22] Liu J, Singh H, White PF. Electroencephalographic bispectral index correlates with intraoperative recall and depth of propofol-induced sedation [abstract]. Anesth Analg 1997;84(1):185–90.

[23] Liu SS. Effects of bispectral index monitoring on ambulatory anesthesia. Anesthesiology 2004;101(2):311–5.

ELSEVIER
SAUNDERS

SURGICAL
CLINICS OF
NORTH AMERICA

Surg Clin N Am 85 (2005) 1091–1102

Perioperative Issues:
Myocardial Ischemia and
Protection — Beta-Blockade

Paul M. Maggio, MD*, Paul A. Taheri, MD

*Department of Surgery, University of Michigan Health System, University Hospital,
Room 1C421, 1500 East Medical Center Drive, Ann Arbor, MI 48109-0033, USA*

Approximately one third of patients undergoing noncardiac surgery have coronary artery disease (CAD), and cardiovascular complications are an important cause of perioperative morbidity and mortality [1,2]. Several algorithms are available to assess the risk for perioperative cardiac events. The American College of Cardiology (ACC) and the American Heart Association (AHA) guidelines for perioperative cardiovascular risk assessment, first published in 1996 and updated in 2002, provide an eight-step algorithm to determine the most appropriate cardiovascular workup and treatment based on clinical assessment, cardiac testing, and the nature of the surgery (Fig. 1) [3,4]. The Revised Cardiac Risk Index, developed by Lee et al. [5], identified six independent factors associated with major cardiac complications: high-risk surgery, history of ischemic heart disease, history of congestive heart failure, history of cerebrovascular disease, insulin-requiring diabetes mellitus, and serum creatinine level >2.0 mg/dL (Box 1). Although preoperative risk assessment is useful in identifying patients at greatest risk for cardiac complications, recent investigations have provided additional guidance in choosing interventions to improve perioperative outcomes.

The results of the Coronary Artery Revascularization Prophylaxis (CARP) trial were recently published [6]. This trial, a prospective study, randomized 510 patients with stable coronary disease to either coronary revascularization (coronary artery bypass grafting (CABG) or percutaneous coronary intervention (PCI)) or medical therapy before undergoing major vascular surgery. Two thirds of the enrolled patients had either one- or two-vessel disease. Excluded from the study were patients who had unstable

---

* Corresponding author.
E-mail address: pmaggio@umich.edu (P.M. Maggio).

0039-6109/05/$ - see front matter © 2005 Elsevier Inc. All rights reserved.
doi:10.1016/j.suc.2005.09.016
surgical.theclinics.com

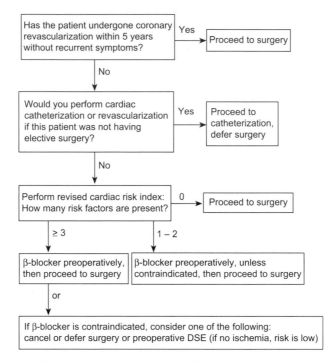

Fig. 1. Proposed clinical algorithm for risk stratification. DSE, dobutamine stress echocardiography. (*From* Grayburn PA, Hillis LD. Cardiac events in patients undergoing noncardiac surgery: shifting the paradigm from noninvasive risk stratification to therapy. Ann Intern Med 2003;138(6):506–11; with permission.)

coronary disease, left main coronary artery stenosis, severe left-ventricular dysfunction, or severe aortic stenosis. Potentially beneficial medications, including beta-blockers, antiplatelet agents, angiotensin-converting-enzyme inhibitors, and statins, were widely used in both groups. For example, 84% of the patients in the revascularization group and 86% of the patients in the medical therapy group received beta-blockers. The study found no significant difference in long-term outcome. After 2.7 years, mortality was 22% in the revascularization group and 23% in the non-revascularized group. These data support the current ACC/AHA perioperative cardiovascular recommendations that the decision to perform coronary revascularization should be based on the same well-proven indications used in the nonoperative setting [4,7,8]. When adequate perioperative medical therapy is provided, patients who have stable coronary disease, specifically those without left main coronary disease, severe left-ventricular dysfunction, or severe aortic stenosis, do as well as patients treated with coronary revascularization.

Coronary revascularization by CABG or PCI appears to be equally effective in the preoperative setting, although the timing of the subsequent surgery is less well defined. Most PCI procedures entail coronary stent

---

Box 1. Factors associated with major cardiac complications

1. *High-risk surgical procedure, including:*
a. Intraperitoneal vascular reconstruction
b. Intrathoracic vascular reconstruction
c. Suprainguinal vascular reconstruction

2. *History of ischemic cardiac disease[a], as indicated by any of the following:*
a. History of myocardial infarction
b. History of a positive exercise test
c. Current complaints of chest pain considered to be secondary to myocardial ischemia
d. Use of nitrate therapy
e. ECG with pathological Q waves
f. Preoperative ECG ST-T wave changes (ST segment elevation, depression or T-wave inversion) not associated with worse cardiac outcomes

3. *History of congestive heart failure defined as the presence of any of the following:*
a. History of congestive heart failure
b. Paroxysmal nocturnal dyspnea
c. Physical examination showing bilateral rales or S3 gallop
d. Chest radiograph showing pulmonary vascular redistribution

4. *History of cerebrovascular disease, defined as either of the following:*
a. Stroke
b. Transient ischemic attack

5. *Preoperative insulin therapy*

6. *Preoperative serum creatinine level >2.0 mg/dL*

---

[a] Prior coronary vascularization alone is not a criterion for ischemic heart disease.

Data from Lee TH, Marcantonio ER, Mangione CM, et al. Derivation and prospective validation of a simple index for prediction of cardiac risk of major noncardiac surgery. Circulation 1999;100(10):1043–9.

---

placement and require antiplatelet therapy to prevent stent thrombosis [9]. The stent is at higher risk of thrombosis until re-endothelialized. This risk may be exacerbated by the need to hold antiplatelet therapy during the perioperative period and the hemostatic changes incurred by surgery [10].

Indeed, retrospective studies have found a higher incidence of cardiovascular complications when surgery is performed shortly after stenting [11–13]. In the largest study by Wilson et al. [12], 4% of patients undergoing noncardiac surgery after coronary stenting suffered myocardial infarctions, stent thrombosis, or death. All complications occurred in patients undergoing surgery within 6 weeks of coronary stenting. The current ACC/AHA guidelines recommend waiting for a minimum of 2 weeks and ideally 4 to 6 weeks before proceeding to noncardiac surgery after coronary stenting [4]. Based on the limited available data, a 6-week interval when feasible seems appropriate.

Perioperative beta-blockers

Pathophysiology

Although the role of cardiac revascularization before elective surgery in high-risk patients remains to be defined, increasing evidence shows that perioperative medical management, particularly beta-adrenergic antagonists, significantly reduces the risk and the incidence of cardiac complications. Plaque disruption and prolonged ischemia are presumed mechanisms of perioperative myocardial infarctions, and the incidence of cardiac events is strongly associated with tachycardia and the presence and duration of perioperative ischemia [14–16]. In one study, perioperative ischemia was associated with as much as a 21-fold increase in adverse cardiac events [17]. Episodes of ischemia peak early during the postoperative period, often while the patient is emerging from general anesthesia, and perioperative myocardial infarctions often occur within the following 48 hours. This finding differs from findings in earlier surgical literature suggesting that myocardial infarctions most commonly occur between postoperative days 3 and 5 [17,18]. Perioperative myocardial ischemia results from physiologic stresses and elevated catecholamines that worsen the myocardial oxygen balance because increased heart rate and cardiac contractility lead to greater myocardial oxygen demand while the decreased time of diastole diminishes coronary blood flow.

A beneficial role of beta-adrenergic blockade has been well documented in patients who have CAD [19]. Beta-blockers decrease heart rate and cardiac contractility, thereby improving the myocardial oxygen balance. In addition, they limit mechanical stresses, which may lead to vulnerable plaque disruption, and decrease the incidence of cardiac arrhythmias, particularly in the face of myocardial ischemia [20]. Apart from their hemodynamic effects, beta-blockers may also limit inflammation, prevent platelet aggregation, modulate the coagulation cascade, and decrease nociception [20–22]. These latter effects have been less well studied but may offer additional mechanisms through which beta-blockers benefit patients who have CAD.

Clinical studies

In the landmark study by Mangano et al., [23] from which the original recommendations for beta-blockade by the ACC/AHA were based, 200 patients at risk or with documented coronary artery disease were randomized to receive atenolol or placebo 30 minutes before surgery. Patients considered to be at risk had at least two of the following risk factors: age over 65, hypertension, serum cholesterol concentration ≥ 240 mg/dL, current smoking, and diabetes mellitus. Treatment with atenolol or placebo was continued for 7 days or until hospital discharge. Patient follow-up evaluations were performed at 6 months, 1 year, and 2 years from the time of surgery. After 2 years, 9 deaths occurred in the atenolol group versus 21 deaths in the placebo group, although the greatest treatment benefit was noted over the first 6 to 8 months. Overall, perioperative treatment with atenolol resulted in a long-term relative risk reduction of 55% ($P = 0.019$). An important criticism of this study is that the investigators chose not to include deaths that occurred during the perioperative treatment period when beta-blockers theoretically may offer the most benefit. Six patients died during the initial hospitalization and were not included in the outcome study; 4 deaths occurred in the atenolol group; and 2 in the placebo group. Therefore, if the study were examined in a true intention-to-treat analysis, the outcome differences would no longer be significant ($P = 0.1$) [24].

The Dutch Echocardiographic Cardiac Risk Evaluation Applying Stress Echocardiography (DECREASE) study by Poldermans et al. [25] found the most significant treatment effect using perioperative beta-blockers. One hundred twelve vascular patients at high cardiac risk (positive dobutamine echocardiography) were randomized to receive bisoprolol or standard care. This was an unblinded study and no placebo was given. Treatment was started at least 1 week before surgery and continued for 30 days postoperatively. At 30 days follow-up from the time of surgery, two cardiac-related deaths (3.4%) occurred in the bisoprolol treatment group and nine (17%) in the control group. No patients in the bisoprolol group suffered nonfatal myocardial infarctions versus nine (17%) in the control group. Overall, patients with left ventricular failure, diabetes, and renal insufficiency benefited most from treatment. This study demonstrated a relative risk reduction for cardiac death and nonfatal myocardial infarction of 80% and 100%, respectively. In a subsequent report by the DECREASE group, the beneficial effects of bisoprolol were maintained during 2 years of follow-up. Here the incidence of cardiac events (cardiac death and nonfatal myocardial infarction) was 12% in the bisoprolol group versus 32% in the standard care group [26]. These results suggest a greater effect of beta-blockers than has been reported in other randomized controlled trials and can partly be attributed to the high-risk patient population studied. The incidence of cardiac events in the control group was 34% during the perioperative period [26]. The DECREASE trial ended early after interim analysis from the first 100 patients found significant improvement in the treatment group. Therefore, the results of this study are dramatic and encouraging but should be confirmed through larger, well-designed randomized controlled trials.

A meta-analysis of trials examining perioperative beta-blockade was recently reported by Stevens et al. [27]. The meta-analysis included 866 patients from 11 randomized controlled trials, from which were 15 nonfatal myocardial infarctions and 18 cardiac-related deaths. This analysis demonstrated a significant improvement in cardiac events during the first 30 post-operative days with perioperative beta-blockade. Beta-blockers reduced the risk of myocardial infarction (0.9% versus 5.2%) and cardiac death (0.8% versus 3.9%). However, the analysis relied heavily on the results from a single study. Of the 33 reported adverse cardiac events in the meta-analysis, 20 (9 nonfatal myocardial infarctions and 11 cardiac-related deaths) were from the DECREASE trial. The DECREASE trial studied only high-risk patients and found a much greater treatment benefit than the other studies included in the meta-analysis. Although this finding in the DECREASE trial may reflect a greater treatment benefit in high-risk patients, the variations in the studies used in the meta-analysis limits the usefulness of the meta-analysis in predicting which patients benefit from perioperative beta-blockade [28].

Perioperative beta-blockers appear to offer the most significant benefit to high-risk patients (those who have documented ischemia) and the supporting evidence is categorized as class I by the current ACC/AHA guidelines. In patients at moderate risk (those who have significant risk factors, untreated hypertension, or a history of CAD) the evidence suggests benefits, but is less conclusive. The low cardiac event rate in this population requires larger, well-designed trials to achieve statistical significance. One such study is the Perioperative Ischemic Evaluation (POISE) trial. The POISE trial is an ongoing international study examining perioperative metoprolol versus placebo in moderate and high-risk cardiac patients. The study began in 2004 and plans for the recruitment of 10,000 patients.

A recent large retrospective cohort study (n = 782,969) assessed the use of perioperative beta-blockers and their association with in-hospital mortality in routine clinical practice in noncardiac surgery in the United States [29]. The study used propensity-score matching to adjust for differences between patients. The relationship between perioperative beta-blocker treatment and the risk of death varied directly with cardiac risk. Among high-risk patients with a Revised Cardiac Risk Index score of greater than two, perioperative beta-blocker therapy was associated with a reduced risk of in-hospital death. In patients with a Revised Cardiac Risk Index score of two, three, or four, the adjusted odds ratio for death were 0.88, 0.71, and 0.58, respectively. In contrast, among patients with a Revised Cardiac Risk Index score of zero or one, treatment was associated with no benefit and possible harm. This study was limited, however, in its retrospective nature. The study contained no data regarding cardiac adverse events and did not explain why patients were receiving beta-blockade. The authors of this cohort study concluded that increasing the use of beta-blockers in high-risk patients might enhance patient safety.

Who should receive perioperative beta-blockade?

Criteria for identifying patients that may benefit from perioperative beta-blockers have varied between trials, but in general recommendations have been based on multi-factorial indices designed to predict cardiac risk. The Revised Cardiac Risk Index, proposed by Lee et al. [5], is a simple and well-studied method of perioperative risk assessment. This system uses six clinical variables and has been incorporated into several proposed treatment algorithms for using perioperative beta-blockers (Tables 1 and 2) [30,31]. Patients at low risk (class I; 0 risk factors) receive little benefit from perioperative beta-blockers, and the reported cardiac complication rate in this population was 0.4% with beta-blockers and 1.0% without beta-blockers. These patients should proceed to the operating room without beta-blocker therapy. These results contrast with those for high-risk populations, where the benefit is most apparent. For high-risk patients (class IV; ≥3 risk factors), the cardiac complication rate ranged from 3.4% to 14% with beta-blockers and 9.8% to 32% without beta-blockers [32]. Patients at intermediate risk with one or two risk factors may also benefit from beta-blockers but the effects are less pronounced. Therefore, all patients with a significant risk factor are candidates for beta-blocker therapy unless contraindicated. Despite evidence supporting the use of perioperative beta-blockers, they are still poorly used. Based on current recommendations for using perioperative beta-blockers, studies have found a compliance rate of only 40% in patients meeting the proposed criteria [33,34]. Improving clinician awareness regarding the use of beta-blockers and instituting guidelines are relatively simple methods to improve outcome and have been shown to improve compliance [35].

Table 1
Likelihood of cardiac complications in noncardiac surgery

Risk factor	Odds ratio (95% CI)
High-risk surgery[a]	2.8 (1.6–4.9)
Ischemic heart disease	2.4 (1.3–4.2)
History of congestive heart failure	1.9 (1.1–3.5)
History of cerebrovascular disease	3.2 (1.8–6.0)
Diabetes (insulin dependent)	3.0 (1.3–7.1)
Renal insufficiency (serum creatinine >2.0 mg/dL)	3.0 (1.4–6.8)

[a] High-risk surgery is defined as intrathoracic, intraperitoneal, or suprainguinal vascular procedures. Ischemic heart disease is defined as history of myocardial infarction, positive exercise test, chest pain consistent with ischemia, use of nitrates, and pathological Q waves on ECG.

Data from Lee TH, Marcantonio ER, Mangione CM, et al. Derivation and prospective validation of a simple index for prediction of cardiac risk of major noncardiac surgery. Circulation 1999;100(10):1043–9.

Table 2
Indications for beta-blocker therapy

Revised cardiac risk index	Cardiac event rate (95% CI) (+/− beta-blockers)	Beta-blocker therapy?
Class I (0 risk factor)	0.4 (0.1–0.9) and 1.0 (0.6–1.9)	No benefit
Class II (1 risk factor)	0.8 (03.–1.7) and 2.2 (1.4–3.3)	Probable benefit
Class III (2 risk factors)	1.6 (0.8–3.3) and 4.5 (3.2–6.3)	Yes
Class IV (3 risk factors)	3.4 (1.7–6.7) and 9.2 (6.5–13)	Yes
(4 risk factors)	7.0 (3.4–14) and 18 (12–26)	
(≥5 risk factors)	14 (6.5–27) and 32 (19–47)	

Data from Boersma E, Poldermans D, Bax JJ, et al. Predictors of cardiac events after major vascular surgery: role of clinical characteristics, dobutamine echocardiography, and beta-blocker therapy. JAMA 2001;285(14):1865–73.

Which beta-blockers should be used?

Several beta-blockers have been studied and proven to be effective, but treatment should be initiated with β_1 selective agents (eg, atenolol, bisoprolol, and metoprolol). Beta$_1$ selective agents have a lower potential for adverse side effects, and recent evidence suggests that they can safely be used for most patients who have reactive airway disease and insulin-diabetes mellitus, generally considered contraindications. Greater caution should be exercised in patients who have uncompensated congestive heart failure, aortic stenosis, severe and active reactive airway disease, and severe cardiac conduction abnormalities. In randomized trials, the most common adverse reaction was bradycardia, which was as high as 10% in the trial by Mangano et al. These episodes had minor clinical significance and required no additional treatment. Although less well studied, other potentially beneficial medications include alpha$_2$-adrenergic agonists, statins, and nitrates [36,37]. These medications have not been shown to be as effective, but may offer an alternative for patients who have contraindications to treatment with beta-blockers.

Timing and duration of beta-blockade

Treatment with beta-blockers should be initiated before anesthetic induction, but no one has yet determined the best timing. The recommended timing for the first dose varies in treatment algorithms, with suggested initiation ranging from 30 days before surgery to immediately before surgery when the patient is in the preanesthesia holding area. The most important principle is that adequate beta-blockade be achieved by the time of surgery. Initiating treatment with short-acting medications may facilitate rapid achievement of this goal. One strategy for initiation of beta-blockade preoperatively is listed in Box 2. Most studies report that a resting heart rate of about 60 beats per minute (bpm) is effective. A single study that failed to achieve this level of beta-blockade also failed to demonstrate significant treatment

---

Box 2. Recommendations for initiation of β-blockade

- Initiation is best 1–2 weeks prior to surgery.
- Goal heart rate is within 60–80 bpm range.
- Evaluate patient's baseline heart rate and blood pressure.
- Start administration of metoprolol 25 to 50 mg by mouth twice daily based on baseline heart rate and blood pressure. Use lower dose (25 mg twice daily) if heart rate in 70–80 bpm range and systolic blood pressure in 110–140 mm Hg range.
- If patient already taking β-blockade, consider increase in dose to achieve goal heart rate of 60–80 bpm preoperatively.
- Continue administering β-blockade postoperatively for at least 1 week.
- Consider continued long-term administration of β-blockade if patient has two or more cardiac risk factors. Long-term administration of β-blockade has been associated with reduced cardiac complications and mortality.
- Do not initiate in patients with severe left-ventricular dysfunction or in decompensated heart failure. Consult cardiology if ejection fraction <20%.

---

effect [38]. The ACC/AHA recommends beginning treatment days to weeks before surgery and maintaining a resting heart rate between 50 and 60 bpm [4]. The appropriate duration of treatment is also unknown, but one study has shown continued benefit up to 2 years, and many patients would likely benefit from long-term treatment. Therefore, although the most benefit may be obtained during the perioperative period, longer treatment may also be warranted.

Summary

Perioperative beta-blockers significantly reduce morbidity and mortality in noncardiac surgery and appear to offer the greatest benefit to high-risk patients. Because of the lower complication rate in intermediate- and low-risk patients and the absence of large randomized controlled trials, the role of beta-blockers in this population is less well defined. Larger studies, such as the POISE study, may offer some clarity, and the optimal timing, duration, and form of beta-blockade continues to be investigated. Even so, in view of the current evidence and the low complication risk of cardio-selective beta-blockers, treatment should be offered to moderate- and high-risk patients. The ACC, the AHA, the American College of Physicians, and the Agency for Health Care Research and Quality currently recommend perioperative beta-blockers in this population.

Despite the supporting evidence and national recommendations, beta-blockers continue to be underused. The reason for poor physician compliance with these guidelines is unclear, but the benefit of using beta-blockers appears to far outweigh the reasons not to use them. In suitable patients, cardioselective beta-blockade is a simple and cost-effective intervention that may greatly improve patient outcomes and should be a standard component in perioperative care.

References

[1] Mangano DT, Goldman L. Preoperative assessment of patients with known or suspected coronary disease. N Engl J Med 1995;333(26):1750–6.

[2] Mangano DT. Perioperative cardiac morbidity. Anesthesiology 1990;72(1):153–84.

[3] Eagle KA, Brundage BH, Chaitman BR, et al. Guidelines for perioperative cardiovascular evaluation for noncardiac surgery. Report of the American College of Cardiology/American Heart Association Task Force on Practice Guidelines. Committee on Perioperative Cardiovascular Evaluation for Noncardiac Surgery. Circulation 1996;93(6):1278–317.

[4] Eagle KA, Berger PB, Calkins H, et al. ACC/AHA guideline update for perioperative cardiovascular evaluation for noncardiac surgery—executive summary: a report of the American College of Cardiology/American Heart Association Task Force on Practice Guidelines (Committee to Update the 1996 Guidelines on Perioperative Cardiovascular Evaluation for Noncardiac Surgery). Circulation 2002;105(10):1257–67.

[5] Lee TH, Marcantonio ER, Mangione CM, et al. Derivation and prospective validation of a simple index for prediction of cardiac risk of major noncardiac surgery. Circulation 1999;100(10):1043–9.

[6] McFalls EO, Ward HB, Moritz TE, et al. Coronary-artery revascularization before elective major vascular surgery. N Engl J Med 2004;351(27):2795–804.

[7] Eagle KA, Guyton RA, Davidoff R, et al. ACC/AHA 2004 guideline update for coronary artery bypass graft surgery: a report of the American College of Cardiology/American Heart Association Task Force on Practice Guidelines (Committee to Update the 1999 Guidelines for Coronary Artery Bypass Graft Surgery). Circulation 2004;110(14):e340–437.

[8] Smith SC Jr, Dove JT, Jacobs AK, et al. ACC/AHA guidelines of percutaneous coronary interventions (revision of the 1993 PTCA guidelines)—executive summary. A report of the American College of Cardiology/American Heart Association Task Force on Practice Guidelines (committee to revise the 1993 guidelines for percutaneous transluminal coronary angioplasty). J Am Coll Cardiol 2001;37(8):2215–39.

[9] Anderson HV, Shaw RE, Brindis RG, et al. A contemporary overview of percutaneous coronary interventions. The American College of Cardiology-National Cardiovascular Data Registry (ACC-NCDR). J Am Coll Cardiol 2002;39(7):1096–103.

[10] Bradbury A, Adam D, Garrioch M, et al. Changes in platelet count, coagulation and fibrinogen associated with elective repair of asymptomatic abdominal aortic aneurysm and aortic reconstruction for occlusive disease. Eur J Vasc Endovasc Surg 1997;13(4):375–80.

[11] Reddy PR, Vaitkus PT. Risks of noncardiac surgery after coronary stenting. Am J Cardiol 2005;95(6):755–7.

[12] Wilson SH, Fasseas P, Orford JL, et al. Clinical outcome of patients undergoing non-cardiac surgery in the two months following coronary stenting. J Am Coll Cardiol 2003;42(2):234–40.

[13] Kaluza GL, Joseph J, Lee JR, et al. Catastrophic outcomes of noncardiac surgery soon after coronary stenting. J Am Coll Cardiol 2000;35(5):1288–94.

[14] Dawood MM, Gutpa DK, Southern J, et al. Pathology of fatal perioperative myocardial infarction: implications regarding pathophysiology and prevention. Int J Cardiol 1996;57(1):37–44.

[15] Wallace A, Layug B, Tateo I, et al. Prophylactic atenolol reduces postoperative myocardial ischemia. McSPI Research Group. Anesthesiology 1998;88(1):7–17.

[16] Raby KE, Brull SJ, Timimi F, et al. The effect of heart rate control on myocardial ischemia among high-risk patients after vascular surgery. Anesth Analg 1999;88(3):477–82.

[17] Landesberg G, Luria MH, Cotev S, et al. Importance of long-duration postoperative ST-segment depression in cardiac morbidity after vascular surgery. Lancet 1993;341(8847): 715–9.

[18] Landesberg G. The pathophysiology of perioperative myocardial infarction: facts and perspectives. J Cardiothorac Vasc Anesth 2003;17(1):90–100.

[19] Gibbons RJ, Chatterjee K, Daley J, et al. ACC/AHA/ACP-ASIM guidelines for the management of patients with chronic stable angina: executive summary and recommendations. A report of the American College of Cardiology/American Heart Association Task Force on Practice Guidelines (Committee on Management of Patients with Chronic Stable Angina). Circulation 1999;99(21):2829–48.

[20] London MJ, Zaugg M, Schaub MC, et al. Perioperative beta-adrenergic receptor blockade: physiologic foundations and clinical controversies. Anesthesiology 2004;100(1):170–5.

[21] Zaugg M, Schaub MC, Pasch T, et al. Modulation of beta-adrenergic receptor subtype activities in perioperative medicine: mechanisms and sites of action. Br J Anaesth 2002;88(1): 101–23.

[22] Ohtsuka T, Hamada M, Hiasa G, et al. Effect of beta-blockers on circulating levels of inflammatory and anti-inflammatory cytokines in patients with dilated cardiomyopathy. J Am Coll Cardiol 2001;37(2):412–7.

[23] Mangano DT, Layug EL, Wallace A, et al. Effect of atenolol on mortality and cardiovascular morbidity after noncardiac surgery. Multicenter study of Perioperative Ischemia Research Group. N Engl J Med 1996;335(23):1713–20.

[24] Devereaux PJ, Yusuf S, Yang H, et al. Are the recommendations to use perioperative beta-blocker therapy in patients undergoing noncardiac surgery based on reliable evidence? CMAJ 2004;171(3):245–7.

[25] Poldermans D, Boersma E, Bax JJ, et al. The effect of bisoprolol on perioperative mortality and myocardial infarction in high-risk patients undergoing vascular surgery. Dutch Echocardiographic Cardiac Risk Evaluation Applying Stress Echocardiography Study Group. N Engl J Med 1999;341(24):1789–94.

[26] Poldermans D, Boersma E, Bax JJ, et al. Bisoprolol reduces cardiac death and myocardial infarction in high-risk patients as long as 2 years after successful major vascular surgery. Eur Heart J 2001;22(15):1353–8.

[27] Stevens RD, Burri H, Tramer MR. Pharmacologic myocardial protection in patients undergoing noncardiac surgery: a quantitative systematic review. Anesth Analg 2003;97(3): 623–33.

[28] Egger M, Smith GD, Phillips AN. Meta-analysis: principles and procedures. BMJ 1997; 315(7121):1533–7.

[29] Lindenauer PK, Pekow P, Wang K, et al. Perioperative beta-blocker therapy and mortality after major noncardiac surgery. N Engl J Med 2005;353(4):349–61.

[30] Auerbach AD, Goldman L. Beta-blockers and reduction of cardiac events in noncardiac surgery: scientific review. JAMA 2002;287(11):1435–44.

[31] Fleisher LA, Eagle KA. Clinical practice. Lowering cardiac risk in noncardiac surgery. N Engl J Med 2001;345(23):1677–82.

[32] Boersma E, Poldermans D, Bax JJ, et al. Predictors of cardiac events after major vascular surgery: role of clinical characteristics, dobutamine echocardiography, and beta-blocker therapy. JAMA 2001;285(14):1865–73.

[33] Rapchuk I, Rabuka S, Tonelli M. Perioperative use of beta-blockers remains low: experience of a single Canadian tertiary institution. Can J Anaesth 2004;51(8):761–7.

[34] Siddiqui AK, Ahmed S, Delbeau H, et al. Lack of physician concordance with guidelines on the perioperative use of beta-blockers. Arch Intern Med 2004;164(6):664–7.

[35] Almanaseer Y, Mukherjee D, Kline-Rogers EM, et al. Implementation of the ACC/AHA guidelines for preoperative cardiac risk assessment in a general medicine preoperative clinic: improving efficiency and preserving outcomes. Cardiology 2005;103(1):24–9.

[36] Wijeysundera DN, Naik JS, Beattie WS. Alpha-2 adrenergic agonists to prevent perioperative cardiovascular complications: a meta-analysis. Am J Med 2003;114(9):742–52.

[37] O'Neil-Callahan K, Katsimaglis G, Tepper MR, et al. Statins decrease perioperative cardiac complications in patients undergoing noncardiac vascular surgery: the Statins for Risk Reduction in Surgery (StaRRS) study. J Am Coll Cardiol 2005;45(3):336–42.

[38] Urban MK, Markowitz SM, Gordon MA, et al. Postoperative prophylactic administration of beta-adrenergic blockers in patients at risk for myocardial ischemia. Anesth Analg 2000; 90(6):1257–61.

ELSEVIER
SAUNDERS

Surg Clin N Am 85 (2005) 1103–1114

SURGICAL
CLINICS OF
NORTH AMERICA

Perioperative Cardiac Issues: Postoperative Arrhythmias

Kathleen M. Heintz, DO, Steven M. Hollenberg, MD*

*Division of Cardiology and Critical Care Medicine, Cooper University Hospital,
Robert Wood Johnson Medical School, One Cooper Plaza, Camden, New Jersey 08103, USA*

Postoperative arrhythmias are common and represent a major source of morbidity after surgical procedures. Following cardiac surgery, supraventricular tachycardias (SVTs), most notably atrial fibrillation, may occur in 30% to 40% of patients [1]. Atrial fibrillation following noncardiac surgery occurs less often, in approximately 4% of patients [2]. Findings from studies conducted in the context of perioperative arrhythmias following cardiac surgery may be carefully applied to patients undergoing noncardiac surgery. The patient's underlying cardiac status is the key to management.

Postoperative arrhythmias are most likely to occur in patients with structural heart disease. The initiating factor for an arrhythmia in a patient following surgery is usually a transient imbalance, often related to hypoxia, ischemia, catecholamines, electrolyte abnormalities, or another insult. Management includes correction of the imbalances and therapy directed at the arrhythmia itself.

The physiologic impact of an arrhythmia depends on ventricular response rate, duration of arrhythmia, and underlying cardiac function. Bradyarrhythmias may decrease cardiac output due to heart rate alone in patients with a relatively fixed stroke volume. Loss of atrial contraction may cause a dramatic increase in pulmonary artery pressures in patients with hypertension and diastolic dysfunction. Similarly, tachyarrhythmias can decrease diastolic filling time and reduce cardiac output, resulting in hypotension and possible myocardial ischemia. The impact of a given arrhythmia depends on the patient's cardiac physiology and function. Treatment is determined by the hemodynamic insult.

This article reviews current concepts in the diagnosis and acute management of arrhythmias after surgery. A systematic approach to diagnosis and

* Corresponding author.
  E-mail address: hollenberg-steven@cooperhealth.edu (S.M. Hollenberg).

0039-6109/05/$ - see front matter © 2005 Elsevier Inc. All rights reserved.
doi:10.1016/j.suc.2005.09.003   *surgical.theclinics.com*

evaluation of predisposing factors is presented, followed by consideration of specific arrhythmias.

Diagnosis of postoperative arrhythmias

Basic principles

The first principle in managing arrhythmias is to appropriately treat the patient, not the electrocardiogram. Accordingly, one must first decide whether the observed arrhythmia may be an artifact. If the arrhythmia is real and sustained, it must be determined whether it has important clinical consequences.

The next step is to establish the urgency of treatment. Clinical assessment includes evaluation of pulse, blood pressure, peripheral perfusion, and consideration of myocardial ischemia or congestive heart failure. If the patient loses consciousness or becomes hemodynamically unstable in the presence of a tachyarrhythmia other than sinus tachycardia, prompt cardioversion may be indicated regardless of anticoagulation status. If the patient is stable, time is often available to establish the rhythm diagnosis and decide upon the most appropriate treatment. Bradyarrhythmias produce less of a diagnostic challenge and treatment options are relatively straightforward.

The goals of antiarrhythmic therapy depend on the type of rhythm disturbance. The initial goal for the treatment of an arrhythmia in the critical care setting is to stabilize the hemodynamics and ventricular response. The next goal is to restore sinus rhythm if possible. If restoration of sinus rhythm cannot be achieved, prevention of complications is important.

Classification of arrhythmias

Arrhythmias are usually classified according to anatomic origin, either supraventricular or ventricular. The most common supraventricular arrhythmia is sinus tachycardia, followed by atrial fibrillation, ectopic atrial or junctional tachycardia, multifocal atrial tachycardia, atrioventricular (AV) nodal re-entry tachycardias, and accessory pathway tachycardias. Ventricular arrhythmias are most commonly premature ventricular beats, ventricular tachycardia and ventricular fibrillation.

It is sometimes useful to consider tachyarrhythmias from a treatment standpoint. Tachyarrhythmias that traverse the AV node can often be controlled by pharmacologically altering AV nodal conduction. Rhythms that traverse the AV node include atrial fibrillation and flutter, ectopic atrial and junctional tachycardias, multifocal atrial tachycardia, and AV nodal re-entry tachycardias. Rhythms that do not use the AV node include accessory pathway tachycardias through a bypass tract, ventricular tachycardia, and ventricular fibrillation. When the arrhythmia does not use the AV node, slowing AV nodal conduction can be dangerous.

Rhythm diagnosis

A comprehensive description of the diagnosis of arrhythmias is beyond the scope of this manuscript. A 12-lead electrocardiogram with a long rhythm strip and a previously obtained 12-lead electrocardiogram for comparison are ideal. If a previous EKG is not available, a systematic approach using a current 12-lead EKG is essential. An approach is outlined using the following four steps [3].

Locate the P wave

P waves are often best seen in leads II and V_1. Normal P waves are upright in leads II, III and aVF, and may be biphasic in leads II and V_1. If P waves are present and always followed by a QRS complex, the rhythm is most likely sinus tachycardia, which usually occurs at a rate of between 100 and 180 per minute in adults. Patients with ectopic atrial and junctional tachycardias often present with negative P-waves in leads II, III and aVF. If P waves are present and the rhythm is irregular, the rhythm is most likely atrial fibrillation. If the P wave is buried in the QRS or ST segment, the rhythm is most likely AV nodal re-entry tachycardia, which usually present with atrial rates from 140 to 220 per minute. If there are multiple P waves followed by a single QRS, especially if the atrial rate is near 300 per minute, the rhythm is most likely atrial flutter. If no P waves are present, the rhythm is most likely atrial fibrillation.

Establish the relationship between the P wave and QRS

If there are more P waves than QRS complexes, then AV block is present. If there are more QRS complexes than P waves, the rhythm is likely an accelerated junctional or ventricular rhythm. If the relationship of the P wave and QRS is 1:1, then measurement of the PR interval can yield useful diagnostic clues.

Examine the QRS morphology

A narrow QRS complex (< 0.12 ms) indicates a supraventricular arrhythmia. A wide QRS complex can be either ventricular tachycardia or SVT with either a pre-existing bundle branch block or, less commonly, an aberrant ventricular conduction or an antegrade accessory pathway.

Search for other clues

The clues to guide appropriate therapy depend on the situation. Carotid sinus massage increases AV block and can either break an SVT or bring out previously undetected flutter waves. Any patient with a ventricular rate of exactly 150 beats per minute should be suspected of having atrial flutter with two to one AV-block. A rate greater than 200 beats per minute in an otherwise healthy adult should raise the suspicion of an accessory pathway. Severe left axis deviation ($-60°$ to $120°$) during tachycardia suggests a ventricular origin, as does AV dissociation, fusion beats, which result from simultaneous activation of two foci, one ventricular and one supraventricular, and capture beats, which are beats that capture the ventricles and are conducted with a narrow complex, ruling out fixed bundle branch block. Grouped beating or more P waves than QRS complexes suggests the possibility of second-degree AV-block.

Predisposing factors for postoperative arrhythmias

Postoperative stress makes patients susceptible to developing arrhythmias. Specific factors, including hypoxemia, hypercarbia, myocardial ischemia, catecholamines, electrolyte or acid–base imbalances, may cause the insult. Drug effects and mechanical factors, such as instrumentation, may also be the cause [4]. Atrial fibrillation following cardiac surgery is the most thoroughly studied postoperative arrhythmia. Proposed mechanisms for postoperative atrial fibrillation include acute atrial distension, atrial inflammation from the trauma of surgery, ischemic injury to the atria due to cardioplegia, and electrolyte and volume shifts during bypass that alter atrial repolarization [5]. However, attribution of an arrhythmia to a single predisposing factor may oversimplify a complex situation. For example, hypokalemia may predispose to the development of perioperative ventricular arrhythmias. Catecholamine release, however, increases cellular potassium uptake and may decrease serum potassium levels [6]. In this context, it may not be clear whether the arrhythmia is due to hypokalemia, is catecholamine-mediated, or results from a combination of both.

Regardless of the complexity of the arrhythmogenesis, the identification and correction of potential predisposing factors form the cornerstone to management of postoperative arrhythmias. In conjunction with assessment of cardiac function, this often determines what therapy is needed. Self-terminating arrhythmias in the setting of transient stress often need no therapy at all. The development of a hemodynamically significant arrhythmia in a patient likely to remain stressed for some time points to the need for intervention.

Bradycardias

Sinus node dysfunction

Bradycardias associated with sinus node dysfunction include sinus bradycardia, sinus pause, sinoatrial block, and sinus arrest. In the perioperative setting, these disturbances often result from increased vagal tone due to spinal or epidural anesthesia, laryngoscopy, or surgical intervention [4]. Initial therapy for postoperative bradyarrhythmias does not differ from other acute circumstances. If bradycardia is transient and not associated with hemodynamic compromise, no therapy is necessary. If it is sustained or compromises end-organ perfusion, therapy with antimuscarinic agents, such as atropine, or beta agonists, such as ephedrine, may be initiated. Transcutaneous or transvenous pacing may be necessary in some cases.

Patients with a combination of bradycardia with paroxysmal atrial tachycardias due to preexisting conduction system disease can be challenging to manage pharmacologically. In these cases, insertion of a temporary pacemaker may allow the administration of rate-lowering agents.

Heart block

The most common cause of acquired chronic atrioventricular (AV) heart block is fibrosis of the conducting system. Although pre-existing conduction system disease is a risk factor for the development of complete heart block, no single laboratory or clinical variable identifies patients at risk for progression to high-degree AV block [7]. Acute myocardial infarction is a common cause of transient AV block. Criteria for insertion of temporary and permanent pacemakers in postoperative infarction are the same as the criteria for any infarction [7]. High-grade second- or third-degree AV block persisting for 7 to 14 days after cardiac surgery is an indication for permanent pacing [7]. It is reasonable to extend these recommendations to patients with high-degree AV block persisting after noncardiac surgery. The need for permanent pacing in patients with transient postoperative AV block and residual bifascicular block has not been established. Patients with AV conduction disturbances that return to normal following surgery have a favorable prognosis.

Supraventricular tachycardias

Supraventricular arrhythmias are common after surgery. Their incidence was estimated at 4% in a large registry of patients undergoing major noncardiac procedures [8], 3.2% in a multicenter study of patients undergoing abdominal aortic aneurysm repair [9], and almost 13% in 295 patients undergoing thoracotomy for lung cancer [10]. Supraventricular tachyarrhythmias can be broken down into atrial tachycardias, atrioventricular nodal reentrant tachycardias (AVNRT), and accessory pathway reentrant tachycardias.

Atrial tachycardias can arise from either an ectopic automatic focus or a reentrant pathway. They comprise approximately 8% of paroxysmal SVTs in adults, and are diagnosed by identification of P wave morphology different from that in sinus rhythm. Potential mechanisms include abnormal automaticity, triggered activity or digitalis intoxication [11]. Short bursts of atrial tachycardias do not require specific drug therapy unless they persist.

Multifocal atrial tachycardia (MAT) usually occurs in acutely ill, elderly patients, or in patients with pulmonary disease [12]. MAT is diagnosed by the presence of three or more different P wave morphologies on one EKG with an irregular rhythm. The most useful therapy for MAT is to treat the underlying causes, including hypoxemia and hypercapnia, myocardial ischemia, congestive heart failure, or electrolyte disturbances. Beta blockers and calcium channel blockers can slow an excessive ventricular rate [13]. These agents should be used cautiously in patients with known congestive heart failure or reduced left ventricular function.

AVNRT is the most common paroxysmal supraventricular tachycardia, accounting for about 60% of all supraventricular arrhythmias [11]. Dual AV nodal pathways with different conduction velocities and refractory periods are usually present, setting up the substrate for re-entry. P waves may not be visible on the electrocardiogram due to near simultaneous retrograde atrial and antegrade ventricular activation. Carotid sinus massage or other vagal maneuvers may convert AVNRT to normal sinus rhythm. Adenosine 6 to 12 mg IV is the preferred initial drug treatment because its extremely short half-life reduces side effects. The 12-mg dose may be repeated if necessary. Urgent cardioversion may be necessary with circulatory insufficiency. Beta blockers or calcium channel blockers should be used judiciously due to their negative ionotropic effects and their potential for vasodilation.

Approximately 30% of patients with supraventricular tachycardia have an accessory pathway between the atrium and the ventricle [11]. The bypass tract may be manifest, with a delta wave visible on the baseline EKG, or concealed. When conduction goes down the AV node and back up the by pass tract, the QRS complex is narrow and conduction is termed orthodromic [11]. Therapy for orthodromic accessory pathway reentrant tachycardias entails AV nodal blockade with vagal maneuvers, IV adenosine, and calcium channel blockers. When conduction goes down the bypass tract and back up the AV node, the QRS complex is wide and conduction is termed antidromic [11]. For antidromic accessory pathway reentrant tachycardias, IV procainamide is the drug of choice. In both circumstances, cardioversion is indicated for hemodynamic collapse.

Atrial flutter or fibrillation in the setting of an accessory pathway is dangerous because of the potential for extremely rapid conduction down the accessory pathway with resultant rapid ventricular rates and possible deterioration to ventricular fibrillation. In this situation, competition between AV nodal conduction and conduction down the bypass tract modulates the ventricular rate. AV nodal blockade may increase ventricular rate, and can precipitate ventricular fibrillation [14]. Drugs that slow conduction down the accessory pathway, such as IV procainamide and amiodarone, can be used for acute termination. Urgent cardioversion may be indicated.

Atrial fibrillation and flutter

Supraventricular arrhythmias are common after both cardiac and noncardiac surgery. Of these, atrial fibrillation (AF) is by far the most common arrhythmia, with potentially serious consequences. In one prospective series of 916 patients over 40 years old undergoing major noncardiac surgery, the incidence of SVT was 4%. Atrial flutter and fibrillation represented 63% of these arrhythmias [8].

Atrial fibrillation and flutter are even more common after cardiac surgery, with rates ranging from 30% to 40% after coronary artery bypass surgery [15,16]. The incidence is even higher following valve replacement, and may be as high as 60% [17]. Due to its incidence, potential morbidity, and association with increased length of stay, AF has been well studied after cardiac surgery. Many, if not most, patients who have AF after noncardiac surgery have underlying cardiac disease. It is reasonable to apply findings in patients with AF after cardiac surgery to the setting of noncardiac surgery. The American College of Chest Physicians has recently published "ACCP Guidelines for the Prevention and Management of Postoperative Atrial Fibrillation After Cardiac Surgery." These guidelines are comprehensive and provide evidence-based recommendations for clinical practice [18].

Risk factors associated with an increased risk of postoperative AF after cardiac surgery include increased age, postoperative electrolyte shifts, pericarditis, a history of preoperative atrial fibrillation, a history of congestive heart failure, and chronic obstructive pulmonary disease [5,19,20]. Most of these risk factors are probably predictive after noncardiac surgery, although this has not been well studied. Atrial fibrillation generally occurs 2 to 4 days after open heart surgery and episodes tend to be transient, frequent, and recurrent.

AF with a rapid ventricular response can worsen diastolic filling due to decreased filling time and loss of atrioventricular synchrony. Symptoms can include chest pain, shortness of breath, and dizziness. For unstable patients who have hypotension, pulmonary edema, or unstable angina, urgent cardioversion is indicated. Intravenous ibutilide, a class III antiarrhythmic agent, is effective in stopping atrial fibrillation and flutter. It is an alternative for acute cardioversion in the hemodynamically stable patient [21]. Ibutilide is administered as a 1 mg bolus over 10 minutes, and can be repeated in 10 minutes, provided the QT interval is not excessively prolonged. The QT prolongation induced by ibutilide is associated with a risk of torsade de pointes, and therefore continuous EKG monitoring is recommended after ibutilide administration for 4 hours or until the QT interval returns to normal [5].

For patients who do not have hemodynamic compromise and who have AF lasting for more than 15 minutes, initiation of therapy to control the ventricular rate is recommended. Intravenous beta blockers are a logical choice in postoperative patients with high sympathetic tone. Intravenous calcium channel blockers and intravenous amiodarone are alternatives for rate control (Table 1). Digoxin has a delayed onset of action and works by increasing vagal tone. Thus digoxin is typically ineffective for acute rate control in this setting. Patients will often convert to normal sinus rhythm on their own without antiarrhythmic medications or electrical intervention.

Table 1
Drugs Used for Postoperative Arrhythmias

Drug	Dosing	Indications	Side effects
Adenosine	6 mg; then 12 mg IV	Paroxysmal SVT; diagnosis of wide or narrow QRS tachycardias	Transient heart block, flushing, chest pain
Atropine	0.4–1 mg IV	Bradycardia or AV block	Excessive tachycardia; myocardial ischemia
Diltiazem	10–20 mg IV bolus; then infusion at 5–15 mg/hr	Rate control	Hypotension; CHF
Esmolol	0.5 mg/kg bolus and infusion at 0.05 mg/kg/hr. ↑ by 0.05 mg/kg/hr q 5 min	Rapid rate control	Bronchospasm; hypotension, exacerbation of CHF
Metoprolol	5 mg IV q 5 min × 3	Rate control	Bronchospasm; hypotension, exacerbation of CHF
Digoxin	0.25 mg IV q 4–6 hr up to 1 mg	Chronic AF	Delayed onset; arrhythmias, nausea, vomiting
Ibutilide	1 mg IV over 10 min. May repeat × 1	Conversion of AF	QT prolongation; torsades de pointes
Amiodarone	150 mg IV over 10 min, then 1 mg/min × 6 hr, then 0.5 mg/min	Refractory VT or VF; rate control and conversion of AF	Occasional mild hypotension with bolus; heart block

Abbreviations: CHF, congestive heart failure; VT, ventricular tachycardia; VF, ventricular fibrillation.

Most episodes of atrial fibrillation in the postoperative setting are self-limited, although they tend to be recurrent. Persistent atrial fibrillation is associated with increased risk of stroke or transient ischemic attack after 48 hours [22]. Antiarrhythmic medication is a reasonable choice for recurrent atrial fibrillation in the postoperative period. For persistent, recurrent AF, anticoagulation should be considered, weighing the potential benefits against the risk of postoperative bleeding.

The high incidence of postoperative AF after cardiac surgery, with the observation that its onset is generally late, has fueled interest in prophylactic measures to prevent its development. Beta blockers have been effective at preventing atrial fibrillation and other supraventricular arrhythmias after cardiac surgery [17]. The incidence of atrial fibrillation is much lower following noncardiac surgery, and so prophylactic beta blockers may be reserved for high-risk patients [23]. Prophylactic use of sotalol, a class III antiarrhythmic agent with beta blocking activity, decreases the incidence of atrial fibrillation following bypass surgery [24]. Several studies have examined the effects of amiodarone on the incidence of atrial fibrillation after cardiac surgery. In randomized trials, both oral amiodarone started 1 week before bypass surgery [25] and intravenous amiodarone given shortly after the completion of surgery [26,27] have reduced the rate of postoperative atrial fibrillation following cardiac surgery. These studies support the potential efficacy of these medications when applied to higher risk cardiac patients undergoing noncardiac surgery.

Ventricular tachycardias

Ventricular tachyarrhythmias (VT) can be classified as benign or malignant. The chief distinction, in addition to duration and hemodynamic consequences, is the presence of significant structural heart disease. This distinction is especially important when evaluating premature ventricular contractions (PVCs) and nonsustained ventricular tachycardia. In patients without structural heart disease, the risk of sudden death or hemodynamic compromise is low, and therapy is rarely necessary in the absence of symptoms. In patients with coronary artery disease, a history of myocardial infarction, or cardiomyopathy, PVCs may indicate the potential for malignant ventricular tachyarrhythmias and merit prompt and thorough assessment. Prompt evaluation for and reversal of precipitating factors, such as ischemia and electrolyte abnormalities, are indicated. Although specific antiarrhythmic therapy may not be needed in all cases, empiric beta blockade or nitroglycerin should be considered.

Studies have evaluated empiric beta blockade in patients undergoing noncardiac surgery. In one study, 200 high-risk patients undergoing noncardiac surgery were randomized to atenolol or placebo, starting preoperatively and continuing until hospital discharge [23]. Atenolol produced a 15% absolute reduction in a combined cardiovascular end point at 6 months, and reduced mortality at both 6 months and 2 years [23]. Although this trial does not directly address the use of beta blockade as postoperative antiarrhythmic therapy, the findings tend to support empiric postoperative initiation of atenolol in high-risk patients with arrhythmias.

Serious ventricular arrhythmias are becoming uncommon after cardiac surgery, and are even less common after noncardiac surgery. The incidence of sustained VT and ventricular fibrillation (VF) after coronary artery bypass surgery was reported to be 1.2% in one series [28], with most cases occurring on the first postoperative day. Causes included perioperative infarction, hypoxia, medications, hypokalemia, and hypomagnesemia. Other series have also found similarly low rates of de novo ventricular arrhythmias after cardiac surgery [29].

Data regarding serious ventricular arrhythmias after noncardiac surgery are sparse. The most common setting is postoperative infarction with underlying structural heart disease [30]. In this context, ventricular arrhythmias may be more worrisome than after cardiac surgery because underlying coronary artery disease may not have been addressed preoperatively.

Sustained monomorphic VT is a reentrant rhythm most commonly occurring more than 48 hours after a myocardial infarction, or in the setting of cardiomyopathy. Initial management of sustained monomorphic VT with a history of structural heart disease depends on its rate, duration, and hemodynamic status. Unstable VT is an indication for prompt defibrillation. Hemodynamically stable patients with a risk of imminent circulatory collapse may be treated with an antiarrhythmic, such as IV amiodarone. Current Advanced Cardiovascular Life Support guidelines consider lidocaine and IV procainamide alternative choices.

Polymorphic VT most commonly occurs in the setting of acute myocardial ischemia. Although it is often faster than sustained monomorphic VT and thus can lead to hemodynamic instability, many episodes of polymorphic VT terminate spontaneously. Initial management for polymorphic VT is similar to that for monomorphic VT, with defibrillation and antiarrhythmic drugs [31]. If ischemia is felt to be the cause of polymorphic VT, therapy for unstable angina may be initiated. If VT or VF persists despite treatment, and there is evidence for ongoing coronary artery disease, intra-aortic balloon pumping and coronary revascularization should be considered.

Torsade de pointes is a syndrome consisting of polymorphic VT with QT prolongation. Acquired QT prolongation is most often caused by drugs, including type I antiarrhythmic agents, tricyclic antidepressants, phenothiazines, nonsedating antihistamines, erythromycin, pentamidine, and azole antifungal agents. QT prolongation may also be caused by electrolyte abnormalities, especially hypomagnesemia, and exacerbated by other conditions, such as hypothyroidism, cerebrovascular accident, and liquid protein diets [32]. Empiric magnesium should be given to all patients with suspected torsade de pointes, since the risk is low and the potential benefits high. Since the length of the QT interval is affected by the RR interval, the use of isoproterenol or temporary pacing to increase the heart rate can be effective in patients with acquired QT prolongation and torsade de pointes [33].

References

[1] Maisel WH, Rawn JD, Stevenson WG. Atrial fibrillation after cardiac surgery. Ann Intern Med 2001;135(12):1061–73.
[2] Polanczyk CA, Goldman L, Marcantonio ER, Orav EJ, Lee TH. Supraventricular arrhythmia in patients having noncardiac surgery: clinical correlates and effect on length of stay. Ann Intern Med 1998;129(4):279–85.
[3] Marriott HJL. Practical electrocardiography. Baltimore: Williams & Wilkins; 1988.
[4] Atlee JL. Perioperative cardiac dysrhythmias: diagnosis and management. Anesthesiology 1997;86(6):1397–424.
[5] Ellenbogen KA, Chung MK, Asher CR, Wood MA. Postoperative atrial fibrillation. Adv Card Surg 1997;9:109–30.
[6] Pinski SL. Potassium replacement after cardiac surgery: it is not time to change practice, yet. Crit Care Med 1999;27(11):2581–2.

[7] Gregoratos G, Cheitlin MD, Conill A, et al. ACC/AHA guidelines for implantation of cardiac pacemakers and antiarrhythmia devices: executive summary–a report of the American College of Cardiology/American Heart Association Task Force on Practice Guidelines (Committee on Pacemaker Implantation). Circulation 1998;97(13):1325–35.

[8] Goldman L. Supraventricular tachyarrhythmias in hospitalized adults after surgery. Clinical correlates in patients over 40 years of age after major noncardiac surgery. Chest 1978;73(4): 450–4.

[9] Johnston KW. Multicenter prospective study of nonruptured abdominal aortic aneurysm. Part II. Variables predicting morbidity and mortality. J Vasc Surg 1989;9(3):437–47.

[10] Beck-Nielsen J, Sorensen HR, Alstrup P. Atrial fibrillation following thoracotomy for noncardiac diseases, in particular cancer of the lung. Acta Med Scand 1973;193(5):425–9.

[11] Kastor J. Arrhythmias. Philadelphia: WB Saunders; 1994.

[12] McCord J, Borzak S. Multifocal atrial tachycardia. Chest 1998;113(1):203–9.

[13] Levine JH, Michael JR, Guarnieri T. Treatment of multifocal atrial tachycardia with verapamil. N Engl J Med 1985;312(1):21–5.

[14] Phibbs B. Advanced EKG: boards and beyond: what you really need to know about electrocardiography. Boston: Little, Brown and Co.; 1997.

[15] Favaloro RG, Effler DB, Groves LK, Sheldon WC, Riahi M. Direct myocardial revascularization with saphenous vein autograft. Clinical experience in 100 cases. Dis Chest 1969;56(4): 279–83.

[16] Lauer MS, Eagle KA, Buckley MJ, DeSanctis RW. Atrial fibrillation following coronary artery bypass surgery. Prog Cardiovasc Dis 1989;31(5):367–78.

[17] Andrews TC, Reimold SC, Berlin JA, Antman EM. Prevention of supraventricular arrhythmias after coronary artery bypass surgery. A meta-analysis of randomized control trials. Circulation 1991;84(5 Suppl):III236–44.

[18] McKeown PP. ACCP guidelines for the prevention and management of postoperative atrial fibrillation after cardiac surgery. Chest 2005;128(2 Suppl):1S–5S.

[19] Podrid PJ. Prevention of postoperative atrial fibrillation: what is the best approach? J Am Coll Cardiol 1999;34(2):340–2.

[20] Creswell LL, Schuessler RB, Rosenbloom M, Cox JL. Hazards of postoperative atrial arrhythmias. Ann Thorac Surg 1993;56(3):539–49.

[21] Ellenbogen KA, Stambler BS, Wood MA, et al. Efficacy of intravenous ibutilide for rapid termination of atrial fibrillation and atrial flutter: a dose-response study. J Am Coll Cardiol 1996;28(1):130–6.

[22] Taylor GJ, Malik SA, Colliver JA, et al. Usefulness of atrial fibrillation as a predictor of stroke after isolated coronary artery bypass grafting. Am J Cardiol 1987;60(10): 905–7.

[23] Mangano DT, Layug EL, Wallace A, Tateo I. Effect of atenolol on mortality and cardiovascular morbidity after noncardiac surgery. Multicenter study of Perioperative Ischemia Research Group. N Engl J Med 1996;335(23):1713–20.

[24] Gomes JA, Ip J, Santoni-Rugiu F, et al. Oral d, l sotalol reduces the incidence of postoperative atrial fibrillation in coronary artery bypass surgery patients: a randomized, double-blind, placebo-controlled study. J Am Coll Cardiol 1999;34(2):334–9.

[25] Daoud EG, Strickberger SA, Man KC, et al. Preoperative amiodarone as prophylaxis against atrial fibrillation after heart surgery. N Engl J Med 1997;337(25):1785–91.

[26] Hohnloser SH, Meinertz T, Dammbacher T, et al. Electrocardiographic and antiarrhythmic effects of intravenous amiodarone: results of a prospective, placebo-controlled study. Am Heart J 1991;121(1 Pt 1):89–95.

[27] Guarnieri T, Nolan S, Gottlieb SO, Dudek A, Lowry DR. Intravenous amiodarone for the prevention of atrial fibrillation after open heart surgery: the Amiodarone Reduction in Coronary Heart (ARCH) trial. J Am Coll Cardiol 1999;34(2):343–7.

[28] Abedin Z, Soares J, Phillips DF, Sheldon WC. Ventricular tachyarrhythmias following surgery for myocardial revascularization. A follow-up study. Chest 1977;72(4):426–8.

[29] Steinberg JS, Gaur A, Sciacca R, Tan E. New-onset sustained ventricular tachycardia after cardiac surgery. Circulation 1999;99(7):903–8.

[30] Mahla E, Rotman B, Rehak P, et al. Perioperative ventricular dysrhythmias in patients with structural heart disease undergoing noncardiac surgery. Anesth Analg 1998;86(1):16–21.

[31] Grogin HR, Scheinman M. Evaluation and management of patients with polymorphic ventricular tachycardia. Cardiol Clin 1993;11(1):39–54.

[32] Napolitano C, Priori SG, Schwartz PJ. Torsade de pointes. Mechanisms and management. Drugs 1994;47(1):51–65.

[33] Roden DM. Torsade de pointes. Clin Cardiol 1993;16(9):683–6.

SURGICAL
CLINICS OF
NORTH AMERICA

Surg Clin N Am 85 (2005) 1115–1135

Surgical Site Infections

Philip S. Barie, MD, MBA*, Soumitra R. Eachempati, MD

Division of Critical Care and Trauma, Department of Surgery P713A, Weill Medical College of Cornell University, 525 East 68 Street, New York, NY 10021, USA

There has been a change in vernacular with respect to infections relating to surgical procedures, owing to confusion between infections of surgical incisions and those of traumatic wounds. Infections of surgical incisions are now referred to as surgical site infections (SSIs) [1]. Surgical site infections are recognized as a common surgical complication, occurring in about 3% of all surgical procedures and in up to 20% of patients undergoing emergency intra-abdominal procedures [2]. Potential complications include tissue destruction, failure or prolongation of proper wound healing, incisional hernias, and occasionally bacteremia. Additionally, recurrent pain and disfiguring and disabling scars may also result. Surgical site infections result in substantial morbidity, prolonged hospital stays, and increased direct patient costs. All of these factors have a substantial impact on patients and hospitals, and create a huge economic burden on the United States health care system [3]. Minimizing SSIs is a top priority for surgeons and hospitals to ensure the safest environment for patients undergoing surgery.

Definitions

What constitutes an SSI? Even experts disagree with respect to the appearance of the incision [2]. Is it cellulitis of the incision without drainage, or nonpurulent drainage without cellulitis? Is any incision infected that must be reopened, or is the requirement for antimicrobial therapy the best indicator? Most experts agree that surgical sites that do not harbor purulent fluid are not infected, but the lack of agreement otherwise means that any retrospective study of SSI is essentially unreliable and useless if it relied upon observation or antibiotic administration as diagnostic criteria.

---

* Corresponding author.
E-mail address: pbarie@med.cornell.edu (P.S. Barie).

0039-6109/05/$ - see front matter © 2005 Elsevier Inc. All rights reserved.
doi:10.1016/j.suc.2005.09.006   *surgical.theclinics.com*

Infection may occur within the surgical site at any depth, starting from the skin itself and extending to the deepest cavity that remains after resection of an organ. Superficial SSI involves tissues down to the fascia (Fig. 1), whereas deep SSI extends beneath the fascia but not intracavitary. Organ/space infections are subfascial or intracavitary, but if related directly to an operation, are considered to be SSIs.

Cellulitis is infection-related erythema of skin (although other tissues may be affected) without drainage or fluctuance. Abscess refers to localized collections of purulent material within tissue. Necrotizing soft tissue infections (NSTIs) invade tissue widely and rapidly, causing widespread tissue necrosis. When fascia is involved, the infection is referred to correctly as necrotizing fasciitis. Myonecrosis refers to involvement of underlying muscle. However, NSTIs are exceedingly unusual in the postoperative period. Two rare but dangerous examples are SSIs caused by *Streptococcus pneumoniae* or *Clostridium perfringens,* which should be managed as would other NSTIs.

Epidemiology

Issues related to bacterial contamination of the surgical site have been well defined [2]. Clean surgical procedures are those where the operation has affected only integumentary and musculoskeletal soft tissues. Clean-contaminated procedures are those where a hollow viscus (eg, alimentary, biliary, genitourinary, respiratory tract) has been opened under controlled circumstances (eg, elective colon surgery). Contaminated procedures are those where bacteria has been introduced extensively into a normally sterile body cavity, but for a period of time too brief to allow infection to become established during surgery (eg, penetrating abdominal trauma, enterotomy during adhesiolysis for mechanical bowel obstruction). Dirty procedures are those where the surgery is performed to control established infection (eg, colon resection for complicated diverticulitis).

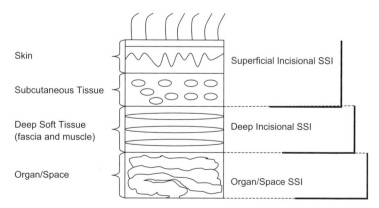

Fig. 1. Surgical site infections. (*Adapted from* Mangram AJ, Horan TC, Pearson ML, et al. The Hospital Infection Control Practices Advisory Committee. Guideline for the prevention of surgical site infection, 1999. Infect Control Hosp Epidemiol 1999;20:247–80.)

Box 1. Risk factors for the development of surgical site infections

Patient factors
Ascites
Chronic inflammation
Corticosteroid therapy (controversial)
Obesity
Diabetes
Extremes of age
Hypocholesterolemia
Hypoxemia
Peripheral vascular disease (especially for lower extremity surgery)
Postoperative anemia
Prior site irradiation
Recent operation
Remote infection
Skin carriage of staphylococci
Skin disease in the area of infection (eg, psoriasis)
Undernutrition

Environmental factors
Contaminated medications
Inadequate disinfection/sterilization
Inadequate skin antisepsis
Inadequate ventilation

Treatment factors
Drains
Emergency procedure
Hypothermia
Inadequate antibiotic prophylaxis
Oxygenation (controversial)
Prolonged preoperative hospitalization
Prolonged operative time

Data from National Nosocomial Infections Surveillance System (NNIS) System Report: Data summary from January 1992–June 2001, issued August 2001. Am J Infect Control 2001;29:404–21.

Numerous factors determine whether a patient will develop an SSI, including factors contributed by the patient, the environment, and the treatment (Box 1) [4]. As incorporated in the National Nosocomial Infections Surveillance System (NNIS) [4–6] (Table 1), the most recognized factors

Table 1
National Nosocomial Infections Surveillance System (NNIS) risk index for surgical site infections

Traditional class	0	1	2	3	All
Clean	1.0%	2.3%	5.4%	NA	2.1%
Clean/contaminated	2.1%	4.9%	9.5%	NA	3.3%
Contaminated	NA	3.4%	6.6%	13.2%	6.4%
Dirty	NA	3.1%	8.1%	12.8%	7.1%
All	1.5%	2.9%	6.8%	13.0%	2.8%

Abbreviation: NA, not applicable.

Data from National Nosocomial Infections Surveillance System (NNIS) system report: data summary from January 1992–June 2001, issued August 2001. Am J Infect Control 2001;29:404–21.

are the wound classification, American Society of Anesthesiology Class 3 or higher (chronic active medical illness; Box 2), and prolonged operative time, where time is longer than the 75th percentile for each such procedure. According to the NNIS classification, the risk of SSI increases with an increasing number of risk factors present, irrespective of the contamination of the incision (Table 2) and almost without regard for the type of operation (see Table 1, Fig. 2) [4].

Laparoscopic surgery is associated with a decreased incidence of SSI under certain circumstances, which has led to modifications of the NNIS risk classification [1]. For laparoscopic biliary, gastric, and colon surgery, one risk factor is subtracted if the operation is performed via the laparoscope. Thus, a new category has been created specifically for the circumstance, representing essentially a minus-1 risk factor. Laparoscopic surgery decreases the risk of SSI for several reasons. These include the smaller wound size, the limited use of cautery in the abdominal wall, and a diminished stress response to tissue injury. Laparoscopic appendectomy, however, is a special case. When no risk factors are present, the incidence of SSI after laparoscopic appendectomy is reduced significantly, but if any risk factor is present (as would be the case with either a perforated appendicitis or a procedure that lasts longer than one hour), then the advantage is lost.

More than 70% of surgical procedures are now performed on an outpatient basis, which poses major problems for surveillance of SSI [7]. Although many SSIs will develop in the first 5 to 10 days after surgery, an SSI may develop as long as 30 days after surgery. Estimates of the incidence of SSI thus depend upon voluntary self-reporting by surgeons, which is unreliable. Therefore, estimates of the incidence of SSI in NNIS are probably underestimates, although the data are the best that are available.

Host-derived factors may contribute to the risk of SSI. Factors of importance include advanced age [8], obesity, malnutrition, diabetes mellitus [9,10], hypocholesterolemia [11], and numerous other factors that are not accounted for specifically by the NNIS system. In one study of 2345 patients undergoing cardiac surgery, the overall incidence of SSI was 8.5% (199/2,345) [12]. The

---

Box 2. American Society of Anesthesiology (ASA) physical status score

ASA 1
A normal healthy patient.

ASA 2
A patient with mild to moderate systemic disturbance that results in no functional limitations. Examples: Hypertension, diabetes mellitus, chronic bronchitis, morbid obesity, extremes of age.

ASA 3
A patient with severe systemic disturbance that results in functional limitations. Examples: Poorly controlled hypertension, diabetes mellitus with vascular complications, angina pectoris, prior myocardial infarction, pulmonary disease that limits activity.

ASA 4
A patient with a severe systemic disturbance that is life-threatening with or without the planned procedure. Examples: Congestive heart failure, unstable angina pectoris, advanced pulmonary, renal or hepatic dysfunction.

ASA 5
A morbid patient not expected to survive with or without the operative procedure. Examples: Ruptured abdominal aortic aneurysm, pulmonary embolism, head injury with increased intracranial pressure.

ASA 6
Any patient in whom the procedure is an emergency. Example: ASA 4E.

Data from National Nosocomial Infections Surveillance System (NNIS) system report: data summary from January 1992–June 2001, issued August 2001. Am J Infect Control 2001;29:404–21; with permission.

---

relative risk for the development of SSI among diabetic patients was 2.29 (95% confidence interval (CI) 1.15–4.54), and the relative risk among obese patients (body mass index > 30) was 1.78 (1.24–2.55). Malone and colleagues studied 5031 patients who underwent noncardiac surgery at a Veterans Affairs hospital over a six-year period ending in 1990. The overall incidence of SSI was 3.2%. Independent risk factors for the development of infection included ascites, diabetes mellitus, postoperative anemia, and recent weight loss, but not chronic obstructive pulmonary disease, tobacco use, or

Table 2
Surgical site infection rates (percent) for selected procedures, National Nosocomial Infections
Surveillance Program, 1992 to 2004

Procedure	Time cutpoint (h)	Number of risk factors			
		0	1	2	3
CABG chest/leg	5	1.25	3.39	5.43	9.76
Laparotomy	2	1.71	3.08	4.71	7.19
ORIF	2	0.79	1.41	2.81	4.97

Abbreviations: CABG, coronary artery bypass grafting (composite incidence for both incisions); ORIF, open reduction and internal fixation of fracture.

Data from National Nosocomial Infections Surveillance System (NNIS) system report: data summary from January 1992–June 2004, issued October 2004. Am J Infect Control 2004;32:470–85.

corticosteroid use [13]. In a prospective study of 9016 patients, 12.5% of patients developed a postoperative infection of some type within 28 days after surgery [14]. The likelihood of readmission for infection management and of death was 2.5% within the period. Multivariate analysis revealed that decreased serum albumin concentration, increased age, tracheostomy, and amputations were associated with an increased probability of an early infection, whereas factors associated with readmission due to infection included a dialysis shunt, vascular repair, and an early infection. Factors associated with 28-day mortality included advanced age, low serum albumin concentration, increased serum creatinine concentration, and an early infection [14].

Microbiology

Inoculation of the surgical site occurs during surgery, either inward from the skin or outward from the internal organ being operated on, hence the rationale for skin preparation and bowel preparation with antiseptics or

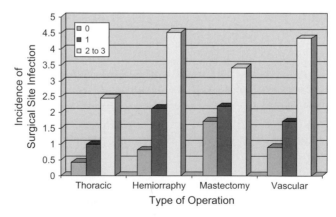

Fig. 2. Incidence of surgical site infection. (*Data from* CDC NNIS System. National nosocomial infections surveillance (NNIS) system report, data summary from January 1992 to June 2004, issued August 2003. Am J Infect Control 2003;31:481–98.)

antibiotics, and prophylactic oral or parenteral administration of antibiotic prophylaxis. The microbiology of SSI depends on the type of operation being performed, with an increased likelihood of infection caused by gram-negative bacilli after gastrointestinal surgery. However, most SSI are caused by gram-positive cocci (Table 3) [15], including *Staphylococcus aureus*, coagulase-negative staphylococci (usually *Staphylococcus epidermidis*), and *Enterococcus* sp., organisms that for the most part are skin-derived. With surgery of the head and neck, (when pharyngoesophageal structures are entered) or intestinal surgery, enteric aerobic (eg, *Escherichia coli*) and anaerobic (eg, *Bacteroides fragilis*) bacteria may cause SSI.

Preoperative preparation

The patient should be assessed for factors that can be corrected in the preoperative period before elective surgery. Open skin lesions should be allowed to heal if possible, and the patient should be free of bacterial infections of any kind. The patient should quit smoking if possible, preferably one month before surgery. The patient should shower with an antibacterial soap the night before the operation. The patient must not be shaved the night before, as the risk of SSI is clearly increased by bacteria that colonize the inevitable small cuts and abrasions [16]. Particular attention should be paid to the nutritional status of the patient. Obese patients should lose as much weight as is safely possible. Malnourished patients can benefit from even brief courses of enteral nutritional supplementation. As little as five days of enteral nutrition can reduce the risk of SSI significantly [17,18].

Antibiotic prophylaxis and the risk of surgical site infection

The administration of antibiotics before surgery to reduce postoperative SSI is common and beneficial in many circumstances. However, these

Table 3
Microbiology of surgical site infection

Pathogen	Prevalence (% of isolates)
Staphylococcus	19
Coagulase-negative *Staphylococcus*	14
Enterococcus sp.	12
Escherichia coli	8
Pseudomonas aeruginosa	8
Miscellaneous aerobic gram-negative bacilli	8
Enterobacter sp.	7
Streptococcus sp.	6
Klebsiella sp.	4
Miscellaneous anaerobic bacteria	3
Miscellaneous aerobic gram-positive bacteria	2

Data from Emori TG, Gaynes RP. An overview of nosocomial infections, including the role of the microbiology laboratory. Clin Microbiol Rev 1993;6:428–42.

antibiotics only protect the surgical incision, and antibiotics are not a panacea. If not administered properly, antibiotic prophylaxis will not be effective and may be harmful.

Some patients benefit from antibiotic prophylaxis whereas others may not. An increased risk of SSI occurs with an increasing degree of wound contamination (eg, contaminated versus clean) regardless of other risk factors (see Box 2) [6], and as the number of risk factors increases for a given type of operation (see Table 2). Antibiotic prophylaxis is indicated clearly for most clean-contaminated and contaminated (or potentially contaminated) operations. Antibiotics for dirty operations represent treatment for an infection, not prophylaxis, therefore that therapy will not be considered further. An example of a potentially contaminated operation is lysis of adhesions for mechanical small bowel obstruction. In this case, intestinal ischemia cannot be predicted accurately before surgery, and the possibility exists of an enterotomy during adhesiolysis, which increases the risk of SSI twofold. An example of a clean-contaminated operation where antibiotic prophylaxis is not always indicated is elective cholecystectomy [19]. Antibiotic prophylaxis is indicated only for high-risk biliary surgery; patients at high risk include those over age 70, diabetic patients, and patients whose biliary tract has been instrumented recently (eg, biliary stent) [19]. The vast majority of patients who undergo laparoscopic cholecystectomy do not require antibiotic prophylaxis [20].

Elective colon surgery is a special circumstance among clean-contaminated operations and one where practices are evolving [21]. Historically, mechanical bowel preparation to reduce bowel feces made colon surgery safe. Antibiotic bowel preparation, standardized in the 1970s by the oral administration of nonabsorbable neomycin and erythromycin base, reduced the risk of SSI further to its present rate of approximately 4% to 8%, depending on the number of risk factors. Outpatient mechanical preparation is now common before elective colon surgery, but the three doses of oral antibiotics at approximately 18, 17, and 10 hours preoperatively are no longer given routinely in favor of parenteral antibiotic prophylaxis. A dose of parenteral cefoxitin or ampicillin-sulbactam (or a quinolone or monobactam plus metronidazole for the penicillin-allergic patient) is given within 1 hour before skin incision [21].

Antibiotic prophylaxis of clean surgery is controversial. Where bone is incised (eg, craniotomy, sternotomy) or a prosthesis is inserted, antibiotic prophylaxis is generally indicated. Controversy centers on cases of clean surgery of soft tissues (eg, breast, hernia). A randomized prospective trial has shown some benefit of prophylaxis, but the results are confounded by higher than expected infection rates in the control group [22].

Which antibiotic should be chosen from the plethora of available agents? Four principles should guide selection. First, the agent should be safe. Second, the agent should have an appropriately narrow spectrum of coverage of relevant pathogens. Third, the agent should not be one that is relied upon for clinical treatment of infection, owing to the possibility that resistance may develop if the agent is overused. Finally, the agent must be administered for a defined, brief period of time (ideally, a single dose; certainly no more than 24 h). According to these principles, a third-generation cephalosporin or quinolone should never be used for surgical prophylaxis. Most SSIs are caused by gram-positive cocci. The most common etiologic agent causing SSI after clean surgery is *S. aureus*, followed by *S. epidermidis*. *Enterococcus faecalis*, *Escherichia coli*, and *Bacteroides fragilis* are common pathogens in SSI after clean-contaminated surgery. The antibiotic chosen should be directed primarily against staphylococci for clean cases and high-risk clean-contaminated elective surgery of the biliary and upper gastrointestinal tracts. A first-generation cephalosporin is the preferred agent for most patients, with clindamycin preferred for patients with a history of anaphylaxis to penicillin [23]. Although methicillin-resistant *S. aureus* (MRSA) has been isolated in the community from never-hospitalized patients, vancomycin prophylaxis is appropriate only in institutions where the incidence of MRSA infection is high (> 20% of all SSIs caused by MRSA).

When should parenteral antibiotics be given for optimum effect? The best time to give cephalosporin prophylaxis is within 1 hour before the time of incision [24] (Table 4). Antibiotics given sooner (except possibly for longer half-life agents such as metronidazole) are not effective, nor are agents that are given after the incision is closed. Antibiotics with short half-lives (< 2 h, eg, cefazolin or cefoxitin) should be re-dosed every 3 to 4 hours during surgery if the operation is prolonged or bloody [25]. There is still some benefit if the initial antibiotic dose is given intraoperatively, but none afterward.

Oral antibiotics can be administered for prophylaxis of SSI, provided that the agent is chosen carefully based on spectrum, oral bioavailability, and the potential need for the patients to take nothing orally for several hours before general anesthesia. Considering the ease with which venous

Table 4
Risk of development of surgical site infection relative to timing of antibiotic prophylaxis

Timing	No. patients	No. (%) infections	RR (95% CI)	OR (95% CI)
Early	369	14 (3.80)*	6.7* (2.9–14.7)	4.3* (1.8–10.4)
Preoperative	1,708	10 (0.59)	1.0	
Perioperative	282	4 (1.40)	2.4 (0.9–7.9)	2.1 (0.6–7.4)
Postoperative	488	16 (3.30)*	5.8* (2.6–12.3)	5.8* (2.4–13.8)
All	2,847	44 (1.5)		

Early, administration more than two hours preoperatively, administration during the recommended interval (≤2 h before skin incision); perioperative, administration within 2 hours after the skin incision; postoperative, administration more than 2 hours after the skin incision is made.

* $p < 0.0001$ as compared to preoperative group. RR, relative risk; OR, odds ratio.

Data from Classen DC, Evans RS, Pestotnik SL, et al. The timing of prophylactic administration of antibiotics and the risk of surgical-wound infection. N Engl J Med 1992;326:281–6.

access can be established, there is little need for oral antibiotic prophylaxis except in the case of colon surgery.

For what duration should prophylactic antibiotics be administered? The need for hemostasis of the surgical incision creates an ischemic milieu. Antibiotics may not penetrate properly into the incision immediately following surgery because of hypoperfusion owing to divided and cauterized vessels. Single-dose preoperative prophylaxis should be standard [26], with intraoperative dosing as noted above. Unfortunately, excessively prolonged use is both pervasive and potentially harmful for the patient. A 24-hour regimen is often standard for orthopedic and cardiac/vascular surgery, owing in part to a lack of data to suggest otherwise. Other than for solid-organ transplant surgery, where therapeutic immunosuppression has made 48-hour regimens standard, prolonged antibiotic prophylaxis is not needed. In particular, antibiotics should not be administered to cover indwelling drains or catheters, in lavage fluid, or as a substitute for poor surgical technique.

Preoperative topical antiseptics or antibiotics may also help prevent SSI. A preoperative shower with an antiseptic soap (eg, povidone-iodine) should be a standard part of preoperative preparation, but is omitted often. Topical 2% mupirocin ointment applied to the nares of patients who are chronic carriers of *S. aureus* reduces the increased incidence of SSI that is characteristic of chronic staphylococcal carriage [27,28].

Prolongation of antibiotic prophylaxis beyond 24 hours not only provides no benefit, but also can be associated with several complications. *Clostridium difficile*-associated disease (CDAD) follows disruption of the normal balance of gut flora, resulting in overgrowth of the enterotoxin-producing *C. difficile*. The incidence of nosocomial CDAD is increasing [29]. The spectrum of disease is broad, ranging from asymptomatic illness to life-threatening transmural colitis with infarction or perforation. Although virtually any antibiotic may cause CDAD even after administration of a single dose, prolonged antibiotic prophylaxis clearly increases the risk. Prolonged prophylaxis also increases the risk of later nosocomial infections unrelated to the surgical site, and the emergence of multi-drug resistant pathogens. Both pneumonia and catheter-related infections have been associated with prolonged antibiotic prophylaxis [29,30], as has the emergence of SSI caused by MRSA [31].

Current status of antibiotic prophylaxis in the United States

The current status of antimicrobial prophylaxis for major surgery in the United States has been summarized by Bratzler and colleagues [32]. A retrospective study of 34,133 Medicare inpatients from 2965 acute-care hospitals was conducted among records of patients undergoing open-chest cardiac surgery, vascular surgery, colorectal surgery, hip and knee total-joint arthroplasty, and abdominal and vaginal hysterectomy in 2001. A dose of antibiotics was administered to only 55.7% of patients (54.8%–56.6%) within 1 hour of surgery, although the agents chosen were consistent with published guidelines 92.6% (92.3%–92.8%) of the time. Disconcertingly, antimicrobial prophylaxis was discontinued within 24 hours of surgery only 40.7% (40.2%–41.2%) of the time, and within 12 hours only 14.5% of the time. Clearly, large numbers of patients are put at increased risk every day by excessive administration of prophylactic antibiotics.

Antibiotic prophylaxis of trauma-related infections

Traumatic injury is profoundly immunosuppressive, and injured patients are at high risk for the development of infection. The overall incidence of infection after trauma is approximately 25% [33], with infection of a wound (or an incision made as treatment) and nosocomial infection equally likely. Certain patterns of injury in particular are independently associated with infectious morbidity, including hemorrhagic shock, the need for blood transfusion, heavy wound contamination, central nervous system injury, colon injury, combined thoracoabdominal injuries, injuries to four or more organs, and increasing injury severity [34].

Certain characteristics of trauma add complexity. Obviously, antibiotics must be administered following injury and injured tissues are vulnerable. Patients in shock are hypotensive and vasoconstricted, and tissue penetration of antibiotics may be decreased. Ongoing blood loss may result in antibiotic loss in shed blood, especially if the agent is highly protein-bound or if the antibiotic is administered before hemorrhage is controlled. Postinjury fluid shifts and hypoalbuminemia can cause major fluctuations in volume of distribution, which can be difficult to estimate. As a result, it has been postulated that higher doses of antibiotics should be administered for the prophylaxis of post-traumatic infection.

Despite the high risk, the basic principles of antibiotic prophylaxis still apply: Use of a safe, narrow-spectrum agent for a defined brief period (certainly no more than 24 hours), preferably one that has a limited role in the therapy of infection (ie, first- or second-generation cephalosporin) [27]. Multiple studies indicate unequivocally that 24 hours of prophylaxis with a second-generation cephalosporin is all that is necessary following penetrating abdominal trauma, even in the presence of a colon injury or shock [35]. Although the severity of injury increases the risk of infection, severe injury is not a justification for prolonged surgical prophylaxis [29]. To do so is to increase the risk of subsequent antibiotic-resistant infection without benefit to the patient.

The operating room environment

Much of what is taken for granted in the modern operating room can, if lapses occur, result in increased rates of SSI. The elements of proper operating room design, management, and comportment have been reviewed with a close look at supporting evidence [16].

Although such factors as proper sterilization technique and ventilation should not be the everyday concern of the surgeon, operating room personnel must remain vigilant. The surgeon must be attentive to his or her personal hygiene (eg, hand scrubbing, hair) and that of the entire team. Recent data indicate that a brief rinse with soap and water followed by use of an alcohol gel hand rub is equivalent to the prolonged (and ritualized) session at the scrub sink [36].

Careful preparation of the skin with an appropriate antiseptic is essential. No evidence has shown that one method (eg, alcohol-based versus povidone-iodine) is superior to another, nor has evidence been found to raise concerns about lack of efficacy of the new quick-drying gel formulations. However, there are also no data to show that untreated or iodine-impregnated adhesive plastic drapes reduce the risk of SSI, so routine use of such products may be foregone.

About 20% of surgical gloves fail during an operation, so contamination of the surgical field, as well as contact between surgeon and the patient's body fluids, are possible. Therefore, attention must be paid to regular inspection of gloves during a procedure. Likewise, most surgical gowns in use offer limited protection (1.5–2 hours at most) against strikethrough of fluids. It may be prudent to change gowns and gloves regularly (every 2 hours or so) during long procedures, and certainly if there is any evidence of loss of integrity of barrier materials.

Although most flora that pose a risk for SSI are skin-derived and inoculated during the procedure, airborne bacteria, especially staphylococci, pose some risk. Surgeons who are chronic nasal carriers of *S. aureus* have higher rates of SSI than do their noncolonized brethren. It is recommended that surgical masks should cover the nose and mouth at all times, and that unnecessary traffic into the operating room and conversation at the operating table be kept to a minimum.

Owing to evaporative water losses, administration of room-temperature fluids, and other factors, patients may become hypothermic during surgery if they are not warmed. Maintenance of normal core body temperature is essential for decreasing the incidence of SSI. Two studies have corroborated a seminal study showing that mild intraoperative hypothermia is associated with an increased rate of SSI following elective colon surgery [37]. In one randomized study, 30 minutes of active preoperative warming reduced the rate of SSI following minor clean operations [38], whereas an observational study of 290 patients showed that those who were allowed to become hypothermic during diverse operations had a significantly higher incidence of SSI [39].

Management of the incision

Cosmesis is important to patients, who naturally want wounds to be closed for the sake of appearance. On the other hand, closure of a contaminated or dirty wound is widely believed to increase the risk of SSI. This conflict poses a dilemma for surgeons. The search goes on for innovative methods or adjuncts to wound closure that will both promote healing and ease cosmetic concerns. Few good studies exist to help sort out the multiplicity of techniques, making this an area where tradition and anecdote seem to prevail over science and wisdom. Tissues should be handled gently, and the use of electrocautery for hemostasis should be minimized [40]. With respect to wound closure, traditional teaching has advised that high-risk incisions should be left open after surgery, with delayed primary closure performed with sutures or adhesives approximately four days after surgery if the incision "looks okay." Incisions that are deemed "not ready" or that fail delayed primary closure are left to heal by secondary intention in a process that takes weeks and consumes precious home care resources. Such an approach could hardly be less satisfying to the scientist or the advocate of evidence-based practice. Patients, assuredly, don't like open incisions either.

Can contaminated incisions be closed primarily? The data that exist are mixed. It appears that muscle-splitting appendectomy incisions can be closed primarily. Pediatric surgeons have been doing so routinely, and decision analysis indicates that primary closure is cost effective if the rate of SSI is less than 27% [41]. However, wound management techniques that may be appropriate for appendectomy incisions may not be suitable for the management of larger abdominal incisions. One large prospective study demonstrated that primary closure of contaminated midline abdominal incisions led to more wound failures and greater cost than did delayed primary closure [42].

Drains placed in incisions probably cause more infections than they prevent. Sealing of the wound by epithelialization is prevented and the drain becomes a conduit, holding open a portal for invasion of the wound by pathogens colonizing the skin. Several studies of drains placed into clean or clean-contaminated incisions show that the rate of SSI is not reduced [43,44]; in fact, the rate is increased [45–49]. Considering that drains pose a risk and accomplish little, they should rarely be used and removed as soon as possible [50]. Under no circumstances should prolonged antibiotic prophylaxis be administered to "cover" indwelling drains.

Wound irrigation remains controversial as a means of reducing the risk of SSI. There is little information to suggest that routine low-pressure washing of an incision with saline reduces the risk of SSI [51], but high pressure (ie, pulse-irrigation) may be beneficial [52]. An increasing body of knowledge suggests that topical antibiotics placed into the incision during surgery can minimize the risk of SSI [53–55], but it might be desirable to accomplish the same result with topical antiseptics rather than antibiotics to minimize the possibility of the development of resistance.

The postoperative period

Blood transfusion

In surgery and trauma, blood transfusions are common and may be life-saving. Alternatives to transfusions in the acute setting are few. However, for hemodynamically stable postoperative patients, hemoglobin concentrations of >7 g/dL are well tolerated [56]. An expanding body of evidence suggests that blood transfusion should be avoided, if possible. Blood transfusions have been associated with increased rates of nosocomial infection following penetrating abdominal trauma independent of related factors such as shock or acute blood loss [57]. Furthermore, blood transfusions have been associated with increased injury severity and increasing transfusion volume in unselected trauma patients [58]. Blood transfusion therapy of 6 to 20 units in the first 12 hours following multiple trauma was associated with an increased risk of nosocomial infection [59], and even a single-unit transfusion carried demonstrable risk in another study [60]. The risk of infection increased as the total transfusion volume increased, especially when units were transfused after more than 14 days of storage [59]. A recent meta-analysis estimated that transfusion of any volume of red blood cell concentrates more than triples the risk of nosocomial infection compared with no transfusion [61]. The postulated "storage lesion" is complex, but includes changes in oxygen affinity, decreased membrane fluidity and red blood cell deformability, shortened circulation time, and the biologic consequences of cytokine generation and release. Recently, observational studies have suggested that transfusion of critically ill patients increases the risk of nosocomial infection [62], may worsen organ dysfunction, and increases mortality [63].

Hyperglycemia, nutrition, and control of blood sugar

Hyperglycemia has several deleterious effects upon host immune function, most notably impaired function of neutrophils and mononuclear phagocytes. Hyperglycemia may also be a marker of the catabolism and insulin resistance associated with the surgical stress response, and that exogenous insulin administration may ameliorate the catabolic state.

Poor control of blood glucose during surgery and in the perioperative period increases the risk of infection, and worsens outcome from sepsis. Diabetic patients undergoing cardiopulmonary bypass surgery have a higher risk of infection of both the sternal incision and the vein harvest incisions on the lower extremities [64]. Tight control of blood glucose by the anesthesiologist during surgery decreases the risk. Moderate hyperglycemia (>200 mg/dL) at any time on the first postoperative day increases the risk of SSI fourfold after noncardiac surgery [65]. In a large randomized trial of critically ill postoperative patients, exogenous insulin administration to keep blood glucose concentrations <110 mg/dL was associated with a 40% decrease of mortality, fewer nosocomial infections, and less organ dysfunction [66]. Meta-analysis of the approximately 35 existing trials indicates that the risk of postoperative infection decreases significantly by tight glucose control, regardless of whether or not the patients had diabetes mellitus [67].

The need to manage carbohydrate metabolism carefully has important implications for the nutritional management of surgical patients. Gastrointestinal surgery may render the gastrointestinal tract unusable for feeding, sometimes for prolonged periods. Ileus is common in surgical ICUs, whether from traumatic brain injury, narcotic analgesia, prolonged bed rest, inflammation near the peritoneal envelope (eg, lower lobe pneumonia, retroperitoneal hematoma, fractures of the thoraco-lumbar spine, pelvis or hip), or other causes. Parenteral nutrition is used frequently for feeding, despite evidence of a lack of efficacy [68] and the possibility of hepatic dysfunction; hyperglycemia may be an important complication as well. Every effort should be made to provide enteral feedings, including the use of promotility agents such as erythromycin [69]. Early enteral feeding (within 36 hours) reduces the risk of nosocomial infection by more than one half among critically ill and injured patients [70].

Oxygenation

It seems logical that the administration of oxygen in the postoperative period should be beneficial for wound healing and the prevention of infection [71,72]. The ischemic milieu of the fresh surgical incision is vulnerable; vasodilation of local tissue beds to improve nutrient blood flow to an incision may help maintain normal body temperature for prevention of surgical site infection. Moreover, oxygen has been postulated to have a direct antibacterial effect [72]. However, clinical trials have had conflicting results [73,74]. In a study of 500 patients undergoing elective colorectal surgery, administration of 80% oxygen (versus 30% oxygen) during surgery and for two hours thereafter decreased the incidence of surgical site infection by more than 50% (5.2% versus 11.2%) [73], whereas another prospective trial of the utility of 80% versus 35% oxygen administered to 165 patients undergoing major intraabdominal procedures showed that the infection rate was twice as high (25.0% versus 11.3%) after 80% oxygen [74]. Although the latter trial can be criticized for the high overall rate of SSI (18.1%) and possible underpowering, controversy now surrounds the administration of supplemental oxygenation specifically to reduce the incidence of surgical site infection.

New active device platforms for prevention of surgical site infection

Innovative technologies can be combined with established surgical practice to possibly decrease further the risk of SSI. Recognizing that two thirds of SSIs are superficial and stem from bacterial inoculation during surgery, and that interventions to decrease SSI after surgery have little impact, surgical device manufacturers are introducing new dual-action or "active platform" devices. Such devices may soon reduce incidence of SSI.

To reduce the infection rates associated with plastic surgery, researchers are studying the use of implantable tissue expander shells impregnated with antimicrobial agents [75]. Dermabond (Ethicon, Somerville, NJ), an oc-tylcyanoacrylate tissue adhesive, is an effective barrier to gram-positive and gram-negative motile and nonmotile bacterial species [76]. The adhesive is noninvasive, easy to apply, and seals the incision rapidly compared with other wound-healing adjuncts. An antibacterial suture, VICRYL Plus Antibacte-rial (Ethicon), can inhibit *S. aureus*, *S. epidermidis* and methicillin-resistant strains of *Staphylococcus* (MRSA and MRSE) [77]. Polyglactin suture is coated with triclosan (2,2,4'-trichloro-2'-hydroxy-diphenyl ether), an anti-septic agent that has been used in many commercial products, and that has activity against the common gram-positive bacteria known to cause SSIs. Triclosan appears to suppress the adherence of viable gram-positive bacteria to the suture, and to diffuse into adjacent tissues to provide a long-lasting antibacterial effect. Higher concentrations of triclosan may inhibit gram-negative bacteria, as well. Addition of triclosan to the coating does not alter the handling properties and performance characteristics of the suture [78,79].

Kerlix Antimicrobial Dressing, (Tyco Health Care, Mansfield, MA), con-tains polyhexamethylene biguanide, an antimicrobial component that resists bacterial colonization within the dressing and reduces bacterial penetration through the dressing [80]. This component may provide protection against gram-positive, gram-negative, and fungal microorganisms [80]. Native skin flora is not affected, promoting the maintenance of host defenses [80]. However, any benefit is questionable after incision epithelization occurs (by about 24 hours).

Acticoat with Silcryst Nanocrystals (Smith & Nephew, Largo, FL) is an effective antimicrobial barrier dressing. The nanocrystalline coating of silver kills a broad spectrum of bacteria in as little as 30 minutes and is effective for at least 3 days [81]. Acticoat dressing consists of three layers: An absorbent inner core sandwiched between outer layers of silver-coated, low-adherence polyethylene net. Nanocrystalline silver protects the wound site from bacte-rial contamination, whereas the inner core helps maintain the moist environ-ment best for wound healing. Acticoat 7 (Smith & Nephew), another antimicrobial barrier dressing, consists of five layers: Two layers of an absor-bent inner core alternating with three layers of silver-coated, low-adherent polyethylene net. Acticoat and Acticoat 7 can be used to manage chronic wounds and burn wounds as an antimicrobial barrier layer, but the benefit for a vulnerable surgical incision is unknown.

Treatment of surgical site infection

Only one constant has guided the management of an established SSI: In-cise and drain the incision. Often, opening the incision and applying basic wound care (eg, topical saline-soaked wet-to-dry cotton gauze dressings) are sufficient, provided that the incision is opened wide enough to facilitate wound care and the diagnosis of associated conditions. Making an incision too small may fail to bring the infection under control. Most nostrums other than physiologic saline applied to gauze dressings (eg, modified Dakin's solution, 0.25% acetic acid solution) actually suppress fibroblast proliferation and may delay secondary wound healing.

Opening the incision adequately is essential not only to gain control of the infection, but also to diagnose and treat any associated conditions, such as skin, subcutaneous tissue, or fascial necrosis that requires debridement; fascial dehiscence or evisceration that requires formal abdominal wall reconstruction; or drainage from beneath the fascia that could signal an organ/space infection or an enteric fistula. Without control of complicating factors, an SSI is difficult or impossible to control.

Antibiotic therapy is not required for uncomplicated SSIs that are opened and drained adequately and that receive appropriate local care. Likewise, if antibiotic therapy is unwarranted, then culture and susceptibility testing of wound drainage are of no value and can be omitted. Even if cultures are taken, routine swabs of drainage are not recommended because the risk of contamination by commensal skin flora is high, reducing utility. Rather, tissue specimens or an aliquot of pus collected aseptically and anaerobically into a syringe are recommended for analysis.

Antibiotics may be indicated if there is systemic evidence of toxicity (eg, fever, leukocytosis) or cellulitis that extends more than 2 cm beyond the incision. Antibiotics are also indicated as adjunctive management of several of the complications mentioned above. The choice of antibiotic is defined by the operation performed through the incision and the likely infecting organism, as discussed. Coverage against gram-positive cocci is indicated in most circumstances.

Wound closure by secondary intention can be protracted and disfiguring. Reports of vacuum-assisted wound closure (VAC) proliferate. Putative benefits of VAC dressings include reduced inflammation, increased fibroblast activity, improved wound hygiene as fluid is aspirated continuously from the field, and more rapid wound contraction and closure [82]. However, these benefits remain conjectural in the absence of definitive Class 1 data.

Summary

Promoting the healing process is an important consideration for both surgeons and patients. Certain timeless principles remain important, including preparation of the patient, careful adherence to sterile technique and infection control, judicious short-term use of antibiotics, and minimization of interventions that impair host defenses. Growth factors, silver hydrocolloid dressings, and the application of negative-pressure dressings can promote healing of chronic wounds, while suture materials, dressings, and coated prosthetic devices may reduce the incidence of SSI. However, adherence to established guidelines has been demonstrated to reduce the incidence of SSI by 27% [83]. Reducing SSIs as much as possible should be the goal of all surgical practitioners and health systems.

References

[1] Horan TC, Gaynes RP, Martone WJ, et al. CDC definitions of nosocomial surgical site infections, 1992: A modification of CDC definitions of surgical wound infections. Infect Control Hosp Epidemiol 1992;13:606–8.

[2] Barie PS. Surgical site infections: Epidemiology and prevention. Surg Infect (Larchmt) 2002; 3(Suppl 1):S9–21.

[3] Fry DE. The economic costs of surgical site infection. Surg Infect (Larchmt) 2002;3(Suppl 1): S37–43.

[4] National Nosocomial Infections Surveillance System (NNIS) System Report. Data summary from January 1992–June 2001, issued August 2001. Am J Infect Control 2001;29:404–21.

[5] National Nosocomial Infections Surveillance (NNIS) System Report, data summary from January 1992 to June 2004, issued October 2004. Am J Infect Control 2004;32:470–85.

[6] Garibaldi RA, Cushing D, Lerer T. Risk factors for post-operative infection. Am J Med 1991;91(Suppl 3B):158S–63S.

[7] Emori TG, Gaynes RP. An overview of nosocomial infections, including the role of the microbiology laboratory. Clin Microbiol Rev 1993;6:428–42.

[8] Raymond DP, Pelletier SJ, Crabtree TD, et al. Surgical infection and the ageing population. Am Surg 2001;67:827–32.

[9] Latham R, Lancaster AD, Covington JF, et al. The association of diabetes and glucose control with surgical-site infections among cardiothoracic surgery patients. Infect Control Hosp Epidemiol 2001;22:607–12.

[10] Pomposelli JJ, Baxter JK III, Babineau TJ, et al. Early postoperative glucose control predicts nosocomial infection rate in diabetic patients. JPEN J Parenter Enteral Nutr 1998;22:77–81.

[11] Delgado-Rodriguez M, Medina-Cuadros M, Martinez-Gallego G, et al. Total cholesterol, HDL cholesterol, and risk of nosocomial infection: a prospective study in surgical patients. Infect Control Hosp Epidemiol 1997;18:9–18.

[12] Malone DL, Genuit T, Tracy JK, et al. Surgical site infections: Reanalysis of risk factors. J Surg Res 2002;103:89–95.

[13] Page CP, Bohnen JM, Fletcher JR, et al. Antimicrobial prophylaxis for surgical wounds. Guidelines for clinical care. Arch Surg 1993;128:79–88.

[14] Scott JD, Forrest A, Feuerstein S, et al. Factors associated with postoperative infection. Infect Control Hosp Epidemiol 2001;22:347–51.

[15] American College of Surgeons. Manual on control of infection in surgical patients. New York: J.B. Lippincott; 1984.

[16] Mangram AJ, Horan TC, Pearson ML, et al. Guideline for prevention of surgical site infection, 1999. Hospital Infection Control Practices Advisory Committee. Infect Control Hosp Epidemiol 1999;20:250–78.

[17] Tepaske R, Velthuis H, Oudemans-van Straatan HM, et al. Effect of preoperative oral immune-enhancing nutritional supplement on patients at high risk of infection after cardiac surgery: a randomized placebo-controlled trial. Lancet 2001;358:696–701.

[18] Gianotti L, Braga M, Nespoli L, et al. A randomized controlled trial of preoperative oral supplementation with a specialized diet in patients with gastrointestinal cancer. Gastroenterology 2002;122:1763–70.

[19] Higgins A, London J, Charland S, et al. Prophylactic antibiotics for elective laparoscopic cholecystectomy: are they necessary? Arch Surg 1999;134:611–3.

[20] Harling R, Moorjani N, Perry C, et al. A prospective, randomised trial of prophylactic antibiotics versus bag extraction in the prophylaxis of wound infection in laparoscopic cholecystectomy. Ann R Coll Surg Engl 2000;82:408–10.

[21] Lewis RT. Oral versus systemic antibiotic prophylaxis in elective colon surgery: a randomized study and meta-analysis send a message from the 1990s. Can J Surg 2002;45:173–80.

[22] Platt R, Zaleznik DF, Hopkins CC, et al. Perioperative antibiotic prophylaxis for herniorrhaphy and breast surgery. N Engl J Med 1990;322:153–60.

[23] Bratzler DW, Houck PM. Surgical Infection Prevention Guideline Writers Workgroup. Antimicrobial prophylaxis for surgery: an advisory statement from the National Surgical Infection Prevention Project. Am J Surg 2005;189:395–404.

[24] Classen DC, Evans RS, Pestotnik SL, et al. The timing of prophylactic administration of antibiotics and the risk of surgical-wound infection. N Engl J Med 1992;326:281–6.

[25] Zaneti G, Giardina R, Platt R. Intraoperative redosing of cefazolin and risk for surgical site infection in cardiac surgery. Emerg Infect Dis 2001;7:828–31.

[26] Antimicrobial prophylaxis in surgery. Med Lett Drugs Ther 2001;43:92–7.

[27] Mest DR, Wong DH, Shimoda KJ, et al. Nasal colonization with methicillin-resistant Staphylococcus aureus on admission to the surgical intensive care unit increases the risk of infection. Anesth Analg 1994;78:644–50.

[28] Perl TM, Cullen JJ, Wenzel RP, et al. The Mupirocin and the Risk of Staphylococcus Aureus Study Team. Intranasal mupirocin to prevent postoperative Staphylococcus aureus infections. N Engl J Med 2002;346:1871–7.

[29] Morris AM, Jobe BA, Stoney M, et al. Clostridium difficile colitis: an increasingly aggressive iatrogenic disease? Arch Surg 2002;137:1096–100.

[30] Namias N, Harvill S, Ball S, et al. Cost and morbidity associated with antibiotic prophylaxis in the ICU. J Am Coll Surg 1999;188:225–30.

[31] Fukatsu K, Saito H, Matsuda T, et al. Influences of type and duration of antimicrobial prophylaxis on an outbreak of methicillin-resistant Staphylococcus aureus and on the incidence of wound infection. Arch Surg 1997;132:1320–5.

[32] Bratzler DW, Houck PM, Richards C, et al. Use of antimicrobial prophylaxis for major surgery. Baseline results from the National Surgical Infection Prevention Project. Arch Surg 2005;140:174–82.

[33] Barie PS. Infections of trauma patients. Surg Infect (Larchmt), in press.

[34] Bozorgzadeh A, Pizzi WF, Barie PS, et al. The duration of antibiotic administration for penetrating abdominal trauma. Am J Surg 1999;177:125–31.

[35] Velmahos GC, Toutouzas KG, Sarkysian G, et al. Severe trauma is not an excuse for prolonged antibiotic prophylaxis. Arch Surg 2002;137:537–41.

[36] Parienti JJ, Thibon P, Heller R, et al. Hand-rubbing with an aqueous alcoholic vs. traditional surgical hand-scrubbing and 30-day surgical site infection rates: a randomized equivalence study. JAMA 2002;288:722–7.

[37] Kurz A, Sessler DI, Lenhardt R. Perioperative normothermia to reduce the incidence of surgical-wound infection and shorten hospitalization, Study of Wound Infection and Temperature Group. N Engl J Med 1996;334:1209–15.

[38] Melling AC, Ali B, Scott EM, et al. Effects of preoperative warming on the incidence of wound infection and clean surgery: a randomized controlled trial. Lancet 2001;358:876–80.

[39] Flores-Maldonado A, Medina-Escobedo CE, Rios-Rodriguez HM, et al. Mild hypothermia and the risk of wound infection. Arch Med Res 2001;32:227–31.

[40] Janik J. Electric cautery lowers contamination threshold for infection by laparotomies. Am J Surg 1998;175:263–6.

[41] Brasel KJ, Borgstrom DC, Weigelt JA. Cost-utility analysis of contaminated appendectomy wounds. J Am Coll Surg 1997;184:23–30.

[42] Cohn SM, Giannotti G, Ong AW, et al. Prospective randomized trial of two wound management strategies for dirty abdominal wounds. Ann Surg 2001;233:409–13.

[43] Al-Inany H, Youssef G, Abd ElMaguid A, et al. Value of subcutaneous drainage system in obese females undergoing cesarean section using Pfannenstiel incision. Gynecol Obstet Invest 2002;53:75–8.

[44] Magann EF, Chauhan SP, Rodts-Palenik D, et al. Subcutaneous stitch closure versus subcutaneous drain to prevent wound disruption after cesarean delivery: a randomized clinical trial. Am J Obstet Gynecol 2002;186:1119–23.

[45] Siegman-Igra Y, Rozin R, Simchen E. Determinants of wound infection in gastrointestinal operations, the Israeli study of surgical infections. J Clin Epidemiol 1993;46:133–40.

[46] Noyes LD, Doyle DJ, McSwain NE. Septic complications associated with the use of peritoneal drains in liver trauma. J Trauma 1998;28:337–46.

[47] Magee C, Rodeheaver GT, Golden GT, et al. Potentiation of wound infection by surgical drains. Am J Surg 1976;131(5):547–9.

[48] Vilar-Compote D, Mohar A, Sandoval S, et al. Surgical site infections at the National Cancer Institute in Mexico: a case-control study. Am J Infect Control 2002;28:14–20.

[49] Manian FA. Vascular and cardiac infections in end-stage renal disease. Am J Med Sci 2003; 325:243–50.

[50] Barie PS. Are we draining the life from our patients? Surg Infect (Larchmt) 2002;3:159–60.

[51] Platell C, Papadimitriou JM, Hall JC. The influence of lavage on peritonitis. J Am Coll Surg 2000;191:672–80.

[52] Cervantes-Sanchez CR, Gutierrez-Vega R, Vasquez-Carpizio JA, et al. Syringe pressure irritation of subdermic tissue after appendectomy to decrease the incidence of postoperative wound infection. World J Surg 2000;24:38–41.

[53] Andersen B, Bendtsen A, Holbraad L, et al. Wound infections after appendectomy. I. A controlled trial on the prophylactic efficacy of topical ampicillin in non-perforated appendicitis. Acta Chir Scand 1972;138:531–6.

[54] Yoshii S, Hosaka S, Suzuki S, et al. Prevention of surgical site infection by antibiotic spraying in the operating field during cardiac surgery. Jpn J Thorac Cardiovasc Surg 2001;49: 279–81.

[55] O'Connor LT Jr, Goldstein M. Topical perioperative antibiotic prophylaxis for minor clean inguinal surgery. J Am Coll Surg 2002;194:407–10.

[56] Hebert PC, Wells G, Blajchman MA, et al. A multi-center, randomized, controlled clinical trial of transfusion requirements in critical care. Transfusion Requirements in Critical Care Investigators, Canadian Critical Care Trials Group. N Engl J Med 1999;340:409–17.

[57] Nichols RL, Smith JW, Klein DB, et al. Risk of infection after penetrating abdominal trauma. N Engl J Med 1984;311:1065–70.

[58] Agarwal N, Murphy JG, Cayten CG, Stahl WM. Blood transfusion increases the risk of infection after trauma. Arch Surg 1993;128:171–6.

[59] Offner PJ, Moore EE, Biffl WL, et al. Increased rate of infection associated with transfusion of old blood after severe injury. Arch Surg 2002;137:711–7.

[60] Claridge JA, Sawyer RG, Schulman AM, et al. Blood transfusions correlate with infections in trauma patients in a dose-dependent manner. Am Surg 2002;68:566–72.

[61] Hill GE, Frawley WH, Griffith KE, et al. Allogeneic blood transfusion increases the risk of postoperative bacterial infection: a meta-analysis. J Trauma 2003;54:908–14.

[62] Taylor RW, Manganaro L, O' Brian J, et al. Impact of allogenic packed red blood cells transfusion on nosocomial infection rates in the critically ill patient. Crit Care Med 2002;30: 2249–54.

[63] Vincent JL, Baron J-F, Reinhart K, et al. Anemia and blood transfusion in critically ill patients. JAMA 2002;288:1499–507.

[64] Latham R, Lancaster AD, Covington JF, et al. The association of diabetes and glucose control with surgical-site infections among cardiothoracic surgery patients. Infect Control Hosp Epidemiol 2001;22:607–12.

[65] Pomposelli JJ, Baxter JK III, Babineau TJ, et al. Early postoperative glucose control predicts nosocomial infection rate in diabetic patients. JPEN J Parenter Enteral Nutr 1998;22:77–81.

[66] van den Berghe G, Wouters P, Weekers F, et al. Intensive insulin therapy in the critically ill patients. N Engl J Med 2001;345:1359–67.

[67] Pittas AG, Siegel RD, Lau J. Insulin therapy for critically ill hospitalized patients: a meta-analysis of randomized controlled trials. Arch Intern Med 2004;164:2005–11.

[68] Heyland DK, MacDonald S, Keefe L, et al. Total parenteral nutrition in the critically ill patient: a meta-analysis. JAMA 1998;280:2013–9.

[69] Berne JD, Norwood SH, McAuley CE, et al. Erythromycin reduces delayed gastric emptying in critically ill trauma patients: a randomized, controlled trial. J Trauma 2002;53:422–5.

[70] Marik PE, Zaloga GP. Early enteral nutrition in acutely ill patients: a systematic review. Crit Care Med 2001;29:2264–70.

[71] Gottrupp F. Oxygen in wound healing and infection. World J Surg 2004;28:312–5.

[72] Knighton DR, Halliday B, Hunt TK. Oxygen as an antibiotic. A comparison of the effects of inspired oxygen concentration and antibiotic administration on in vivo bacterial clearance. Arch Surg 1986;121:191–5.

[73] Greif R, Akca O, Horn EP, et al. Supplemental perioperative oxygen to reduce the incidence of surgical-wound infection. Outcomes Research Group. N Engl J Med 2000;342:161–7.

[74] Pryor KO, Fahey TJ 3rd, Lien CA, et al. Surgical site infection and the routine use of perioperative hyperoxia in a general surgical population: a randomized controlled trial. JAMA 2004;291:79–87.

[75] Darouiche RO, Netscher DT, Mansouri MD, et al. Activity of antimicrobial-impregnated silicone tissue expanders. Ann Plast Surg 2002;49:567–71.

[76] Bhende S, Rothernburger S, Spangler D, et al. *In Vitro* assessment of microbial barrier properties of Dermabond topical skin adhesive. Surg Infect (Larchmt) 2002;3:251–7.

[77] Rothenberger S, Spangler D, Bhende S, et al. In vitro antimicrobial evaluation of coated VICRYL Plus antimicrobial suture using zone of inhibition assays. Surg Infect (Larchmt) 2002;3(Suppl 1):S79–87.

[78] Storch M, Perry LC, Davidson JM, et al. A 28 day study of the effect of Coated VICRYL Plus antibacterial suture (coated polyglactin 910 suture with triclosan) on wound healing in guinea pig linear incisional skin wounds. Surg Infect (Larchmt) 2002;3(Suppl 1):S89–98.

[79] Storch M, Scalzo H, Van Lue S, et al. Physical and functional comparison of Coated VICRYL* Plus Antibacterial Suture (coated polyglactin 910 suture with triclosan) with Coated VICRYL* Plus Suture (coated polyglactin 910 suture). Surg Infect (Larchmt) 2002; 3(Suppl 1):S65–77.

[80] Reitsma AM, Rodeheaver GT. Effectiveness of a new antimicrobial gauze dressing as a bacterial barrier. Document H-5273. Mansfield, MA. Tyco Healthcare, 2001.

[81] Thomas S, McCubbin P. A comparison of the antimicrobial effects of four silver-containing dressings on three organisms. J Wound Care 2003;12:101–7.

[82] Fuchs U, Zittermann A, Stuettgen B, et al. Clinical outcome of patients with deep sternal wound infection managed by vacuum-assisted closure compared to conventional therapy with open packing: a retrospective analysis. Ann Thorac Surg 2005;79:526–31.

[83] Dellinger EP, Hausmann SM, Bratzler DW, et al. Hospitals collaborate to decrease surgical site infections. Am J Surg 2005;190:9–15.

ELSEVIER
SAUNDERS

Surg Clin N Am 85 (2005) 1137–1152

SURGICAL
CLINICS OF
NORTH AMERICA

Health-Care–Associated Infections and Prevention

Traci L. Hedrick, MD*, Robert G. Sawyer, MD

*Surgical Infectious Disease Laboratory, PO Box 801380, Department of Surgery,
University of Virginia Health System, Charlottesville, Virginia 22908, USA*

Health-care–associated infections (HAIs) remain a leading cause of perioperative morbidity and mortality, contributing substantially to rising health-care costs. Currently, one out of every 10 surgical patients develops an HAI [1]. Several factors predispose surgical patients to the development of infection. One is the insult of surgery, which causes corticosteroid and catecholamine release resulting in transient immunodeficiency [2]. Another is postsurgical pain, which leads to immobility and facilitates the development of atelectasis and subsequently pneumonia. Additionally, surgical patients often require the placement of indwelling devices, promoting infection through barrier compromise and biofilm formation. The authors will briefly review three of the most commonly acquired HAIs, focusing predominantly on preventive strategies specific to each infection.

Health-care–associated pneumonia

A. Epidemiology

Health-care–associated pneumonia (HAP) is defined as any case of pneumonia beginning 48 hours or more following admission. In the case of ventilated patients, this is referred to as ventilator-associated pneumonia (VAP). Although HAP is the second most frequent HAI, it accounts for most HAIs in intensive care unit (ICU) patients and is the most lethal [3,4]. Aspiration of oropharyngeal and gastric contents is the leading cause of HAP. The time of acquisition determines the causative organism. Early-onset pneumonia (≤96 hours following admission) is caused by *Escherichia coli*, *Klebsiella* spp, *Streptococcus pneumoniae*, *Haemophilus influenzae*, and

* Corresponding author.
E-mail address: th8q@virginia.edu (T.L. Hedrick).

Staphylococcus aureus, while late-onset pneumonia is associated with methicillin-resistant *S. aureus* (MRSA) and *Pseudomonas aeruginosa* [5]. Box 1 lists the most common risk factors associated with HAP.

B. Diagnosis and treatment

Traditionally, diagnosis of HAP relied on the presence of fever, cough, or purulent sputum, with a new or progressive infiltrate on a chest radiograph [6]. Over the past decade, efforts have been made to improve diagnostic utility through the use of quantitative culture and lower airway sampling via bronchoalveolar lavage or protected brush specimen. Currently, high-level evidence is insufficient to suggest definitively that either improves outcome [7,8]. But the invasive approach to VAP diagnosis provides a more accurate microbiologic diagnosis. Whether these techniques will prove superior in multicenter prospective trials is yet to be determined. Treatment of HAP requires early initiation of empiric broad-spectrum antibiotics narrowed once microbiological profiles become available. Past recommendations for treatment duration have been 14 to 21 days [5]. However, a recent randomized trial by Chastre et al. [9] suggests 8 days is equivalent to 15 days for the treatment of VAP.

Box 1. Risk factors associated with health-care–associated pneumonia

Administration of antacids or histamine type-2 antagonists
Supine positioning
Coma
Paralytics
Enteral nutrition
Nasogastric tube
Reintubation
Tracheostomy
Patient transport
Acute respiratory distress syndrome
Prior antibiotic exposure
Age greater than 60 years
Admitting diagnosis of burns, trauma, or coagulase-negative
    staphylococcus disease
Presence of intracranial pressure monitoring

Data from Cook DJ, Kollef MH. Risk factors for ICU-acquired pneumonia. JAMA 1998;279(20):1605–6.

C. Prevention

The Centers for Disease Control (CDC) recently published evidence-based guidelines for the prevention of HAP (Boxes 2 and 3) [6]. Preventive strategies are categorized below into four groups as they pertain to surgical patients.

1. Factors related to endotracheal intubation

The incidence of pneumonia in ventilated patients increases at a rate of 1% to 3% per day of mechanical ventilation [10]. Several studies support the use of noninvasive positive-pressure ventilation to avoid intubation in patients with cardiogenic pulmonary failure [11] and the use of weaning and sedation protocols to reduce the incidence of VAP [12,13]. Avoidance of nasotracheal intubation can prevent the development of VAP through prevention of sinusitis [14–16]. A randomized trial demonstrated that a systematic search for sinusitis in nasotracheally intubated patients decreased incidence of VAP and improved mortality [17].

2. Factors related to mechanical ventilation

Condensate within the ventilator circuit forms at a rate of 30mL/h and is rapidly colonized, serving as a route of contamination [18]. By frequently draining condensate and avoiding routine changes of ventilator tubing, incidence of VAP can be reduced [18–20]. Heat and moisture exchangers for humidification may slightly reduce the incidence of VAP and are more cost-effective while less labor-intensive than conventional methods [21–23]. The type of endotracheal suctioning system (open versus closed) does not affect the incidence of VAP [24–27]. However, with elimination of routine in-line catheter changes, the closed system is more cost-effective [28]. Subglottic suctioning reduces the incidence of VAP and shortens the duration of mechanical ventilation. However, such suctioning does not affect mortality [29–31].

3. Pharmacologic intervention

Medical experts have not reached a consensus on the best method to prevent stress ulcers in patients at risk for HAP. Whether gastric acid suppression leads to increased aerodigestive colonization and higher rates of HAP is yet to be determined [32–36]. Selective gut decontamination involves combination oral and enteral antimicrobials with a short course of parenteral antibiotics to reduce the colonization of the aerodigestive tract with pathogenic microorganisms. Multiple randomized trials demonstrate that selective gut decontamination reduces incidence of VAP and mortality, particularly in surgical and trauma patients. However, this practice has yet to gain acceptance in the United States because of fear that such treatment will lead to antimicrobial resistance [37–41]. Chlorhexidine gluconate oral rinse in critically ill ventilated patients is a safe and effective way to reduce the incidence of VAP [42,43].

Box 2. CDC guidelines for preventing health-care–associated pneumonia

Staff education
1. Educate staff on epidemiology and infection-control measures related to HAP.

Surveillance
1. Conduct surveillance of HAP in ICU and return data to personnel.
2. Avoid routine culture in absence of clinical suspicion.

Transmission
1. Thoroughly clean all equipment to be sterilized.
2. Sterilize equipment properly.
3. Rinse sterile equipment with sterile water if needed.
4. Do not sterilize or disinfect internal machinery of ventilators or anesthesia equipment. However, clean and sterilize reusable components of the system between patients, according to guidelines from the manufacturer.
5. Change breathing circuits, heat moisture exchangers, or humidifier tubing only when visibly soiled or nonfunctioning.
6. Drain tubing condensate away from the patient.
7. Use sterile water with bubbling humidifiers.
8. Between treatments, clean, disinfect, and rinse small-volume nebulizers with sterile water.
9. Use sterile fluid for nebulization and dispense it aseptically.
10. Use aerosolized medication in single-dose vials when possible.
11. When using mist tents, replace all disposable parts between each use on different patients with sterilized or highly disinfected equipment.
12. Subject mist-tent nebulizers, reservoirs, and tubing used on the same patient to daily low-level disinfection or pasteurization followed by air-drying.
13. Subject resuscitation bags, respirometers, and ventilator thermometers to sterilization or high-level disinfection between uses on different patients.
14. Do not use large-volume room-air humidifiers unless they can be sterilized or subjected to high-level disinfection.
15. Adhere to standard precautions.
16. Perform and change tracheostomy tube under aseptic conditions.

17. If an open-system suction catheter is used for suctioning of respiratory tract secretions, use a sterile, single-use catheter.
18. Use only sterile fluid to flush the suction catheter.

Modifying host
1. Administer the pneumococcal vaccine to persons 65 years or older, those with chronic medical conditions, all transplant patients, and those in long-term care facilities.
2. Use noninvasive ventilation initially or for weaning from mechanical ventilation whenever feasible to reduce the need for endotracheal intubation.
3. Avoid reintubation.
4. Perform orotracheal, rather than nasotracheal, intubation, unless contraindicated.
5. Use an endotracheal tube with dorsal lumen above the cuff to allow intermittent or continuous suctioning of subglottic secretions.
6. Clear all subglottic secretions before deflating the cuff.
7. Elevate the head of the bed 30–45° unless contraindicated.
8. Routinely verify appropriate placement of the feeding tube.
9. Develop and implement an oral-hygiene program for ICU patients.
10. Preoperatively instruct high-risk surgical patients about the importance of taking deep breaths and ambulating in the immediate postoperative period.
11. Encourage all postoperative patients to take deep breaths and ambulate unless contraindicated.
12. Use incentive spirometry on postoperative patients at high risk for pneumonia.

From Guidelines for preventing health-care–associated pneumonia. 2003 Recommendations of the CDC and the Healthcare Infection Control Practices Advisory Committee. Respir Care 2004;49(8):926–39.

4. Miscellaneous

Semi-recumbent positioning prevents pneumonia in ventilated patients [44–46]. However, the effectiveness of kinetic therapy and prone positioning in preventing VAP is not firmly established [47,48]. Based on several small randomized clinical trials, the use of epidural anesthesia for perioperative pain control may lead to fewer postoperative cases of pneumonia [49–52]. Data is scant regarding feeding of mechanically ventilated patients, especially surgical patients, at risk for VAP. Today, the evidence does not support the use of small bore feeding tubes, the practice of measuring gastric residual volumes, or postpyloric feeding in the prevention of VAP [53–60].

Box 3. Relevant CDC unresolved issues for preventing HAP

1. Placement of filter to collect condensate from mechanical ventilator breathing circuit
2. Use of closed, continuous-feed humidification system
3. Use of heat moisture exchangers or heated humidifiers in patients receiving mechanical ventilation
4. Daily application of topical antimicrobial agents to the tracheostoma
5. Use of closed- or open-system suction catheters for suctioning of respiratory tract secretions in ventilated patients
6. Wearing of sterile or clean gloves when endotracheal suctioning
7. Frequent changing the in-line suction catheter of a closed-suction system in use on one patient
8. Administration of granulocyte-colony stimulating factor or intravenous gamma globulin for prophylaxis
9. Enteral administration of glutamine
10. Preferential use of small-bore enteral feeding tubes
11. Continuous versus intermittent enteral feedings
12. Postpyloric versus gastric enteral tubes
13. Routine use of oral chlorhexidine rinse in postoperative or high-risk patients
14. Oral decontamination with topical antimicrobial agents
15. Preferential use of sucralfate, H2-antagonists, or antacids for stress ulcer prophylaxis in ventilated patients
16. Selective decontamination of the digestive tract
17. Routinely conduct acidifying gastric feeding
18. Systemic antibiotic prophylaxis
19. Scheduled changes in the class of antimicrobial agents used for empiric therapy
20. Rotational therapy, either by "kinetic" therapy or by continuous lateral rotational therapy

---

From Guidelines for preventing health-care–associated pneumonia. 2003 Recommendations of the CDC and the Healthcare Infection Control Practices Advisory Committee. Respir Care 2004;49(8):926–39.

Health-care–associated urinary tract infection

A. Epidemiology

Catheter-associated urinary-tract infection (CAUTI) is the most common health-care–associated infection worldwide [61]. CAUTIs are problematic not only for their attributable morbidity and mortality. They also can harbor resistant organisms and have been linked to the development of surgical-site infections [62,63]. Traditionally, *E coli* has been the most commonly isolated organism from patients with bacteriuria [64]. However, the most common isolates among patients at our institution are now *Candida* spp (35%), *Enterococcus* spp (30%), and *E coli* (16%). Pathogenic microorganisms typically gain access to the urinary system through extraluminal ascent and less frequently through intraluminal contamination from reflux through the drainage system.

B. Diagnosis and treatment

Up to 90% of patients with a CAUTI lack symptoms, making diagnosis difficult [65]. The most accepted definition of a urinary-tract infection is a urine specimen growing greater than 10^5 colony forming units (CFUs) per milliliter for noncatheterized patients [66]. However, data suggest that once normally sterile urine is inoculated through an indwelling catheter, progression to concentrations greater than 10^5 CFU/mL occurs within 72 hours [67]. Therefore, many clinicians consider concentrations greater than 10^3 CFU/mL in a properly collected specimen to be clinically relevant in a catheterized patient with symptoms [68].

Management of CAUTI should include removal or replacement of the urinary catheter. Because causative microorganisms are often multiresistant, broad-spectrum antibiotics should be initiated and narrowed accordingly. Treatment duration for CAUTI has scarcely been addressed. One small study in women with CAUTI demonstrated single-dose therapy to be as effective as 10 days of therapy for asymptomatic patients and those with lower-tract symptoms alone [69]. Current Infectious Diseases Society of America (IDSA) guidelines recommend 3-day treatment for uncomplicated cystitis [70]. Therefore, the best treatment for patients with CAUTI is likely between 3 and 14 days, but the exact number of days is yet to be determined. The question of whether it is useful to treat patients with asymptomatic candiduria is also unresolved [71].

C. Prevention

Eight risk factors are associated with increased rates of CAUTI [64,116]. These factors are listed in Box 4.

The most important risk factor for the development of a urinary-tract infection in a hospitalized patient is the presence of a urinary catheter. Often such catheters are used inappropriately and remain in place unnoticed by clinicians [72]. Daily prompting by the nursing staff to remove unnecessary catheters significantly decreases the duration of catheterization and incidence of CAUTI in an ICU setting [73]. Other effective strategies to prevent CAUTI include catheter insertion by properly trained personnel using

---

Box 4. Risk factors associated with CAUTI

Duration of catheterization
Lack of systemic antibiotic during short catheter courses
Lack of urimeter drainage
Female sex
Diabetes mellitus
Microbial colonization of the drainage bag
Serum creatinine greater than 2 mg/dl at the time of
  catheterization
Severity of illness

---

aseptic technique and sterile equipment, maintenance of closed sterile drainage, and maintenance of unobstructed urine flow [74].

Through regression analysis, the use of antibiotic therapy was found to be a protective factor in preventing CAUTI [75]. Methodological concerns plague the few randomized trials evaluating prophylactic antimicrobial use and overall do not provide sufficient evidence to support such practice [76–78]. Multiple studies have failed to demonstrate the efficacy of daily regimented metal cleaning, bladder irrigation with antiseptic or antibiotic solution, or the addition of a disinfectant to the collection system in the prevention of CAUTI [79–84]. Alternatives to transurethral catheterization, including condom catheters and suprapubic catheters, may reduce the incidence of CAUTI [85–90]. However, suprapubic catheters are associated with mechanical problems and may be best suited for patients with long-term catheters [85].

Results are mixed with regard to the use of silver-coated urinary catheters. Two large randomized trials demonstrate no benefit with silver-oxide–impregnated catheters in preventing CAUTI [91,92]. Silver-alloy–coated catheters and hydrogel-silver-ion–coated catheters may be beneficial. However, the evidence about the effectiveness of their use is conflicting [93–96].

Intravascular-catheter–related infections

A. Epidemiology

Intravascular-catheter–related infections (CRIs) account for many HAIs acquired by surgical patients. Causative organisms include Coagulase-negative *Staphylococcus* (CNS), *S aureus*, gram negative bacilli and *Candida* spp. MRSA now accounts for 60% of all *S aureus* isolates acquired from ICUs [97]. CRI stems most commonly from contamination of the extraluminal catheter surface with skin flora. The intraluminal surface may also become contaminated from infusates or through hematogenous spread. Risk factors associated with CRIs are given in Box 5:

Box 5. Risk factors for intravascular catheter related infections

Internal jugular catheterization
Duration of catheterization $\geq$8 days
Polyvinyl or polyethylene catheters
Frequent manipulations
Improper aseptic technique during insertion
Increasing number of catheter lumens
Povidone-iodine skin antisepsis
Use of the catheter for TPN

Data from Oncu S, Ozsut H, Yildirim A, et al. Central venous catheter related infections: Risk factors and the effect of glycopeptide antibiotics. Annals of Clinical Microbiology and Antimicrobials 2003;2(1):3.

B. Diagnosis and treatment

Local signs of infection at the catheter site are normally absent. However, in the presence of local or systemic signs of infection, the isolation of more than 15 CFUs or 10^2 CFUs from a catheter by means of semiquantitative or quantitative culture, respectively, indicates a CRI [98]. Two sets of percutaneous blood cultures may confirm the presence of a bloodstream infection. However, the authors have previously observed that bloodstream infection in the setting of a CRI is not an independent predictor of outcome [99].

Treatment of CRIs involves empiric antibiotic therapy with vancomycin or linezolid that targets the most likely pathogens, CNS and MRSA. In the presence of severe sepsis or immunosuppression, empiric coverage for gram-negative bacilli and *Candida* spp may be necessary. In general, the catheter should be removed and antibiotic treatment continued for 10 to 14 days if blood cultures are positive. For patients with septic thrombosis or endocarditis, treatment should be continued for 4 to 6 weeks. All patients with *S aureus* CRI with bloodstream infection or associated valvular heart disease should undergo transesophageal echocardiogram in the absence of contraindication to evaluate for vegetations. In uncomplicated cases of CNS infection, the catheter sometimes may be retained with 7 to 14 days of antibiotic treatment and antibiotic lock therapy. Antibiotics need only be continued for 5 to 7 days in patients with uncomplicated CRI caused by CNS if the catheter is removed [98].

C. Prevention

Practices that decrease the rate of CRI include proper hand hygiene and sterile barrier precautions (eg, large drape, hat, mask, and sterile gown) during central venous catheter (CVC) insertion, skin antisepsis with 2%

chlorhexidine gluconate rather than povidone-iodine, and the use of polyurethane catheters rather than polyvinyl chloride or polyethylene catheters [100–103]. The subclavian position is the preferred site for temporary CVCs in preventing CRI when feasible [104]. While catheters impregnated with chlorhexidine and silver sulfadiazine or with minocycline and rifampin have reduced infectious complications, considerations for using such catheters must be balanced against potential risks of antimicrobial resistance [105–107]. CDC guidelines recommend the use of "an antimicrobial or antiseptic-impregnated CVC in adults whose catheter is expected to remain in place more than 5 days if, after implementing a comprehensive strategy to reduce rates of CRI, the CRI rate remains above the goal set by the individual institution" [104]. It is recommended that peripheral catheters be rotated every 72 to 96 hours [104]. However, the routine replacement or rewiring of CVCs does not prevent CRI and is associated with increased mechanical complications [108]. Finally, staff education for all providers inserting, maintaining, and using intravascular catheters cannot be overemphasized in the prevention of CRI. For a complete description of CRI preventative strategies, the reader may refer to CDC Intravascular Catheter Guidelines [104].

Hand hygiene

Semmelweis demonstrated in 1847 that maternal mortality significantly improved following implementation of a hand-hygiene policy [109]. Since that time, numerous studies have demonstrated the cost-effectiveness and efficacy of hand washing in reducing the incidence of HAI [110–112]. Yet, on average, medical professionals adhere to basic hand hygiene recommendations only 40% of the time [109]. Adherence to recommended hand-hygiene practices can be improved through education, feedback, and the use of waterless alcohol-based hand-rub solutions in pocketsize and bedside dispensers [109,113].

Summary

Over the last 30 years the medical community has witnessed a significant reduction in the incidence of bloodstream infections, urinary tract infections, HAPs, and surgical-site infections [114–117]. This improvement is the cumulative result of many of the novel preventative strategies highlighted in this review. In recent years, technological advances have led to better outcomes. Even so, future improvements may still depend on increasing compliance with the simplest interventions, such as correct hand hygiene. Only through a multifaceted approach involving basic science and clinical research, practice improvement, and continuous outcomes monitoring will the rates of health-care–associated infections be reduced to the absolute minimum.

References

[1] Vazquez-Aragon P, Lizan-Garcia M, Cascales-Sanchez P, et al. Nosocomial infection and related risk factors in a general surgery service: a prospective study. J Infect 2003;46(1): 17–22.

[2] Ogawa K, Hirai M, Katsube T, et al. Suppression of cellular immunity by surgical stress. Surgery 2000;127(3):329–36.

[3] McEachern R, Campbell GD Jr. Hospital-acquired pneumonia: epidemiology, etiology, and treatment. Infect Dis Clin North Am 1998;12(3):761–79.

[4] Richards MJ, Edwards JR, Culver DH, et al. Nosocomial infections in medical intensive care units in the United States. Crit Care Med 1999;27(5):887–92.

[5] Hospital-acquired pneumonia in adults: diagnosis, assessment of severity, initial antimicrobial therapy, and preventive strategies. A consensus statement, American Thoracic Society, November 1995. Am J Respir Crit Care Med 1996;153(5):1711–25.

[6] Guidelines for preventing health-care-associated pneumonia, 2003 recommendations of the CDC and the Healthcare Infection Control Practices Advisory Committee. Respir Care 2004;49(8):926–39.

[7] Grossman RF, Fein A. Evidence-based assessment of diagnostic tests for ventilator-associated pneumonia. Executive summary. Chest 2000;117(4, Suppl 2):177S–81S.

[8] Shorr AF, Sherner JH, Jackson WL, et al. Invasive approaches to the diagnosis of ventilator-associated pneumonia: a meta-analysis. Crit Care Med 2005;33(1):46–53.

[9] Chastre J, Wolff M, Fagon JY, et al. Comparison of 8 vs 15 days of antibiotic therapy for ventilator-associated pneumonia in adults: a randomized trial. JAMA 2003;290(19): 2588–98.

[10] George DL. Epidemiology of nosocomial pneumonia in intensive care unit patients. Clin Chest Med 1995;16(1):29–44.

[11] Keenan SP. Noninvasive positive pressure ventilation in acute respiratory failure. JAMA 2000;284(18):2376–8.

[12] Schweickert WD, Gehlbach BK, Pohlman AS, et al. Daily interruption of sedative infusions and complications of critical illness in mechanically ventilated patients. Crit Care Med 2004;32(6):1272–6.

[13] Dries DJ, McGonigal MD, Malian MS, et al. Protocol-driven ventilator weaning reduces use of mechanical ventilation, rate of early reintubation, and ventilator-associated pneumonia. J Trauma 2004;56(5):943–51 [discussion 951–2].

[14] Holzapfel L. Nasal vs oral intubation. Minerva Anestesiol 2003;69(5):348–52.

[15] Bach A, Boehrer H, Schmidt H, et al. Nosocomial sinusitis in ventilated patients. Nasotracheal versus orotracheal intubation. Anaesthesia 1992;47(4):335–9.

[16] Salord F, Gaussorgues P, Marti-Flich J, et al. Nosocomial maxillary sinusitis during mechanical ventilation: a prospective comparison of orotracheal versus the nasotracheal route for intubation. Intensive Care Med 1990;16(6):390–3.

[17] Holzapfel L, Chastang C, Demingeon G, et al. A randomized study assessing the systematic search for maxillary sinusitis in nasotracheally mechanically ventilated patients. Influence of nosocomial maxillary sinusitis on the occurrence of ventilator-associated pneumonia. Am J Respir Crit Care Med 1999;159(3):695–701.

[18] Craven DE, Goularte TA, Make BJ. Contaminated condensate in mechanical ventilator circuits. A risk factor for nosocomial pneumonia? Am Rev Respir Dis 1984;129(4):625–8.

[19] Kollef MH, Shapiro SD, Fraser VJ, et al. Mechanical ventilation with or without 7-day circuit changes. A randomized controlled trial. Ann Intern Med 1995;123(3):168–74.

[20] Fink JB, Krause SA, Barrett L, et al. Extending ventilator circuit change interval beyond 2 days reduces the likelihood of ventilator-associated pneumonia. Chest 1998;113(2):405–11.

[21] Kollef MH, Shapiro SD, Boyd V, et al. A randomized clinical trial comparing an extended-use hygroscopic condenser humidifier with heated-water humidification in mechanically ventilated patients. Chest 1998;113(3):759–67.

[22] Kirton OC, DeHaven B, Morgan J, et al. A prospective, randomized comparison of an in-line heat moisture exchange filter and heated wire humidifiers: rates of ventilator-associated early-onset (community-acquired) or late-onset (hospital-acquired) pneumonia and incidence of endotracheal tube occlusion. Chest 1997;112(4):1055–9.

[23] Memish ZA, Oni GA, Djazmati W, et al. A randomized clinical trial to compare the effects of a heat and moisture exchanger with a heated humidifying system on the occurrence rate of ventilator-associated pneumonia. Am J Infect Control 2001;29(5):301–5.

[24] Deppe SA, Kelly JW, Thoi LL, et al. Incidence of colonization, nosocomial pneumonia, and mortality in critically ill patients using a Trach Care closed-suction system versus an open-suction system: prospective, randomized study. Crit Care Med 1990;18(12):1389–93.

[25] Combes P, Fauvage B, Oleyer C. Nosocomial pneumonia in mechanically ventilated patients, a prospective randomised evaluation of the Stericath closed suctioning system. Intensive Care Med 2000;26(7):878–82.

[26] Topeli A, Harmanci A, Cetinkaya Y, et al. Comparison of the effect of closed versus open endotracheal suction systems on the development of ventilator-associated pneumonia. J Hosp Infect 2004;58(1):14–9.

[27] Lorente L, Lecuona M, Martin MM, et al. Ventilator-associated pneumonia using a closed versus an open tracheal suction system. Crit Care Med 2005;33(1):115–9.

[28] Kollef MH, Prentice D, Shapiro SD, et al. Mechanical ventilation with or without daily changes of in-line suction catheters. Am J Respir Crit Care Med 1997;156(2 Pt 1):466–72.

[29] Valles J, Artigas A, Rello J, et al. Continuous aspiration of subglottic secretions in preventing ventilator-associated pneumonia. Ann Intern Med 1995;122(3):179–86.

[30] Kollef MH, Skubas NJ, Sundt TM. A randomized clinical trial of continuous aspiration of subglottic secretions in cardiac surgery patients. Chest 1999;116(5):1339–46.

[31] Smulders K, van der Hoeven H, Weers-Pothoff I, et al. A randomized clinical trial of intermittent subglottic secretion drainage in patients receiving mechanical ventilation. Chest 2002;121(3):858–62.

[32] Kantorova I, Svoboda P, Scheer P, et al. Stress ulcer prophylaxis in critically ill patients: a randomized controlled trial. Hepatogastroenterology 2004;51(57):757–61.

[33] Cook DJ, Reeve BK, Guyatt GH, et al. Stress ulcer prophylaxis in critically ill patients. Resolving discordant meta-analyses. JAMA 1996;275(4):308–14.

[34] Cook D, Guyatt G, Marshall J, et al. A comparison of sucralfate and ranitidine for the prevention of upper gastrointestinal bleeding in patients requiring mechanical ventilation. N Engl J Med 1998;338(12):791–7.

[35] Messori A, Trippoli S, Vaiani M, et al. Bleeding and pneumonia in intensive care patients given ranitidine and sucralfate for prevention of stress ulcer: meta-analysis of randomised controlled trials. BMJ 2000;321(7269):1103–6.

[36] Simms HH, DeMaria E, McDonald L, et al. Role of gastric colonization in the development of pneumonia in critically ill trauma patients: results of a prospective randomized trial. J Trauma 1991;31(4):531–6 [discussion 536–7].

[37] Kollef MH. Selective digestive decontamination should not be routinely employed. Chest 2003;123(5 Suppl):464S–8S.

[38] Gastinne H, Wolff M, Delatour F, et al. A controlled trial in intensive care units of selective decontamination of the digestive tract with nonabsorbable antibiotics. N Engl J Med 1992; 326(9):594–9.

[39] Sanchez Garcia M, Cambronero Galache JA, Lopez Diaz J, et al. Effectiveness and cost of selective decontamination of the digestive tract in critically ill intubated patients.

A randomized, double-blind, placebo-controlled, multicenter trial. Am J Respir Crit Care Med 1998;158(3):908–16.

[40] Verwaest C, Verhaegen J, Ferdinande P, et al. Randomized, controlled trial of selective digestive decontamination in 600 mechanically ventilated patients in a multidisciplinary intensive care unit. Crit Care Med 1997;25(1):63–71.

[41] de La Cal MA, Cerda E, Garcia-Hierro P, et al. Survival benefit in critically ill burned patients receiving selective decontamination of the digestive tract: a randomized, placebo-controlled, double-blind trial. Ann Surg 2005;241(3):424–30.

[42] Houston S, Hougland P, Anderson JJ, et al. Effectiveness of 0.12% chlorhexidine gluconate oral rinse in reducing prevalence of nosocomial pneumonia in patients undergoing heart surgery. Am J Crit Care 2002;11(6):567–70.

[43] Genuit T, Bochicchio G, Napolitano LM, et al. Prophylactic chlorhexidine oral rinse decreases ventilator-associated pneumonia in surgical ICU patients. Surg Infect (Larchmt) 2001;2(1):5–18.

[44] Torres A, Serra-Batlles J, Ros E, et al. Pulmonary aspiration of gastric contents in patients receiving mechanical ventilation: the effect of body position. Ann Intern Med 1992;116(7): 540–3.

[45] Orozco-Levi M, Torres A, Ferrer M, et al. Semirecumbent position protects from pulmonary aspiration but not completely from gastroesophageal reflux in mechanically ventilated patients. Am J Respir Crit Care Med 1995;152(4 Pt 1):1387–90.

[46] Drakulovic MB, Torres A, Bauer TT, et al. Supine body position as a risk factor for nosocomial pneumonia in mechanically ventilated patients: a randomised trial. Lancet 1999; 354(9193):1851–8.

[47] Ahrens T, Kollef M, Stewart J, et al. Effect of kinetic therapy on pulmonary complications. Am J Crit Care 2004;13(5):376–83.

[48] Guerin C, Gaillard S, Lemasson S, et al. Effects of systematic prone positioning in hypoxemic acute respiratory failure: a randomized controlled trial. JAMA 2004;292(19): 2379–87.

[49] Ballantyne JC, Carr DB, deFerranti S, et al. The comparative effects of postoperative analgesic therapies on pulmonary outcome: cumulative meta-analyses of randomized, controlled trials. Anesth Analg 1998;86(3):598–612.

[50] Ryan P, Schweitzer SA, Woods RJ. Effect of epidural and general anaesthesia compared with general anaesthesia alone in large bowel anastomoses. A prospective study. Eur J Surg 1992;158(1):45–9.

[51] Cuschieri RJ, Morran CG, Howie JC, et al. Postoperative pain and pulmonary complications: comparison of three analgesic regimens. Br J Surg 1985;72(6):495–8.

[52] Scott NB, Turfrey DJ, Ray DA, et al. A prospective randomized study of the potential benefits of thoracic epidural anesthesia and analgesia in patients undergoing coronary artery bypass grafting. Anesth Analg 2001;93(3):528–35.

[53] Kearns PJ, Chin D, Mueller L, et al. The incidence of ventilator-associated pneumonia and success in nutrient delivery with gastric versus small intestinal feeding: a randomized clinical trial. Crit Care Med 2000;28(6):1742–6.

[54] Montecalvo MA, Steger KA, Farber HW, et al. Nutritional outcome and pneumonia in critical care patients randomized to gastric versus jejunal tube feedings. Crit Care Med 1992;20(10):1377–87.

[55] Montejo JC, Grau T, Acosta J, et al. Multicenter, prospective, randomized, single-blind study comparing the efficacy and gastrointestinal complications of early jejunal feeding with early gastric feeding in critically ill patients. Crit Care Med 2002;30(4): 796–800.

[56] Strong RM, Condon SC, Solinger MR, et al. Equal aspiration rates from postpylorus and intragastric-placed small-bore nasoenteric feeding tubes: a randomized, prospective study. JPEN J Parenter Enteral Nutr 1992;16(1):59–63.

[57] McClave SA, DeMeo MT, DeLegge MH, et al. North American summit on aspiration in the critically ill patient: consensus statement. JPEN J Parenter Enteral Nutr 2002; 26(6 Suppl):S80–5.

[58] McClave SA, Snider HL. Clinical use of gastric residual volumes as a monitor for patients on enteral tube feeding. JPEN J Parenter Enteral Nutr 2002;26(6 Suppl):S43–8 [discussion S49–50].

[59] McClave SA, Snider HL, Lowen CC, et al. Use of residual volume as a marker for enteral feeding intolerance: prospective blinded comparison with physical examination and radiographic findings. JPEN J Parenter Enteral Nutr 1992;16(2):99–105.

[60] McClave SA, Lukan JK, Stefater JA, et al. Poor validity of residual volumes as a marker for risk of aspiration in critically ill patients. Crit Care Med 2005;33(2):324–30.

[61] Tambyah PA. Catheter-associated urinary tract infections: diagnosis and prophylaxis. Int J Antimicrob Agents 2004;24(Suppl 1):S44–8.

[62] Bjork DT, Pelletier LL, Tight RR. Urinary tract infections with antibiotic resistant organisms in catheterized nursing home patients. Infect Control 1984;5(4):173–6.

[63] Krieger JN, Kaiser DL, Wenzel RP. Nosocomial urinary tract infections cause wound infections postoperatively in surgical patients. Surg Gynecol Obstet 1983;156(3):313–8.

[64] Leone M, Albanese J, Garnier F, et al. Risk factors of nosocomial catheter-associated urinary tract infection in a polyvalent intensive care unit. Intensive Care Med 2003;29(7): 1077–80.

[65] Tambyah PA, Knasinski V, Maki DG. The direct costs of nosocomial catheter-associated urinary tract infection in the era of managed care. Infect Control Hosp Epidemiol 2002; 23(1):27–31.

[66] Garner JS, Jarvis WR, Emori TG, et al. CDC definitions for nosocomial infections, 1988. Am J Infect Control 1988;16(3):128–40.

[67] Stark RP, Maki DG. Bacteriuria in the catheterized patient. What quantitative level of bacteriuria is relevant? N Engl J Med 1984;311(9):560–4.

[68] Maki DG, Tambyah PA. Engineering out the risk for infection with urinary catheters. Emerg Infect Dis 2001;7(2):342–7.

[69] Harding GK, Nicolle LE, Ronald AR, et al. How long should catheter-acquired urinary tract infection in women be treated? A randomized controlled study. Ann Intern Med 1991;114(9):713–9.

[70] Warren JW, Abrutyn E, Hebel JR, et al. Guidelines for antimicrobial treatment of uncomplicated acute bacterial cystitis and acute pyelonephritis in women. Clin Infect Dis 1999; 29(4):745–58.

[71] Leone M, Garnier F, Avidan M, et al. Catheter-associated urinary tract infections in intensive care units. Microbes Infect 2004;6(11):1026–32.

[72] Jain P, Parada JP, David A, et al. Overuse of the indwelling urinary tract catheter in hospitalized medical patients. Arch Intern Med 1995;155(13):1425–9.

[73] Huang WC, Wann SR, Lin SL, et al. Catheter-associated urinary tract infections in intensive care units can be reduced by prompting physicians to remove unnecessary catheters. Infect Control Hosp Epidemiol 2004;25(11):974–8.

[74] Guidelines for preventing catheter associated urinary tract infections—on Internet for consultation. Commun Dis Rep CDR Wkly 2000;10(17):149, 152.

[75] Shapiro M, Simchen E, Izraeli S, et al. A multivariate analysis of risk factors for acquiring bacteriuria in patients with indwelling urinary catheters for longer than 24 hours. Infect Control 1984;5(11):525–32.

[76] van der Wall E, Verkooyen RP, Mintjes-de Groot J, et al. Prophylactic ciprofloxacin for catheter-associated urinary-tract infection. Lancet 1992;339(8799):946–51.

[77] Verbrugh HA, Mintjes-de Groot AJ, Andriesse R, et al. Postoperative prophylaxis with norfloxacin in patients requiring bladder catheters. Eur J Clin Microbiol Infect Dis 1988; 7(4):490–4.

[78] Britt MR, Garibaldi RA, Miller WA, et al. Antimicrobial prophylaxis for catheter-associated bacteriuria. Antimicrob Agents Chemother 1977;11(2):240–3.

[79] Thompson RL, Haley CE, Searcy MA, et al. Catheter-associated bacteriuria. Failure to reduce attack rates using periodic instillations of a disinfectant into urinary drainage systems. JAMA 1984;251(6):747–51.

[80] Warren JW, Platt R, Thomas RJ, et al. Antibiotic irrigation and catheter-associated urinary-tract infections. N Engl J Med 1978;299(11):570–3.

[81] Sweet DE, Goodpasture HC, Holl K, et al. Evaluation of H2O2 prophylaxis of bacteriuria in patients with long-term indwelling Foley catheters: a randomized controlled study. Infect Control 1985;6(7):263–6.

[82] Schneeberger PM, Vreede RW, Bogdanowicz JF, et al. A randomized study on the effect of bladder irrigation with povidone-iodine before removal of an indwelling catheter. J Hosp Infect 1992;21(3):223 9.

[83] Burke JP, Garibaldi RA, Britt MR, et al. Prevention of catheter-associated urinary tract infections. Efficacy of daily meatal care regimens. Am J Med 1981;70(3):655–8.

[84] Burke JP, Jacobson JA, Garibaldi RA, et al. Evaluation of daily meatal care with poly-antibiotic ointment in prevention of urinary catheter-associated bacteriuria. J Urol 1983; 129(2):331–4.

[85] Shapiro J, Hoffmann J, Jersky J. A comparison of suprapubic and transurethral drainage for postoperative urinary retention in general surgical patients. Acta Chir Scand 1982; 148(4):323–7.

[86] Sethia KK, Selkon JB, Berry AR, et al. Prospective randomized controlled trial of urethral versus suprapubic catheterization. Br J Surg 1987;74(7):624–5.

[87] O'Kelly TJ, Mathew A, Ross S, et al. Optimum method for urinary drainage in major abdominal surgery: a prospective randomized trial of suprapubic versus urethral catheterization. Br J Surg 1995;82(10):1367–8.

[88] Hirsh DD, Fainstein V, Musher DM. Do condom catheter collecting systems cause urinary tract infection? JAMA 1979;242(4):340–1.

[89] Ouslander JG, Greengold B, Chen S. External catheter use and urinary tract infections among incontinent male nursing home patients. J Am Geriatr Soc 1987;35(12): 1063–70.

[90] Warren JW. Urethral catheters, condom catheters, and nosocomial urinary tract infections. Infect Control Hosp Epidemiol 1996;17(4):212–4.

[91] Johnson JR, Roberts PL, Olsen RJ, et al. Prevention of catheter-associated urinary tract infection with a silver oxide-coated urinary catheter: clinical and microbiologic correlates. J Infect Dis 1990;162(5):1145–50.

[92] Riley DK, Classen DC, Stevens LE, et al. A large randomized clinical trial of a silver-impregnated urinary catheter: lack of efficacy and staphylococcal superinfection. Am J Med 1995;98(4):349–56.

[93] Liedberg H, Lundeberg T. Silver alloy coated catheters reduce catheter-associated bacteriuria. Br J Urol 1990;65(4):379–81.

[94] Karchmer TB, Giannetta ET, Muto CA, et al. A randomized crossover study of silver-coated urinary catheters in hospitalized patients. Arch Intern Med 2000;160(21):3294–8.

[95] Bologna RA, Tu LM, Polansky M, et al. Hydrogel/silver ion-coated urinary catheter reduces nosocomial urinary tract infection rates in intensive care unit patients: a multicenter study. Urology 1999;54(6):982–7.

[96] Thibon P, Le Coutour X, Leroyer R, et al. Randomized multi-centre trial of the effects of a catheter coated with hydrogel and silver salts on the incidence of hospital-acquired urinary tract infections. J Hosp Infect 2000;45(2):117–24.

[97] National Nosocomial Infections Surveillance (NNIS) System report. Data summary from January 1992 through June 2004, issued October 2004. Am J Infect Control 2004;32(8): 470–85.

[98] Mermel LA, Farr BM, Sherertz RJ, et al. Guidelines for the management of intravascular catheter-related infections. Clin Infect Dis 2001;32(9):1249–72.

[99] Pelletier SJ, Crabtree TD, Gleason TG, et al. Bacteremia associated with central venous catheter infection is not an independent predictor of outcomes. J Am Coll Surg 2000; 190(6):671–80 [discussion 680–1].

[100] Eggimann P, Harbarth S, Constantin MN, et al. Impact of a prevention strategy targeted at vascular-access care on incidence of infections acquired in intensive care. Lancet 2000; 355(9218):1864–8.

[101] Raad II, Hohn DC, Gilbreath BJ, et al. Prevention of central venous catheter-related infections by using maximal sterile barrier precautions during insertion. Infect Control Hosp Epidemiol 1994;15(4 Pt 1):231–8.

[102] Maki DG, Ringer M, Alvarado CJ. Prospective randomised trial of povidone-iodine, alcohol, and chlorhexidine for prevention of infection associated with central venous and arterial catheters. Lancet 1991;338(8763):339–43.

[103] Sheth NK, Franson TR, Rose HD, et al. Colonization of bacteria on polyvinyl chloride and Teflon intravascular catheters in hospitalized patients. J Clin Microbiol 1983;18(5): 1061–3.

[104] O'Grady NP, Alexander M, Dellinger EP, et al. Guidelines for the prevention of intravascular catheter-related infections. MMWR Recomm Rep 2002;51(RR-10):1–29.

[105] Veenstra DL, Saint S, Sullivan SD. Cost-effectiveness of antiseptic-impregnated central venous catheters for the prevention of catheter-related bloodstream infection. JAMA 1999; 282(6):554–60.

[106] Maki DG, Stolz SM, Wheeler S, et al. Prevention of central venous catheter-related bloodstream infection by use of an antiseptic-impregnated catheter. A randomized, controlled trial. Ann Intern Med 1997;127(4):257–66.

[107] Hanna HA, Raad II, Hackett B, et al. Antibiotic-impregnated catheters associated with significant decrease in nosocomial and multidrug-resistant bacteremias in critically ill patients. Chest 2003;124(3):1030–8.

[108] Cobb DK, High KP, Sawyer RG, et al. A controlled trial of scheduled replacement of central venous and pulmonary-artery catheters. N Engl J Med 1992;327(15):1062–8.

[109] Boyce JM, Pittet D. Guideline for hand hygiene in health-care settings: recommendations of the Healthcare Infection Control Practices Advisory Committee and the HICPAC/SHEA/APIC/IDSA Hand Hygiene Task Force. Infect Control Hosp Epidemiol 2002; 23(12 Suppl):S3–40.

[110] Larson E. A causal link between handwashing and risk of infection? Examination of the evidence. Infect Control 1988;9(1):28–36.

[111] Pittet D, Hugonnet S, Harbarth S, et al. Effectiveness of a hospital-wide programme to improve compliance with hand hygiene. Infection Control Programme. Lancet 2000; 356(9238):1307–12.

[112] Webster J, Faoagali JL, Cartwright D. Elimination of methicillin-resistant *Staphylococcus aureus* from a neonatal intensive care unit after hand washing with triclosan. J Paediatr Child Health 1994;30(1):59–64.

[113] Pittet D. Compliance with hand disinfection and its impact on hospital-acquired infections. J Hosp Infect 2001;48(Suppl A):S40–6.

[114] Jarvis WR. Benchmarking for prevention: the Centers for Disease Control and Prevention's National Nosocomial Infections Surveillance (NNIS) System experience. Infection 2003; 31(Suppl 2):44–8.

[115] Cook DJ, Kollef MH. Risk factors for ICU-acquired pneumonia. JAMA 1998;279(20): 1605–6.

[116] Platt R, Polk BF, Murdock B, et al. Risk factors for nosocomial urinary tract infection. Am J Epidemiol 1986;124(6):977–85.

[117] Oncu S, Ozsut H, Yildirim A, et al. Central venous catheter related infections: risk factors and the effect of glycopeptide antibiotics. Ann Clin Microbiol Antimicrob 2003;2(1):3.

ELSEVIER
SAUNDERS

SURGICAL
CLINICS OF
NORTH AMERICA

Surg Clin N Am 85 (2005) 1153–1161

Impact of Diabetes Mellitus and Metabolic Disorders

Matthias Turina, MD[a], Mirjam Christ-Crain, MD[b],
Hiram C. Polk, Jr, MD[c],*

[a]*Department of Surgery, Price Institute of Surgical Research, 511 South Floyd Street,
MDR Building, Room 312, Louisville, KY 40202, USA*
[b]*Clinic of Endocrinology, Diabetes and Clinical Nutrition, University Hospital Basel,
Petersgraben 4, CH-4031 Basel, Switzerland*
[c]*Department of Surgery, University of Louisville School of Medicine, Ambulatory Care
Building, 550 South Jackson Street, Louisville, KY 40292, USA*

Metabolic disorders are common and relevant in surgical patients. A number of endocrinopathies, electrolyte problems, or metabolic derangements may either preexist or develop during the course of surgical treatment. Left unattended, these disorders may lead to significant morbidity and mortality. Early recognition, adequate diagnostic evaluation, and strict perioperative metabolic control are the mainstays of successful surgical intervention in affected patients.

Diabetes mellitus

The prevalence of diabetes mellitus, the most common endocrine disorder in the United States, rose by 40% among adults between 1990 and 1999. Roughly 16 million Americans were affected by this disease at the turn of the millennium [1,2]. In addition, most estimates suggest a rising incidence in coming years, which is mainly attributed to a rapid increase of type 2 diabetes in recent decades. The lifetime likelihood of developing diabetes is 32% for males and 39% for females born in the year 2000 [2]. Its incidence, by nature, rises with age, and thus pertains to a large percentage of patients admitted to surgical services. Diabetics undergoing surgery or major trauma suffer an increased risk of perioperative complications, mainly because of

This work was supported in part by the Ferguson Research Fund.

* Corresponding author.

E-mail address: Hcpolk01@louisville.edu (H.C. Polk).

a higher infection rate, compromised wound healing, ischemic complications, and longer hospital stays [3,4]. In addition, diabetic patients frequently have undiagnosed atherosclerotic cardiovascular disease, running the risk of potential vascular thrombotic sequelae promoted by the procoagulant effects of transient hyperglycemia [5,6]. Even in previously nondiabetic patients, the occurrence of acute hyperglycemia during critical illness correlates with adverse outcomes [7], demonstrating the importance of precise glucose control in any patient admitted to a surgical intensive care unit (ICU).

Diagnosis and classification

A new classification by the World Health Organization (WHO) and the American Diabetes Association (ADA) was introduced in 2003 [8], defining 4 categories of the diabetes (Box 1). However, of all patients who have diabetes, 95% suffer from diabetes mellitus type 2. It is not uncommon for a diagnosis of diabetes mellitus type 2 to be first made upon routine evaluation of patients admitted for common surgical procedures. Diagnostic criteria include the presence of classic symptoms of diabetes in combination with casual (any time of day without regard to last meal) plasma glucose values exceeding 200 mg/dL (11.1 mmol/L), or fasting plasma glucose values (no caloric intake for at least 8 hours) above 125 mg/dL (7 mmol/L). Any

---

Box 1. WHO and ADA classification of diabetes mellitus

1. *Type 1: characterized as immune-mediated or idiopathic*
2. *Type 2: may range from predominately insulin resistance with relative insulin deficiency to a predominately secretory defect with insulin resistance*
3. *Other types. Caused by or related to any of the following:*
   - Genetic defects of β-cell function
   - Genetic defects in insulin action
   - Diseases of the exocrine pancreas
   - Endocrinopathies
   - Drug- or chemical-induced
   - Infections
   - Uncommon immune-mediated forms
   - Other genetic syndromes associated with diabetes
4. *Gestational diabetes mellitus*

Adapted from The report of the expert committee on the diagnosis and classification of diabetes mellitus. Diabetes Care 2003;26(Suppl 1):S5–20; with permission.

positive measurement needs to be confirmed on the following day to allow for a firm diagnosis of diabetes mellitus [8].

Perioperative metabolic control in diabetic patients

Regarding perioperative management of diabetic patients, a clear distinction must be made between insulin-deficient diabetic patients, who require insulin at all times, and type 2 diabetics on oral antidiabetic drugs, who are often able to maintain normoglycemia despite discontinuation of their antidiabetic medication upon surgical treatment. In latter patients, oral hypoglycemic agents are routinely withheld on the day of surgery and resumed later along with a normal diet. The administration of metformin, which has a potential to alter perioperative renal function, should be discontinued until normal renal parameters are confirmed 48 to 72 hours postoperatively. When treated with insulin, type 2 diabetic patients often exhibit near-normal blood glucose values upon diet-restriction alone, and require only supplemental short-acting insulin by sliding scale [5]. Their previous insulin regimen should be withheld until normal dietary intake is resumed.

In insulin-dependent diabetic patients, perioperative insulin replacement is more elaborate, and clinicians are faced with several options. Ideally, subcutaneous insulin is replaced by continuous intravenous insulin perioperatively, begun on the morning of surgery at a rate of 1 to 2 U/h in combination with intravenous dextrose [9]. This method allows for exact regulation of plasma glucose values by adjusting the ratio of insulin/dextrose and should be continued until normal dietary uptake is established postoperatively. If continuous intravenous insulin is not an option, glycemic control can be achieved using reduced doses of subcutaneous intermediate- and short-acting insulin combinations with a background intravenous dextrose infusion that can be titrated [9]. Patients using long-acting insulin regimens should either be shifted to shorter-acting agents or be given two thirds of their bedtime dose in the evening before surgery and half their usual morning dose on the morning of surgery. Another option is the use of combined glucose-insulin-potassium infusions as first proposed by Alberti in 1979 [10]. The choice of which perioperative insulin strategy to use depends largely on the expertise of hospital and nursing staffs to correctly monitor and adjust blood glucose values, the general condition of the patient, and the extent of the planned surgical procedure. Short, less-invasive operations, or those performed with local, regional, or epidural anesthesia, do not require continuous intravenous insulin. This method is proven superior in most cases that require general anesthesia, as long as medical personnel are adequately trained to safely handle and monitor a continuous intravenous insulin regimen [3]. If in doubt about which method to choose, or in the case of any long-standing diabetic patient with a history of frequent glycemic excursions, an interdisciplinary approach with specialized endocrinologists or diabetologists should be sought. These patients require exact preoperative evaluation and frequent follow-up visits throughout their hospitalization to avoid metabolic derangements and increased mortality.

Hyperglycemia in previously non-diabetic individuals

Critical illness and severe surgical stress each trigger a metabolic response that invariably causes a transient increase in plasma glucose concentrations, creating stress hyperglycemia. Its occurrence is common in surgical ICUs, with almost 75% of previously admitted patients exceeding 110 mg/dL and 12% exceeding 200 mg/dL in a mixed surgical ICU population [7]. In previous years, a cutoff value of 200 mg/dL was used both as a diagnostic marker and a threshold above which to initiate insulin treatment. However, more recent, well-performed clinical trials have demonstrated that blood glucose levels already above the physiologic threshold of 110 mg/dL are associated with higher ICU morbidity and mortality rates. Thus, most clinicians today no longer consider 200 mg/dL an adequate threshold to initiate insulin therapy.

Stress hyperglycemia is caused and sustained by a variety of factors. Activation of the hypothalamic-pituitary-adrenal (HPA) axis, increased circulating levels of epinephrine, norepinephrine, glucagon, and growth hormone all promote hepatic glycogenolysis, gluconeogenesis, and the release of glucose into the circulation. Insulin levels are usually normal or decreased, presumably by a release-inhibiting effect of interleukin-1 (IL-1) and tumor necrosis factor-α (TNF-α). Both IL-1 and TNF-α, but also IL-6, are known to further induce a state of peripheral insulin resistance, which combined with the above-mentioned endocrine changes, relative insulin deficiency, and the common iatrogenic dextrose and nutritional support, all work together to keep blood glucose levels supranormal [11,12].

Once established, stress hyperglycemia in critical illness serves as a strong predictor of adverse outcome. Many large clinical trials have demonstrated a direct association between blood glucose levels and increased rates of infectious complications, organ dysfunction or failure, and death rates on the ICU [7,13–17]. Table 1 gives an overview of the most recent clinical trials. In 2001, van den Berghe and colleagues conducted a randomized controlled trial on 1548 surgical ICU patients, comparing strict blood glucose control aimed at restoration of physiologic concentrations (80–110 mg/dL) with a control group receiving insulin only above a blood glucose level of 215 mg/dL. After 12 months, ICU mortality fell from 8% with conventional treatment to 4.6% in the intensive insulin group, and total in-hospital mortality declined 34%, an effect mainly attributed to a reduction of infectious complications, organ failure rates, and transfusion requirements. Despite these impressive results, the exact glucose level to be targeted continues to be debated, as not all investigators recorded a difference in outcome between patients kept at physiologic glucose levels and those slightly exceeding this range [18]. In addition, many remain concerned about the potential risk

Table 1
Clinical trials related to surgical patients and diabetes

Author	Study design	Outcome	Issues
Van den Berghe, et al [7]	PRCT. 1548 surgical patients. Randomization to receive either tight glucose control (80–110 mg/dL), or "conventional" control (only <215 mg/dL)	Total mortality: 34%; bloodstream infections: 46%; renal failure: 41%	High percentage of CT surgery patients. Few if any medical patients
Finney, et al [13]	Prospective, observational, 523 surgical patients. Multivariable analysis of insulin treatment and blood glucose levels versus ICU outcome	Lower glucose = better outcome, but high insulin requirements associated with adverse outcome	Mainly CT surgery. No medical patients
Malmberg, et al [14]	PRCT. 620 diabetic AMI patients. Randomized diabetics to tight blood glucose control with an initial insulin/glucose infusion or conventional therapy	Improved survival, most notable in patients with lowest risk and least previous insulin use	Only diabetics. Intervention group with glucose levels still >110mg/dL
Krinsley JS [15]	Retrospective analysis of blood glucose levels vs. clinical outcome in 1826 medical/surgical ICU patients	Lowest mortality with 80–99 mg/dL glucose. Progressive increase in mortality with increasing glycemia	Heterogeneous medical and surgical patient population
Krinsley JS [16]	PNRCT of an intensive glucose management protocol in a heterogeneous population of 800 medical/surgical ICU patients.	29% decrease of mortality, 75% decrease of renal insufficiency	Heterogeneous medical and surgical patient population
Grey, et al [17]	PRCT. 61 surgical ICU patients, randomized to strict (target glucose range 80–120 mg/dL), or "standard" insulin therapy (target glucose range 180–220 mg/dL)	Decreased rate of infections with strict blood glucose control	High rate of hypoglycemia (<60 mg/dL) in treatment group (32%)

Abbreviations: PRCT, prospective randomized controlled trial; PNRCT, prospective, non-randomized controlled trial; CT, cardiothoracic surgery; AMI, acute myocardial infarction.

Adapted from Coursin DB, Connery LE, Ketzler JT. Perioperative diabetic and hyperglycemic management issues. Crit Care Med 2004;32(Suppl):S116–25, with permission.

of iatrogenic hypoglycemia in unresponsive intensive care patients treated in ICUs less well staffed or with less experienced staff [19]. However, no other clinical trial yet approaches van den Berghe's level of evidence with regard to strict randomization and size of study population, rendering direct comparisons technically unjustified.

Other endocrine changes in critical illness

The pituitary-adrenal axis in critical illness

Appropriate adaptation of the HPA axis to stress is essential for survival. Critical illness can impair the proper stress response of the HPA axis [20].

The terms "relative" or "functional" adrenal insufficiency have been proposed for hypotensive, septic critically ill patients who show hemodynamic improvement with cortisol administration. In these patients, the cortisol levels (despite being within the normal reference range or even elevated) are still considered to be inadequate for the severe stress, and the patient may be unable to respond to any additional or protracted stress [20].

An ongoing debate concerns the definition of relative adrenal insufficiency. Corticosteroid insufficiency is difficult to discern clinically and must be actively sought by the treating physician. The diurnal pattern of cortisol secretion together with a large interindividual range of circulating cortisol levels during severe illness and stress make it impossible to define an absolute serum cortisol threshold level that identifies a patient with failure of the HPA-axis in critical illness. A simple and widely used test is stimulation with synthetic corticotropin (synacthen) in hypotensive critically ill patients. A "basal" cortisol of >34 μg/dL (935 nmol/L) combined with an increase of cortisol <9 μg/dL (250 nmol/L) after 250 μg corticotropin stimulation has been associated with a mortality of 80%, arguably pointing to a relative adrenal insufficiency [21]. Because the 250 μg corticotropin stimulation test induces supraphysiological corticotropin concentrations, the 1 μg synthetic corticotropin test has been suggested to be more sensitive to diagnose adrenocortical insufficiency [22].

Up to 75% of patients in septic shock requiring vasopressors manifest relative adrenal insufficiency. The Surviving Sepsis Campaign guidelines for the management of severe sepsis and septic shock, published in 2004, recommend the following: "Intravenous corticosteroids (hydrocortisone 200–300 mg/day, for 7 days in 3 or 4 divided doses or by continuous infusion) are recommended in patients with septic shock who, despite adequate fluid replacement, require vasopressor therapy to maintain adequate blood pressure" [23].

One multi-center, randomized, controlled trial (RCT) with patients in severe septic shock showed a significant shock reversal and reduction of mortality rate in patients with relative adrenal insufficiency (defined as post-corticotropin cortisol increase <9 μg/dL) [24]. Two additional smaller RCTs showed significant effects on shock reversal [25,26]. A recent meta-analysis examined the efficacy of glucocorticoids in sepsis [27] and concluded that a 5- to 7-day course of physiologic hydrocortisone doses with subsequent tapering increases survival rate and shock reversal in patients with vasopressor-dependent septic shock.

Based on the evidence to date, clinicians treating patients with septic shock should consider administering a dose of dexamethasone until a corticotropin stimulation test can be performed. Dexamethasone is recommended because it, unlike hydrocortisone, does not interfere with the cortisol assay. Administration of steroids should be continued to determine if the patient is a responder, as indicated by an increase in blood pressure, and the results of the corticotropin stimulation test are reviewed.

There is little definitive advice to offer concerning the use of pharmacologic doses of glucocorticoids in critical illness in general, especially in patients who do not meet the criteria for relative adrenal insufficiency. The alleged benefits should be weighed against the potential dangers of such therapy, such as hyperglycemia. The marked reduction of harmful hyperglycemia in critically ill patients by insulin should be a further cause for concern. In addition, the ebb and flow of attitudes regarding the usefulness of large-dose steroid treatment in patients with spinal cord injuries further underscores the uncertainty surrounding this issue [28,29].

Thyroid hormones in critical illness

In critical illness, profound changes occur in the hypothalamic-pituitary-thyroid (HPT) axis. Terms for these changes include euthyroid sick syndrome (ESS) or non-thyroid illness (NTI). Typically, a normal level of thyrotropin and free T4 and decreased total T3 suggest a change in the HPT axis setpoint [30]. This change is thought to represent a homeostatic correction by which the body diminishes the effects of the biologically active hormone, T3. It remains controversial whether patients with NTI should be treated [30]. However, the actual evidence is far from compelling, and, in the absence of clear clinical or laboratory evidence for abnormal thyroid function, most investigators currently advise withholding thyroid hormone therapy for NTI in critically ill patients.

Growth hormone in critical illness

The mean concentration of growth hormone (GH) increases sharply in most stress states, such as surgery or trauma. Non-survivors generally have higher levels of GH than do survivors. Despite the increased GH, insulin-like growth factor-1 (IGF-1) levels are consistently low, suggesting a GH-resistant state. Although a multitude of studies have demonstrated that growth hormone supplementation has salutary anabolic effects in a number of different stressful conditions, this therapy may lead to increased mortality in critical illness [31]. In addition, the broad nontherapeutic use of these agents in North American life, especially among athletes, has endangered its availability to many who legitimately benefit from GH therapy.

The pituitary-gonadal axis in critical illness

All acute severe illnesses are capable of producing hypogonadotrophic hypogonadism [32]. This condition is usually temporary and its pattern mimics that of nonthyroidal illness with levels of testosterone or estrogen returning to normal approximately 6 weeks after recovery [33]. Testosterone increases lean body mass, muscle size, strength, and bone density when given in supraphysiological doses in healthy individuals [34]. However, apart from the proven benefit of oxandrolone to restore muscle protein metabolism in severely burned patients [35], little evidence supports the use of replacement therapy or the use of anabolic steroids in hypogonadism associated with acute illness. Further work needs to be done before their supplemental use in critically ill surgical patients is justified.

References

[1] Harris MI. Diabetes in America: epidemiology and scope of the problem. Diabetes Care 1998;21(Suppl 3):C11–4.

[2] Narayan KM, Boyle JP, Thompson TJ, et al. Lifetime risk for diabetes mellitus in the United States. JAMA 2003;290(14):1884–90.

[3] Furnary AP, Gao G, Grunkemeier GL, et al. Continuous insulin infusion reduces mortality in patients with diabetes undergoing coronary artery bypass grafting. J Thorac Cardiovasc Surg 2003;125(5):1007–21.

[4] Zerr KJ, Furnary AP, Grunkemeier GL, et al. Glucose control lowers the risk of wound infection in diabetics after open heart operations. Ann Thorac Surg 1997;63(2):356–61.

[5] Inzucchi SE. Glycemic management of diabetes in the perioperative setting. Int Anesthesiol Clin 2002;40(2):77–93.

[6] Rao AK, Chouhan V, Chen X, et al. Activation of the tissue factor pathway of blood coagulation during prolonged hyperglycemia in young healthy men. Diabetes 1999;48(5): 1156–61.

[7] Van Den BG, Wouters P, Weekers F, et al. Intensive insulin therapy in the critically ill patients. N Engl J Med 2001;345(19):1359–67.

[8] Report of the expert committee on the diagnosis and classification of diabetes mellitus. Diabetes Care 2003;26(Suppl 1):S5–20.

[9] Glister BC, Vigersky RA. Perioperative management of type 1 diabetes mellitus. Endocrinol Metab Clin North Am 2003;32(2):411–36.

[10] Alberti KG, Thomas DJ. The management of diabetes during surgery. Br J Anaesth 1979; 51(7):693–710.

[11] McCowen KC, Malhotra A, Bistrian BR. Stress-induced hyperglycemia. Crit Care Clin 2001;17(1):107–24.

[12] Ogawa H, Nielsen S, Kawakami M. Cachectin/tumor necrosis factor and interleukin-1 show different modes of combined effect on lipoprotein lipase activity and intracellular lipolysis in 3T3–L1 cells. Biochim Biophys Acta 1989;1003(2):131–5.

[13] Finney SJ, Zekveld C, Elia A, et al. Glucose control and mortality in critically ill patients. JAMA 2003;290(15):2041–7.

[14] Malmberg K, Norhammar A, Wedel H, et al. Glycometabolic state at admission: important risk marker of mortality in conventionally treated patients with diabetes mellitus and acute myocardial infarction: long-term results from the Diabetes and Insulin-Glucose Infusion in Acute Myocardial Infarction (DIGAMI) study. Circulation 1999;99(20):2626–32.

[15] Krinsley JS. Association between hyperglycemia and increased hospital mortality in a heterogeneous population of critically ill patients. Mayo Clin Proc 2003;78(12):1471–8.

[16] Krinsley JS. Effect of an intensive glucose management protocol on the mortality of critically ill adult patients. Mayo Clin Proc 2004;79(8):992–1000.

[17] Grey NJ, Perdrizet GA. Reduction of nosocomial infections in the surgical intensive-care unit by strict glycemic control. Endocr Pract 2004;10(Suppl 2):46–52.

[18] Laird AM, Miller PR, Kilgo PD, et al. Relationship of early hyperglycemia to mortality in trauma patients. J Trauma 2004;56(5):1058–62.

[19] Murrary MJ, Brull SJ, Coursin DB. Strict blood glucose control in the ICU: panacea or Pandora's box? J Cardiothorac Vasc Anesth 2004;18(6):687–9.

[20] Cooper MS, Stewart PM. Corticosteroid insufficiency in acutely ill patients. N Engl J Med 2003;348(8):727–34.

[21] Annane D, Sebille V, Troche G, et al. A 3-level prognostic classification in septic shock based on cortisol levels and cortisol response to corticotropin. JAMA 2000;283(8):1038–45.

[22] Dickstein G, Spigel D, Arad E, et al. One microgram is the lowest ACTH dose to cause a maximal cortisol response. There is no diurnal variation of cortisol response to submaximal ACTH stimulation. Eur J Endocrinol 1997;137(2):172–5.

[23] Dellinger RP, Carlet JM, Masur, et al. Surviving Sepsis Campaign guidelines for management of severe sepsis and septic shock. Crit Care Med 2004;32(3):858–73.

[24] Annane D, Sebille V, Charpentier C, et al. Effect of treatment with low doses of hydrocortisone and fludrocortisone on mortality in patients with septic shock. JAMA 2002;288(7): 862–71.

[25] Briegel J, Forst H, Haller M, et al. Stress doses of hydrocortisone reverse hyperdynamic septic shock: a prospective, randomized, double-blind, single-center study. Crit Care Med 1999; 27:723–32.

[26] Bollaert PE, Charpentier C, Levy B, et al. Reversal of late septic shock with supraphysiologic doses of hydrocortisone. Crit Care Med 1998;26:645–50.

[27] Minneci PC, Deans KJ, Banks SM, et al. Meta-analysis: the effect of steroids on survival and shock during sepsis depends on the dose. Ann Intern Med 2004;141(1):47–56.

[28] Galandiuk S, Raque G, Appel S, et al. The two-edged sword of large-dose steroids for spinal cord trauma. Ann Surg 1993;218(4):419–25.

[29] Spencer MT, Bazarian JJ. Evidence-based emergency medicine/systematic review abstract. Are corticosteroids effective in traumatic spinal cord injury? Ann Emerg Med 2003;41(3): 410–3.

[30] Fliers E, Alkemade A, Wiersinga WM. The hypothalamic-pituitary-thyroid axis in critical illness. Best Pract Res Clin Endocrinol Metab 2001;15(4):453–64.

[31] Takala J, Ruokonen E, Webster NR, et al. Increased mortality associated with growth hormone treatment in critically ill adults. N Engl J Med 1999;341(11):785–92.

[32] Semple CG, Gray CE, Beastall GH. Male hypogonadism—a non-specific consequence of illness. Q J Med 1987;64(243):601–7.

[33] Turner HE, Wass JA. Gonadal function in men with chronic illness. Clin Endocrinol (Oxf) 1997;47(4):379–403.

[34] Bhasin S, Storer TW, Berman N, et al. The effects of supraphysiologic doses of testosterone on muscle size and strength in normal men. N Engl J Med 1996;335(1):1–7.

[35] Hart DW, Wolf SE, Ramzy PI, et al. Anabolic effects of oxandrolone after severe burn. Ann Surg 2001;233(4):556–64.

ELSEVIER
SAUNDERS

SURGICAL
CLINICS OF
NORTH AMERICA

Surg Clin N Am 85 (2005) 1163–1177

Thrombosis and Coagulation: Deep Vein Thrombosis and Pulmonary Embolism Prophylaxis

Daniel A. Anaya, MD[a,b],
Avery B. Nathens, MD, MPH[a,b,*]

[a]Division of General and Trauma Surgery, Harborview Medical Center,
325 Ninth Avenue, Seattle, WA 98104, USA
[b]Department of Surgery, University of Washington,
1959 North East Pacific Street, Seattle, WA 98195, USA

Venous thromboembolism (VTE, ie, deep vein thrombosis [DVT] or pulmonary embolism [PE]) is a common complication affecting approximately 25% of all hospitalized patients. The burden of disease is significant, with an estimated 450,000 patients affected annually in the United States [1]. The major health risk associated with VTE is PE. PE affects approximately 1% of all hospitalized patients and is thought to be responsible for at least 10% of all inpatient deaths [2–4]. It is the primary cause of preventable deaths in hospitalized patients and has first priority in patient-safety strategies being developed by different governmental and nongovernmental agencies. Patients who have VTE are at significant risk for long-term sequelae including postthrombotic syndrome, recurrent DVT, and pulmonary hypertension [5,6].

The natural history of VTE has been well characterized. In one third of patients, the DVT is proximal to the calf, which is associated with a higher risk of PE. In the residual two thirds of patients who have calf DVT, 10% to 20% may extend toward the more proximal veins, particularly if the predisposing conditions persist. Clinical studies indicate a strong association between DVT and PE. As many as 50% of patients who have a proximal DVT develop a PE, and among those who have a clinically significant PE, 70% have evidence of DVT. Further, the long-term sequelae of DVT,

* Corresponding author.
E-mail address: anathens@u.washington.edu (A.B. Nathens).

0039-6109/05/$ - see front matter © 2005 Elsevier Inc. All rights reserved.
doi:10.1016/j.suc.2005.10.015   *surgical.theclinics.com*

irrespective of location, are significant, with as many as 30% of patients developing either postthrombotic syndrome or recurrent DVT [7,8].

The rationale for VTE prophylaxis is based on multiple principles. First, the incidence of VTE among hospitalized patients is high, and in some cases a fatal PE might be its first and only manifestation. Screening strategies for VTE have significant limitations and are not thought to be effective. Most importantly, prophylaxis has been proven to be highly effective in preventing VTE and in reducing the costs associated with its diagnosis and management. Despite its benefits, VTE prophylaxis remains underused. Multiple studies have shown that appropriate prophylaxis is used in only one third of patients who have clear identifiable risk factors and that in many patients who develop PE, prophylaxis was never given. This underuse is probably driven by an incorrect perception of a low risk of VTE, a high risk of perioperative bleeding, and no apparent benefit when individual practitioners examine their own practice experience [9–11].

This article describes an approach to identify surgical patients at high risk for VTE and reviews options for VTE prophylaxis. Data are derived from evidence-based guidelines for thromboprophylaxis in specific clinical settings.

Risk factors for venous thromboembolism

The pathophysiology of venous thrombosis was first described by Rudolph Virchow in 1884, who identified three main etiologic factors: venous stasis, endothelial damage, and hypercoagulability. During the next century a large number of clinical risk factors were identified, all of which fit into one of these three categories. Knowledge of the risk factors for VTE can help identify high-risk patients and guide prophylactic measures. Box 1 lists the most common risk factors associated with VTE. Although not all are considered to have the same predictive value, it is well accepted that the interaction between multiple coexistent risk factors leads to a higher risk of venous thrombosis [12–14].

In the general surgical practice, major surgery (defined as abdominal or thoracic operations lasting longer than 30 minutes and requiring general anesthesia) is considered to be a significant risk factor for VTE. Studies from the 1970s and 1980s, in which screening fibrinogen uptake studies were used to diagnose DVT, showed an incidence of DVT of 15% to 30% in surgical patients in the absence of thromboprophylaxis. The incidence of fatal PE in the same cohort of patients was between 0.2% and 0.9%. It is difficult to estimate the current risk of DVT/PE in surgical patients not receiving prophylaxis. It is likely that that the risk is considerably higher now than previously reported, given that surgical patients are older and have greater degrees of comorbidity than in the past [12,15,16].

The actual risk of DVT/PE is difficult to determine for any specific patient. It is well recognized, however, that risk factors seem to have

---

Box 1. Major general risk factors for venous thromboembolism

Surgery
Trauma
Immobility, paresis
Malignancy
Cancer therapy (hormonal, chemotherapy, or radiotherapy)
Previous VTE
Increasing age
Pregnancy and postpartum period
Estrogen-containing contraceptives or hormonal replacement
    therapy
Selective estrogen receptor modulators
Acute medical illness
Heart or respiratory failure
Inflammatory bowel disease
Nephrotic syndrome
Myeloproliferative disease
Paroxysmal nocturnal hemoglobinuria
Obesity
Smoking
Varicose veins
Central venous catheterization
Inherited or acquired hypercoagulability

---

a cumulative effect on the risk of VTE. Although all these factors are associated with a higher risk of VTE, they do not provide a structure for stratifying individual patients. Taking an alternative approach, Geerts [14] used a prospective cohort design to stratify surgical patients according to the risk of DVT/PE based on age, presence of major risk factors, and clinical setting (related to specific surgical characteristics). This relatively simple classification scheme has the additional advantage of tying thromboprophylaxis recommendations to risk strata. It is simple and easy to apply to patients in everyday practice (Table 1).

General aspects of venous thromboembolism prophylaxis

Many studies have been performed to define the optimal method of thromboprophylaxis in surgical patients. Endpoints or outcomes measured vary across studies; however, the current recommendations are directed toward minimizing the risk of symptomatic DVT/PE, asymptomatic proximal DVT, and fatal PE [14,17]. Several diagnostic modalities have been used to identify DVT in these clinical studies including venography, fibrinogen uptake

Table 1
Stratification of surgical patients according to VTE risk without thromboprophylaxis

Category	Definition	Calf DVT (%)	Proximal DVT (%)	Clinical PE (%)	Fatal PE (%)
Low risk	Age < 40 years, no risk factor, minor surgery	2	0.4	0.2	< 0.01
Moderate risk	Presence of only 1 of the following: Age 40–60 years Major surgery[a] Risk factor present	10–20	2–4	1–2	0.1–0.4
High risk	Age > 60 years Age > 40 years + major surgery + risk factor present	20–40	4–8	2–4	0.4–1.0
Highest risk	Age > 40 years + major surgery and: Previous VTE or Cancer or Hypercoagulable condition Major trauma Spinal cord injury Hip/knee arthroplasty Hip surgery	40–80	10–20	4–10	0.2–5

Abbreviations: DVT, deep vein thrombosis; PE, pulmonary embolism; VTE, venous thrombolism.

[a] Major surgery involves a thoracic or abdominal procedure associated with general anesthesia lasting longer than 30 minutes.

Data from Geerts WH, Pineo GF, Heit JA, et al. Prevention of venous thromboembolism: the seventh ACCP Conference on Antithrombotic and Thrombolytic Therapy. Chest 2004;126(3 Suppl):341S.

tests, and Doppler ultrasonography. Although Doppler ultrasonography has been shown to have limitations in identifying DVT in asymptomatic patients, it is currently the standard diagnostic tool because of its availability, reproducibility, and noninvasive nature. Most of the more recent studies comparing VTE prophylaxis regimens are based on findings identified using this modality.

Mechanisms of prophylaxis

VTE prophylaxis can be accomplished using either mechanical or pharmacologic approaches. Mechanical options include graduated compression stockings, intermittent pneumatic compression, and venous foot pumps. Pharmacologic options include antiplatelet agents (aspirin, dextran), low-dose unfractionated heparin (LDUH), low molecular weight heparin (LMWH), vitamin K antagonists (warfarin), and synthetic pentasaccharide factor Xa inhibitor (fondaparinux).

Mechanical methods prevent venous stagnation in the lower extremities. The main benefit of these methods is the absence of bleeding complications. In general, there are relatively few studies evaluating the role of these mechanical methods in general surgical patients. Graduated compression stockings and intermittent pneumatic compression have shown to decrease the risk of DVT, although neither of these methods has been shown to decrease the risk of PE or death [14,18]. From a practical standpoint, compliance with these devices is relatively low, suggesting that their effectiveness outside clinical trials is probably lower than reported [19–21]. Mechanical prophylaxis should be used when the risk of bleeding precludes the use of pharmacologic prophylaxis or in conjunction with such prophylaxis in the patients at highest risk [22].

Antiplatelet agents act by inhibiting the platelet–related steps in clot formation. Aspirin has been the most studied, although many of the clinical trials have significant methodologic limitations. It has no greater effectiveness than other methods of pharmacologic prophylaxis (LDUH or LMWH) and has a higher bleeding risk. As such, it is not recommended for routine perioperative prophylaxis [16].

Vitamin K antagonists as well as synthetic pentasaccharides have not been well studied in general surgical patients. They have, however, been recommended for prophylaxis of VTE in patients undergoing high-risk orthopedic procedures, in which several randomized, controlled trials have demonstrated their safety and effectiveness [16].

LDUH and LMWH are antithrombotic agents extensively used for VTE prophylaxis in patients undergoing major general surgical procedures. Both have been well studied in different surgical settings and are the mainstay of thromboprophylaxis in this patient population. With both, there is fairly strong evidence of their effectiveness as prophylactic agents and considerable data on the risk of bleeding complications. LMWH has the additional advantage of a lower incidence of heparin-induced thrombocytopenia and once-daily dosing [14–17].

Low-dose unfractionated heparin/low molecular weight heparin and neuraxial anesthesia/analgesia

In 1997 the United States Food and Drug Administration released a public health advisory reporting 41 cases of patients who developed perispinal hematoma after receiving LMWH for VTE prophylaxis [23]. Since then additional cases have been reported with the use of both LMWH and LDUH, although the incidence seems to be lower with LDUH. Unfortunately the actual risk of this complication is not well documented, and although specific predictors are not well defined, in most cases additional risk factors are present (bleeding abnormalities, abnormal anatomy, traumatic tap, continuous epidural catheter, and use of other anticoagulant/antiplatelet medications). Based on the data available, the American Association of

Regional Anesthesia has developed recommendations to minimize the risk of this catastrophic complication in patients receiving anticoagulant prophylaxis with LDUH/LMWH [24]:

1. Avoid neuraxial anesthesia/analgesia in patients who have bleeding disorders.
2. Avoid neuraxial anesthesia/analgesia in patients who have drug-related preoperative impairment of hemostasis.
3. Delay catheter insertion/spinal needle for 8 to 12 hours after a subcutaneous dose of heparin or a twice-daily dose of LMWH.
4. Delay catheter insertion/spinal needle for 18 hours after a once-a-day injection of LMWH.
5. Delay anticoagulant prophylaxis if a hemorrhagic aspirate ("bloody tap") is seen during initial insertion.
6. Remove epidural catheter when the anticoagulant effect is at a minimum (ie, just before next scheduled dose).
7. Delay anticoagulant prophylaxis at least 2 hours after catheter is removed.

In general, the use of spinal/epidural anesthesia/analgesia does not preclude the use of adequate thromboprophylaxis as long as appropriate caution is taken. It is recommended that every hospital that uses neuraxial anesthesia/analgesia develop specific protocols to delineate specific details of its management when combined with pharmacologic thromboprophylaxis and that protocols for close and careful monitoring be put in place to help with the early identification and treatment of complications related to perispinal hematoma [14,24].

Risk and preventive measures in specific clinical settings

Through an extensive review of the literature and expert consensus, the American College of Chest Physicians has provided evidence-based guidelines pertaining to the prevention of VTE in a variety of clinical settings [14]. Much of the data given here is a concise description of the rationale and final recommendations. Additionally, this article highlights specific situations in which the deviation from these recommendations seems to be appropriate. Standardized recommendations for thromboprophylaxis in general surgical patients stratified by their risk of VTE are summarized in Table 2.

General surgery

Many randomized, controlled trials have been performed to evaluate the role of LDUH in VTE prophylaxis in surgical patients. A meta-analysis of 46 randomized, controlled trials in which LDUH was compared with either no prophylaxis or placebo provides clear evidence of the efficacy of LDUH.

Table 2
Guidelines for prophylaxis of venous thromboembolism in surgical patients according to risk category

Category	Definition	Prevention Strategy
Low risk	Age < 40 years, no RF, minor surgery	Aggressive and early mobilization
Moderate risk	Presence of only one of the following: Age 40–60 years Major surgery RF present	LDUH every 12 h or LMWH or GCS/IPC (if bleeding risk)
High risk	Age > 60 years Age > 40 + major surgery + RF present	LDUH every 8 h or LMWH or IPC (if bleeding risk)
Highest risk	Age > 40 years + major surgery and: Previous VTE or Cancer or Hypercoagulable condition Major trauma Spinal cord injury Hip/knee arthroplasty Hip surgery	LMWH (trauma, spinal cord injury) LDUH every 8 h + GCS/IPC or LMWH + GCS/IPC Consider extended prophylaxis for cancer or spinal cord injury

Abbreviations: GCS, graduated compression stockings; IPC, intermittent pneumatic compression; LDUH, low-dose unfractionated heparin; LMWH, low molecular weight heparin; VTE, venous thromboembolism.

Data from Geerts WH, Pineo GF, Heit JA, et al. Prevention of venous thromboembolism: the seventh ACCP Conference on Antithrombotic and Thrombolytic Therapy. Chest 2004; 126(3 Suppl):341S.

The use of LDUH decreased the rate of DVT from 22% to 9%, the rate of symptomatic PE from 2% to 1.3, the rate of fatal PE from 0.8% to 0.3%, and all-cause mortality from 4.2% to 3.2%. In this analysis, the rate of perioperative bleeding increased from 3.8% to 5.9% with the use of LDUH [25]. Another meta-analysis corroborated these findings and demonstrated an increase in the risk of wound hematomas (4.1% versus 6.3%) in patients receiving LDUH. There was, however, no increased risk of major bleeding [26]. In general, for the majority of these studies, LDUH was administered 1 to 2 hours preoperatively followed by 5000 units subcutaneously two or three times per day. It is thought that thrice-daily dosing is associated with a better prophylactic effect without an increased risk of bleeding, although these two regimens have never been directly compared.

Many randomized, controlled trials and meta-analyses have been done comparing LDUH and LMWH for VTE prophylaxis. Pooled results show that LMWH is as effective as LDUH in reducing symptomatic VTE (> 60%–70% reduction rate) [27–29]. Some reports have shown a further decrease in asymptomatic VTE with LMWH as compared with LDUH, although the clinical implications of these results are not clear [30–32]. Much of the variability in effectiveness across trials can be explained by differences in patients and in the VTE prophylaxis regimen. Specifically, there is considerable variability in the precise LMWH agent selected and in the dosing regimen used. In general, rates of perioperative bleeding seem to be similar whether LDUH or LMWH is used. LMWH in excess of 3400 U/d might be associated with higher rates of bleeding, however [28,33]. The effect on overall mortality from prophylaxis with LDUH/LMWH is well documented [34–36]. In randomized, controlled trials, LMWH offers no additional advantage over LDUH in terms of overall mortality or fatal PE [37], although studies evaluating selected high-risk surgical patients have shown a benefit of LMWH over LDUH, as discussed later.

Most published data on VTE prophylaxis are derived from studies comparing LDUH and LMWH. There are limited data on other methods of pharmacologic prophylaxis. In one large, randomized, controlled trial, fondaparinux (a factor Xa inhibitor) was equivalent to LMWH in reducing the risk of VTE [38].

Graduated compression stockings have some documented efficacy, reducing the risk of DVT by approximately 52%, but there are few data documenting a reduction in the risk of either proximal DVT or symptomatic PE. Graduated compression stockings might provide added benefit when combined with LDUH in high-risk patients, with a 75% reduction in the risk of DVT when compared with LDUH alone. Similar results have been documented with the use of intermittent pneumatic compression. Both graduated compression stockings and intermittent pneumatic compression might offer some benefit in high-risk patients when used as adjunct to pharmacologic prophylaxis or in patients at very high risk of perioperative bleeding [22,39].

Extended prophylaxis beyond discharge has been evaluated in selected groups of patients undergoing major general surgery. The rationale for this approach is based on observational studies in which new DVT were detected in up to 25% of patients within 4 weeks of discharge [40]. Extended prophylaxis seems to have a role in patients undergoing major oncologic surgery, as discussed later [41,42].

Laparoscopy

The increasing use of laparoscopic procedures has raised new questions about the value of VTE prophylaxis in this setting. It is thought that both the pneumoperitoneum and the prolonged reverse Trendelenburg positioning are associated with an increased risk of DVT. Many studies of varying methodologic quality have been published with somewhat inconsistent results.

In general, the rates of VTE seem to be lower in patients undergoing laparoscopic procedures. The rate of DVT was only 0.3% in a series of 2384 patients undergoing laparoscopic gastrointestinal surgery who had received a short course of LMWH postoperatively [43]. Another study of more than 153,000 patients undergoing laparoscopic cholecystectomy in which a variety of prophylactic measures were used demonstrated rates of DVT, PE, and fatal PE of 0.03%, 0.06%, and 0.02%, respectively [44]. A recent population based analysis of more than 100,000 patients undergoing laparoscopic cholecystectomy revealed a postoperative (3-month) risk of VTE of 0.2% compared with 0.5% for open cholecystectomy [45]. Two recent, randomized, controlled trials evaluating the role of thromboprophylaxis in patients undergoing laparoscopic procedures showed no difference in VTE rate between placebo and LMWH or between graduated compression stockings and graduated compression stockings plus LMWH [46,47].

Despite a seemingly lower incidence of VTE in patients undergoing uncomplicated laparoscopic procedures, the Society of American Gastrointestinal Endoscopic Surgeons has recommended the use of thromboprophylaxis for laparoscopic procedures following the same guidelines as for equivalent open operations [48]. The European Association for Endoscopic Surgery has also recommended the routine use of intermittent pneumatic compression for all prolonged laparoscopic operations [49]. Clearly, additional data are required to provide directed recommendations for VTE prophylaxis in patients undergoing laparoscopic procedures.

Malignancy

Patients who have malignancy have a sixfold increased risk of VTE, and it is estimated that the incidence of VTE in the cancer population is 1 in 200 patients [50,51]. The actual risk seems to be related to the type of malignancy. Patients who have brain tumors and adenocarcinoma of the ovaries, pancreas, stomach, colon, lung, prostate, and kidney have a higher risk of VTE than those who have other malignancies. In patients undergoing major oncologic surgery, the risk of DVT is at least twice that of patients who do not have cancer, and the risk of fatal PE at least three times greater [45,52]. It is estimated that the incidence of VTE in general surgery patients undergoing cancer surgery is close to 30%. Some of the mechanisms involved with increased risk of VTE in this population include hypercoagulability, cancer as a surrogate for other risk factors (eg, age and comorbidities), hemostatic and hemodynamic abnormalities, and other cancer therapies (hormones, chemotherapy) [16,53].

A lack of response to certain prophylactic regimens has been reported in patients who have malignancy [14]. As a result, the choice of regimen is critically important in these patients. LDUH has proven effective in preventing VTE (DVT and fatal PE) in patients undergoing major oncologic surgery [26,34], and prophylaxis with LMWH is at least as effective as LDUH [33,54,55]. The dose of prophylaxis is particularly important. In a study of patients who had gynecologic cancer undergoing surgery, LDUH given three times per day was more efficacious than a dose given two times per day [56]; hence it is recommended that LDUH be administered three times per day. Similarly a study evaluating the effect of LMWH (dalteparin) at doses of 5000 U versus 2500 U proved that the former was more efficacious

[57]. LMWH is recommended in a dose exceeding 3400 U per day in surgical patients who have cancer.

Extended prophylaxis in patients who have cancer also decreases the incidence of VTE in the postoperative period. An autopsy study showed that in patients undergoing surgery for cancer, death caused by PE occurred in 54.5% of patients. In more than 40% of the cases, the PE occurred after the second postoperative week, highlighting the late occurrence of VTE in many patients who have cancer. Two randomized, controlled trials have shown a reduction in the risk of DVT of approximately 60% in patients receiving LMWH for 3 or 4 additional weeks [41,42]. The ENOXACAN II study compared two groups of patients undergoing abdominal/pelvic surgery for malignancy. One group received 1 week of thromboprophylaxis with LMWH (enoxaparin) followed by 3 weeks of placebo, and the second group received 4 weeks of LMWH (enoxaparin). The rate of VTE was 13.8% in the placebo group versus 5.5% in the enoxaparin group ($P = .01$) at 3-month follow up. No increased complications were seen in this group of patients [42]. Although cost-effectiveness analyses have not yet been performed, extended prophylaxis in surgical patients who have cancer should be considered as a component of the strategy to prevent VTE. LMWH should be the drug of choice, given the available data and the ease of administration (once per day).

Colorectal surgery

A few studies have recently focused on VTE in patients undergoing colorectal surgery. These patients are thought to have a higher risk of VTE, given the pelvic dissection and intraoperative positioning, with a risk of DVT as high as 40%. In general, results of studies of prophylaxis have yielded the same results as for general surgery patients, with LMWH and LDUH having equivalent efficacy in reducing VTE and a similar complication rate. Prophylactic strategies in these patients should follow standard guidelines for general surgery patients. Given the perceived higher risk of VTE in this group of patients, combination of LDUH/LMWH with mechanical measures is reasonable [55,58,59].

Trauma

Patients who have sustained major trauma have a high risk of developing VTE. VTE is the third leading cause of death in those who survive the first day of admission [60,61]. A prospective study evaluated the risk of DVT (using venography) in 443 polytrauma patients not receiving thromboprophylaxis. The incidence of DVT was 58%, with one third of these cases occurring above the calf (proximal DVT) [61]. Another study evaluated the risk of DVT in trauma patients receiving a standard prophylactic regimen and demonstrated an incidence of DVT and proximal DVT of 27% and

7%, respectively (assessed by Doppler ultrasonography) [62]. Independent predictors of VTE in trauma patients have been identified and include spinal cord injury, lower extremity or pelvic fractures, surgery, advanced age, femoral venous line, prolonged immobility, and prolonged length of stay [14].

The use of LDUH has been studied extensively in trauma patients. A recent meta-analysis showed LDUH had no benefit in preventing VTE in high-risk patients as compared with placebo [63]. A large, randomized, controlled trial comparing LDUH and LMWH in major trauma patients who did not have overt bleeding or intracranial injuries showed that LMWH use was associated with a lower risk of DVT and proximal DVT. Bleeding complications were similar with the two treatments and affected less than 2% of patients [64]. Subsequent cost-effectiveness analyses confirm the benefit of LMWH and argue for this approach as the standard of care in injured patients [65,66]. Patients at increased risk of bleeding who have contraindications to pharmacologic prophylaxis should receive some form of mechanical prophylaxis, preferably intermittent pneumatic compression. If appropriate pharmacologic prophylaxis is not possible, duplex ultrasonographic screening should be performed. Routine prophylactic inferior vena caval filters are not recommended and should be placed only when there is some objective evidence of a DVT. In general, mechanical prophylaxis is inadequate as the sole means of prophylaxis in this patient population [14].

Spinal cord injury

Patients who have spinal cord injury have the highest risk of developing VTE. The incidence of proximal DVT and PE are 15% and 5%, respectively [16]. As in trauma patients, LMWH has proven to be a more effective preventive measure than LDUH or mechanical strategies. Patients who have spinal cord injury should receive LMWH as soon as bleeding is controlled; if treatment with LMWH is not possible, mechanical measures should be instituted. If mechanical measures are not possible, screening with duplex ultrasonography to identify patients who have DVT should be pursued, with placement of an inferior vena caval filter once objective data confirm the presence of a DVT. Given their continued risk for VTE, these patients should receive extended prophylaxis with LMWH or warfarin [13–16].

Burns

Burn patients have multiple associated conditions that put them at risk for VTE. These risk factors include hypercoagulability, immobility, concomitant trauma, and femoral venous lines. Retrospective series have reported an incidence of DVT in ranging from 6% to 27% in burn patients. Although no specific trials on thromboprophylaxis have been published, it seems reasonable to administer standard pharmacologic prophylaxis (LDUH/LMWH) in burn patients who have associated risk factors [14].

Summary

Surgical patients have a high risk of developing VTE, but prophylaxis is not used appropriately in more than half of all patients undergoing major operative procedures. Identification of risk factors for VTE and their potential interactions allows accurate stratification and helps match patients to the appropriate prophylaxis strategy. Certain conditions such as cancer, trauma, and spinal cord injury are associated with the highest risk of VTE, and PE constitutes a significant cause of death in these patients. Familiarity with and implementation of the recommended preventive strategies decreases morbidity, mortality, and costs. Clear benefit from VTE prophylaxis has been well established in a variety of clinical settings, and its practice should be the standard of care in the practice of surgery.

References

[1] Silverstein MD, Heit JA, Mohr DN, et al. Trends in the incidence of deep vein thrombosis and pulmonary embolism: a 25-year population-based study. Arch Intern Med 1998;158(6): 585–93.

[2] Sandler DA, Martin JF. Autopsy proven pulmonary embolism in hospital patients: are we detecting enough deep vein thrombosis? J R Soc Med 1989;82(4):203–5.

[3] Lindblad B, Eriksson A, Bergqvist D. Autopsy-verified pulmonary embolism in a surgical department: analysis of the period from 1951 to 1988. Br J Surg 1991;78(7):849–52.

[4] Stein PD, Henry JW. Prevalence of acute pulmonary embolism among patients in a general hospital and at autopsy. Chest 1995;108(4):978–81.

[5] Anderson FA Jr, Wheeler HB, Goldberg RJ, et al. A population-based perspective of the hospital incidence and case-fatality rates of deep vein thrombosis and pulmonary embolism. The Worcester DVT Study. Arch Intern Med 1991;151(5):933–8.

[6] Shojania KGDB, McDonald KM. Making health care safer: a critical analysis of patient safety practices. Evidence Report/Technology Assessment No. 43 (prepared by the University of California at San Francisco-Stanford Evidence-based Practice Center under Contract No. 290–97–0013). University of California at San Francisco-Stanford Evidence-based Practice Center; 2001. p. 332–46.

[7] Bick RL. Current status of thrombosis: a multidisciplinary medical issue and major American health problem-beyond the year 2000. Clin Appl Thromb Hemost 1997;3(Suppl 1):1.

[8] Prandoni P, Lensing AW, Cogo A, et al. The long-term clinical course of acute deep venous thrombosis. Ann Intern Med 1996;125(1):1–7.

[9] Bratzler DW, Raskob GE, Murray CK, et al. Underuse of venous thromboembolism prophylaxis for general surgery patients: physician practices in the community hospital setting. Arch Intern Med 1998;158(17):1909–12.

[10] Arnold DM, Kahn SR, Shrier I. Missed opportunities for prevention of venous thromboembolism: an evaluation of the use of thromboprophylaxis guidelines. Chest 2001;120(6):1964–71.

[11] Gillies TE, Ruckley CV, Nixon SJ. Still missing the boat with fatal pulmonary embolism. Br J Surg 1996;83(10):1394–5.

[12] Anderson FA Jr, Spencer FA. Risk factors for venous thromboembolism. Circulation 2003; 107(23, Suppl 1):I9–16.

[13] Geerts WH, Heit JA, Clagett GP, et al. Prevention of venous thromboembolism. Chest 2001; 119(1 Suppl):132S–75S.

[14] Geerts WH, Pineo GF, Heit JA, et al. Prevention of venous thromboembolism: the seventh ACCP Conference on Antithrombotic and Thrombolytic Therapy. Chest 2004;126(3 Suppl): 338S–400S.

[15] Agnelli G. Prevention of venous thromboembolism in surgical patients. Circulation 2004; 110(24, Suppl 1):IV4–12.

[16] O'Donnell M, Weitz JI. Thromboprophylaxis in surgical patients. Can J Surg 2003;46(2): 129–35.

[17] Bick RL, Haas S. Thromboprophylaxis and thrombosis in medical, surgical, trauma, and obstetric/gynecologic patients. Hematol Oncol Clin North Am 2003;17(1):217–58.

[18] Agu O, Hamilton G, Baker D. Graduated compression stockings in the prevention of venous thromboembolism. Br J Surg 1999;86(8):992–1004.

[19] Comerota AJ, Katz ML, White JV. Why does prophylaxis with external pneumatic compression for deep vein thrombosis fail? Am J Surg 1992;164(3):265–8.

[20] Cornwell EE III, Chang D, Velmahos G, et al. Compliance with sequential compression device prophylaxis in at-risk trauma patients: a prospective analysis. Am Surg 2002;68(5): 470–3.

[21] Haddad FS, Kerry RM, McEwen JA, et al. Unanticipated variations between expected and delivered pneumatic compression therapy after elective hip surgery: a possible source of variation in reported patient outcomes. J Arthroplasty 2001;16(1):37–46.

[22] Amaragiri SV, Lees TA. Elastic compression stockings for prevention of deep vein thrombosis. Cochrane Database Syst Rev 2000;3:CD001484.

[23] Lumpkin MM. FDA public health advisory. Anesthesiology 1998;88(2):27A–8A.

[24] Horlocker TT, Wedel DJ, Benzon H, et al. Regional anesthesia in the anticoagulated patient: defining the risks (the second ASRA Consensus Conference on Neuraxial Anesthesia and Anticoagulation). Reg Anesth Pain Med 2003;28(3):172–97.

[25] Collins R, Scrimgeour A, Yusuf S, et al. Reduction in fatal pulmonary embolism and venous thrombosis by perioperative administration of subcutaneous heparin. Overview of results of randomized trials in general, orthopedic, and urologic surgery. N Engl J Med 1988;318(18): 1162–73.

[26] Clagett GP, Reisch JS. Prevention of venous thromboembolism in general surgical patients. Results of meta-analysis. Ann Surg 1988;208(2):227–40.

[27] Palmer AJ, Schramm W, Kirchhof B, et al. Low molecular weight heparin and unfractionated heparin for prevention of thrombo-embolism in general surgery: a meta-analysis of randomised clinical trials. Haemostasis 1997;27(2):65–74.

[28] Koch A, Bouges S, Ziegler S, et al. Low molecular weight heparin and unfractionated heparin in thrombosis prophylaxis after major surgical intervention: update of previous meta-analyses. Br J Surg 1997;84(6):750–9.

[29] Koch A, Ziegler S, Breitschwerdt H, et al. Low molecular weight heparin and unfractionated heparin in thrombosis prophylaxis: meta-analysis based on original patient data. Thromb Res 2001;102(4):295–309.

[30] Kakkar VV, Murray WJ. Efficacy and safety of low-molecular-weight heparin (CY216) in preventing postoperative venous thrombo-embolism: a co-operative study. Br J Surg 1985;72(10):786–91.

[31] Bergqvist D, Matzsch T, Burmark US, et al. Low molecular weight heparin given the evening before surgery compared with conventional low-dose heparin in prevention of thrombosis. Br J Surg 1988;75(9):888–91.

[32] The European Fraxiparin Study (EFS) Group. Comparison of a low molecular weight heparin and unfractionated heparin for the prevention of deep vein thrombosis in patients undergoing abdominal surgery. Br J Surg 1988;75(11):1058–63.

[33] Mismetti P, Laporte S, Darmon JY, et al. Meta-analysis of low molecular weight heparin in the prevention of venous thromboembolism in general surgery. Br J Surg 2001;88(7):913–30.

[34] Kakkar VV, Corrigan TP, Fossard DP, et al. Prevention of fatal postoperative pulmonary embolism by low doses of heparin. Reappraisal of results of an international multicentre trial. Lancet 1977;1(8011):567–9.

[35] Sagar S, Massey J, Sanderson JM. Low-dose heparin prophylaxis against fatal pulmonary embolism. BMJ 1975;4(5991):257–9.

[36] Pezzuoli G, Neri Serneri GG, Settembrini P, et al. Prophylaxis of fatal pulmonary embolism in general surgery using low-molecular weight heparin Cy 216: a multicentre, double-blind, randomized, controlled, clinical trial versus placebo (STEP). STEP-Study Group. Int Surg 1989;74(4):205–10.

[37] Wolf H, Encke A, Haas S, et al. Comparison of the efficacy and safety of Sandoz low molecular weight heparin and unfractionated heparin: interim analysis of a multicenter trial. Semin Thromb Hemost 1991;17(4):343–6.

[38] Agnelli G, Bergqvist D, Cohen AT, et al. Randomized clinical trial of postoperative fondaparinux versus perioperative dalteparin for prevention of venous thromboembolism in high-risk abdominal surgery. Br J Surg 2005;92(10):1212–20.

[39] Ramos R, Salem BI, De Pawlikowski MP, et al. The efficacy of pneumatic compression stockings in the prevention of pulmonary embolism after cardiac surgery. Chest 1996; 109(1):82–5.

[40] Scurr JH, Coleridge-Smith PD, Hasty JH. Deep venous thrombosis: a continuing problem. BMJ 1988;297(6640):28.

[41] Rasmussen MS. Preventing thromboembolic complications in cancer patients after surgery: a role for prolonged thromboprophylaxis. Cancer Treat Rev 2002;28(3):141–4.

[42] Bergqvist D, Agnelli G, Cohen AT, et al. Duration of prophylaxis against venous thromboembolism with enoxaparin after surgery for cancer. N Engl J Med 2002;346(13):975–80.

[43] Catheline JM, Turner R, Gaillard JL, et al. Thromboembolism in laparoscopic surgery: risk factors and preventive measures. Surg Laparosc Endosc Percutan Tech 1999;9(2): 135–9.

[44] Lindberg F, Bergqvist D, Rasmussen I. Incidence of thromboembolic complications after laparoscopic cholecystectomy: review of the literature. Surg Laparosc Endosc 1997;7(4): 324–31.

[45] White RH, Zhou H, Romano PS. Incidence of symptomatic venous thromboembolism after different elective or urgent surgical procedures. Thromb Haemost 2003;90(3):446–55.

[46] Bounameaux H, Didier D, Polat O, et al. Antithrombotic prophylaxis in patients undergoing laparoscopic cholecystectomy. Thromb Res 1997;86(3):271–3.

[47] Baca I, Schneider B, Kohler T, et al. [Prevention of thromboembolism in minimal invasive interventions and brief inpatient treatment. Results of a multicenter, prospective, randomized, controlled study with a low molecular weight heparin.] Chirurg 1997;68(12):1275–80.

[48] Society of American Gastrointestinal Endoscopic Surgeons. Global statement on deep venous thrombosis prophylaxis during laparoscopic surgery. SAGES position statement. Surg Endosc 1999;13(2):200.

[49] Zacharoulis D, Kakkar AK. Venous thromboembolism in laparoscopic surgery. Curr Opin Pulm Med 2003;9(5):356–61.

[50] Heit JA, Silverstein MD, Mohr DN, et al. Risk factors for deep vein thrombosis and pulmonary embolism: a population-based case-control study. Arch Intern Med 2000;160(6): 809–15.

[51] Lee AY. Epidemiology and management of venous thromboembolism in patients with cancer. Thromb Res 2003;110(4):167–72.

[52] Kakkar AK, Williamson RC. Prevention of venous thromboembolism in cancer patients. Semin Thromb Hemost 1999;25(2):239–43.

[53] Khushal A, Quinlan D, Alikhan R, et al. Thromboembolic disease in surgery for malignancy-rationale for prolonged thromboprophylaxis. Semin Thromb Hemost 2002;28(6):569–76.

[54] ENOXACAN Study Group. Efficacy and safety of enoxaparin versus unfractionated heparin for prevention of deep vein thrombosis in elective cancer surgery: a double-blind randomized multicentre trial with venographic assessment. Br J Surg 1997;84(8):1099–103.

[55] McLeod RS, Geerts WH, Sniderman KW, et al. Subcutaneous heparin versus low-molecular-weight heparin as thromboprophylaxis in patients undergoing colorectal surgery: results of the Canadian colorectal DVT prophylaxis trial: a randomized, double-blind trial. Ann Surg 2001;233(3):438–44.

[56] Clarke-Pearson DL. Prevention of venous thromboembolism in gynecologic surgery patients. Curr Opin Obstet Gynecol 1993;5(1):73–9.

[57] Bergqvist D, Burmark US, Flordal PA, et al. Low molecular weight heparin started before surgery as prophylaxis against deep vein thrombosis: 2500 versus 5000 XaI units in 2070 patients. Br J Surg 1995;82(4):496–501.

[58] Borly L, Wille-Jorgensen P, Rasmussen MS. Systematic review of thromboprophylaxis in colorectal surgery–an update. Colorectal Dis 2005;7(2):122–7.

[59] Wille-Jorgensen P, Rasmussen MS, Andersen BR, et al. Heparins and mechanical methods for thromboprophylaxis in colorectal surgery. Cochrane Database Syst Rev 2003;4: CD001217.

[60] O'Malley KF, Ross SE. Pulmonary embolism in major trauma patients. J Trauma 1990; 30(6):748–50.

[61] Geerts WH, Code KI, Jay RM, et al. A prospective study of venous thromboembolism after major trauma. N Engl J Med 1994;331(24):1601–6.

[62] Meissner MH, Chandler WL, Elliott JS. Venous thromboembolism in trauma: a local manifestation of systemic hypercoagulability? J Trauma 2003;54(2):224–31.

[63] Velmahos GC, Kern J, Chan LS, et al. Prevention of venous thromboembolism after injury: an evidence-based report–part I: analysis of risk factors and evaluation of the role of vena caval filters. J Trauma 2000;49(1):132–8 [discussion: 139].

[64] Geerts WH, Jay RM, Code KI, et al. A comparison of low-dose heparin with low-molecular-weight heparin as prophylaxis against venous thromboembolism after major trauma. N Engl J Med 1996;335(10):701–7.

[65] Devlin JW, Petitta A, Shepard AD, et al. Cost-effectiveness of enoxaparin versus low-dose heparin for prophylaxis against venous thrombosis after major trauma. Pharmacotherapy 1998;18(6):1335–42.

[66] Selby R, Geerts WH. Venous thromboembolism prophylaxis after trauma: dollars and sense. Crit Care Med 2001;29(9):1839–40.

SURGICAL
CLINICS OF
NORTH AMERICA

ELSEVIER
SAUNDERS

Surg Clin N Am 85 (2005) 1179–1189

Thrombosis and Coagulation: Operative Management of the Anticoagulated Patient

Christopher D. Owens, MD*, Mike Belkin, MD

Department of Surgery, Division of Vascular Surgery, Brigham and Women's Hospital, Harvard Medical School, 75 Francis Street, Boston, MA 02115, USA

The literature provides no consensus for the best perioperative management of patients receiving long-term anticoagulant therapy. This lack of agreement is largely because of the many different indications for anticoagulation, the variety of invasive procedures planned, the specific patient and physician preferences, and the wide range of potential costs. Surgeons must weigh the risk of thromboembolism if anticoagulation is discontinued against the risk of bleeding from the procedure if anticoagulation is continued. Another consideration is the original indication for anticoagulation. Finally, efficacy and safety data on different management strategies are lacking. Nevertheless, we as surgeons are frequently faced with issues regarding anticoagulation management before our procedures. For instance, estimates say 2.3 million patients in the United States have atrial fibrillation; 40% of these are receiving oral anticoagulation. As our population ages, we can expect that number to increase. Ultimately, surgeons must use available literature, clinical experience, and practice standards to make judgments. Underlying those judgments should be a sound working knowledge of the fundamentals in coagulation and hemostasis, and an understanding of the mechanisms that cause anticoagulants to work.

Blood coagulation

The practicing surgeon must have a good working knowledge of the coagulation system. Although a detailed discussion of the coagulation process is beyond our scope, an overview is useful to emphasize points of intervention

---

* Corresponding author.
E-mail address: cmowens@partners.org (C.D. Owens).

0039-6109/05/$ - see front matter © 2005 Elsevier Inc. All rights reserved.
doi:10.1016/j.suc.2005.09.008   *surgical.theclinics.com*

with the currently used anticoagulants. Models we most often associate with the coagulation system resemble a cascade, or waterfall, of enzymes divided into extrinsic and intrinsic pathways working independently [1]. However, the three components of hemostasis—platelet activation, clotting cascade, and fibrinolysis—are closely related in vivo. The events initiating coagulation involve tissue factor and collagen. Endothelial disruption exposes the circulating factors to tissue factor (TF), which activates factor VII to form factor VIIa. At the same time, exposed collagen and von Willebrand factor (vWF) bind and activate platelets. The activated platelets change shape and externalize their rich anionic procoagulant phospholipid membranes. A platelet plug forms and this provides the critical membrane surface and receptors that allow the assembly of the clotting enzymes [2].

Tissue factor is the physiologic initiator of clotting in the vascular wound. The TF-VIIa complex activates factor X. Factor Xa, in the presence of the cofactor Va, forms the prothrombinase complex that activates prothrombin to form thrombin. In this key reaction, factor Xa is the protease, factor Va is the cofactor, and prothrombin is the substrate. This complex forms on the activated platelet surface. The enzyme complex bound to the cell surface markedly accelerates the generation of thrombin and ultimately fibrin, while protecting active enzymes from inhibition by their plasma protease inhibitors. The platelets also contain a large amount of plasminogen activator inhibitor 1 (PAI-1). PAI-1 is the physiologic inhibitor of tissue type plasminogen activator (tPA). This inhibitor contributes to the platelet-rich arterial thrombus resistance to lysis by tPA or urokinase.

Thrombin is the final common enzyme of the pathway and therefore a target of most clinically active anticoagulants [3]. Thrombin has many biologically important functions. It activates and aggregates platelets, breaks down fibrinogen to form a fibrin network, and performs downstream feedback amplification in the coagulation system. Thrombin activates factor XIII to form factor XIIIa, which catalyzes the cross linkage of fibrin to form a mature clot, and activates factors V and VIII [3].

While thrombin is central to the coagulation pathway, antithrombin is the key element in the natural anticoagulation pathway. Antithrombin is a glycoprotein, which binds thrombin and prevents the enzymatic breakdown of fibrinogen to fibrin. Antithrombin also prevents the activation of factors V and VIII and inhibits the activation and aggregation of platelets. Protein C inactivation of factors Va and VIIIa comprises the other natural anticoagulant pathway.

Agents that alter coagulation

Aspirin and clopidogrel

Aspirin irreversibly inhibits cyclooxygenase and therefore prevents formation of thromboxane A2 (TxA2), a platelet-aggregating substance.

Aspirin is rapidly absorbed from the proximal intestine and stomach. Aspirin is also absorbed from the rectum, but less reliably. Aspirin is rapidly converted to salicylate, which has peak circulating levels 2 hours after ingestion. The half-life of salicylate is 2 to 15 hours, depending on the dosage.

While aspirin use can increase the incidence of procedure-related hemorrhagic complications, it also reduces thrombotic complications following cardiac and vascular surgery and results in lower mortality [4–6]. Patients undergoing these procedures are usually higher risk patients and have a significant atherosclerotic burden. The Seventh American College of Chest Physicians (ACCP) Conference on Antithrombotic and Thrombolytic Therapy recommended that aspirin be given 6 hours after cardiac surgery [7]. Nevertheless, the use of aspirin should be stopped before procedures that are especially risky for hemorrhage or in procedures during which hemorrhage would have catastrophic consequences, such as neurosurgery. Once the decision has been made to withhold aspirin before a procedure, a period of 7 days should be allowed for new platelets to form. Because aspirin irreversibly inhibits cyclooxygenase, thromboxane synthesis recovers only when new platelets enter circulation.

Clopidogrel hydrogen sulfate is a thienopyridine antithrombotic agent that prevents platelet aggregation caused by adenosine diphosphate (ADP). ADP initiates platelet aggregation by simultaneous activation of two G-protein–coupled receptors, P2Y1 and P2Y12. P2Y12 couples to Gi to reduce adenylyl cyclase activity, which reduces downstream phosphorylation dependant on cyclic adenosine monophosphate (cAMP) [8]. Clopidogrel blocks the binding of fibrinogen to its receptor GPIIb/IIIa on the platelet surface.

Clopidogrel has a half-life of about 8 hours, but its effect can be seen as soon as 2 hours after a 300-mg loading dose. The safety profile of clopidogrel is similar to that of aspirin and, in a large randomized trial, clopidogrel showed no increase in gastrointestinal bleeding [9].

More of our patients come to us on this agent as its indications for use are increasing. The American College of Cardiology/American Heart Association (ACC/AHA) guidelines gave a class 1 recommendation to maintaining clopidogrel for 1 month after implantation of a bare metal stent, 3 months after implantation of a sirolumus-eluting stent, and 6 months after implantation of a paclitaxel-eluting stent in the coronary vasculature to prevent subacute stent thrombosis [10,11]. The trend is to continue clopidogrel for up to 1 year or longer if the risk/safety profile is favorable [11]. This is particularly true if the patient has other systemic manifestations of atherosclerosis, such as cerebrovascular or peripheral vascular disease. Additionally, physicians are increasingly administering clopidogrel after peripheral interventions, such as carotid stenting, although supportive data are currently lacking.

Patients taking clopidogrel should withhold from the drug for 5 to 6 days before the procedure. Following percutaneous coronary intervention, recommendations suggest that elective surgery be delayed until the patient has completed the course of clopidogrel. If this cannot be done, recommendations say to continue the drug with meticulous attention to hemostasis. No antidote exists for the effects of aspirin or clopidogrel because both produce irreversible platelet effects. Platelet transfusion should be considered in patients who take these agents and have hemorrhagic complications.

Warfarin

Warfarin, a coumarin derivative, produces its anticoagulant effect by interfering with the cyclic conversion of vitamin K and its 2,3 epoxide. Vitamin K is a necessary cofactor for the carboxylation of glutamate on the N-terminus of the enzyme coagulation factors II, VII, IX, and X [12]. These factors interact with the plasma membrane via their amino terminal domains that contain γ-carboxyglutamic acid residues. Because warfarin interferes with the formation of these residues, its use results in the loss of the factors' ability to interact with the phospholipid membrane. Warfarin also inhibits glutamate carboxylation on the amino terminus of the anticoagulant proteins C and S. Thrombomodulin, an endothelial cell receptor for thrombin, rapidly accelerates the activation of protein C. Activated protein C inhibits activated factors Va and VIIIa and stimulates fibrinolytic activity. Protein S is a cofactor for protein C and increases its ability to inactivate factors Va and VIIIa [13].

Warfarin is rapidly and completely absorbed, and peak plasma concentrations can be seen within 1 hour of ingestion. Its half-life is about 37 hours. Circulating warfarin is almost completely bound to albumin. It is metabolized in the liver into inactive compounds excreted in the stool and urine.

The measured anticoagulant effect of warfarin results predominantly from reduction in factor II (prothrombin) rather than a cumulative effect of lowering all four vitamin K–dependent factors. Prothrombin has a considerably longer half-life, 96 hours, than the other vitamin K–dependent factors, including protein C, which has a half-life of about 30 minutes. For this reason, recommendations call for heparin to be overlapped with warfarin until the international normalized ratio (INR) is in a therapeutic range [12].

Cutaneous necrosis is a rare but well described complication of warfarin therapy. It is characterized by wide areas of skin necrosis confined to the lower half of the body. Homozygous protein C deficiency is associated with massive venous thrombosis and usually death in infancy. Patients who are heterozygotes have only 50% of circulating levels of protein C. Administration of warfarin in these patients drops the circulating levels down to near homozygote deficiency states causing a hypercoagulable state to develop. If patients are not treated with heparin concomitantly, skin necrosis can develop from thrombosis of cutaneous nutrient vessels [14].

The American College of Chest Physicians has recommended an INR of 2.0 to 3.0 for most indications [15]. The exceptions are for some types of mechanical heart valves (see below) and patients with the antiphospholipid antibody syndrome. Cases involving these valves or these patients may require higher INRs.

After the use of warfarin is stopped, the INR in almost all patients reaches 1.5 in about four days [16]. There is theoretical concern and some biochemical evidence of rebound hypercoagulability owing to increased thrombin production or platelet activation if the use of warfarin is abruptly discontinued [17]. However, this rebound has not been proven clinically [18] and warfarin is routinely withdrawn before surgery without a taper.

Bleeding caused by warfarin can be corrected by transfusing fresh frozen plasma (FFP). FFP contains all of the coagulation proteins, including factors II, VII, IX, and X, and can be used to rapidly lower the INR. Recombinant activated factor VIIa can also lower INR quickly and effectively [19], but this should be reserved for uncontrollable hemorrhage. For supratherapeutic INRs that require correction, the Seventh American College of Chest Physicians Conference on Oral Anticoagulation recommends that Vitamin K1 (phytonadione) be given orally at a dose of 1 to 5 mg [20]. Vitamin K1 can be given at a dose of 10 mg by slow IV infusion if there is serious bleeding.

Heparin and low-molecular-weight heparin

Heparin is an indirect thrombin inhibitor that exerts its anticoagulation effect by binding to antithrombin (AT). Heparin binds to AT by unique pentasaccharide chains randomly distributed throughout the molecule [21]. While only about one third of circulating heparin binds to antithrombin, this fraction is enough to produce heparin's anticoagulant effect [22]. The heparin-antithrombin complex inactivates thrombin, as well as factors IIa, Xa, IXa, XIa, and XIIa. However, of all these, thrombin is the most sensitive to inactivation. The inactivation of thrombin requires a complex between heparin, antithrombin, and thrombin. This complex requires a saccharide chain of at least 18 residues. Because most low-molecular-weight heparin (LMWH) molecules do not have chains this long, LMWH has more anti-Xa activity than anti-IIa activity. One of the significant limitations of heparin is its inability to inactivate thrombin bound to fibrin or endothelial surfaces.

Heparin is used for the treatment of venous thrombosis or thromboembolism, and acute myocardial infarction, and for patients undergoing cardiopulmonary bypass, vascular surgery, and percutaneous coronary and peripheral vascular procedures. A weight-adjusted bolus of 70 U/kg can achieve therapeutic levels in most individuals. For those patients undergoing cardiac or vascular procedures, intraoperative measurement of the activated clotting time, ACT, is used to maintain an adequate circulating level to achieve anticoagulation. An ACT of 200 to 300 seconds is recommended for cross clamping during vascular surgery. During coronary bypass surgery where the blood is run through a heparin-bonded circuit, the ACT is kept at 300 seconds to prevent thrombosis.

Protamine, a cationic protein derived from fish sperm, can be used to neutralize the anticoagulant effect of heparin [22]. Dosing is usually based on a ratio of one milligram of protamine per 100 U of unfractionated heparin. Dosing consideration is given to the half-life of heparin, 1 hour. Therefore, 30 mg of protamine would be required to neutralize the anticoagulant effect of 3000 U of heparin. To avoid potential side effects such as hypotension or bradycardia, protamine should be given as a slow infusion over 3 minutes with a test dose.

Although laboratory monitoring of LMWH therapy is usually not necessary, monitoring for certain patient populations is advisable. Patients with morbid obesity or renal failure are two such populations. The College of American Pathologists recommends the anti-Xa assay [23]. This recommendation is based on the recognition that high circulating levels of anti-Xa levels have been associated with clinical bleeding [24].

The rationale for bridging periprocedural oral anticoagulation with either unfractionated IV heparin or LMWH is to reduce the time that the patient is without anticoagulation and therefore reduce the likelihood of thromboembolic complications. Traditionally, a patient is admitted to the hospital several days before the planned procedure, the use of warfarin is stopped and IV heparin is administered. The use of heparin is typically discontinued 3 or 4 hours (four half-lives) before the procedure, restarted 12 hours following the procedure, and continued until the INR climbs to a therapeutic range. Two advantages of unfractionated heparin are its relatively short half-life and its ability to be rapidly and completely reversed with protamine should a bleeding complication occur. The use of warfarin can be restarted on postoperative day 0 or 1, depending on the nature of the procedure. LMWH is an attractive alternative because it can be administered on an outpatient basis. However, its safety after major vascular or general surgery has not been established. In an attempt to answer these questions, Douetis and colleagues determined that in patients undergoing low-risk procedures and requiring temporary interruption of anticoagulation, LMWH could serve as a bridge until oral anticoagulation was established with a low risk of either arterial thromboembolism or postoperative hemorrhage [25]. These low-risk procedures include endoscopy, percutaneous catheter therapy, and minor surgery. However, the investigators recognized the need for additional studies in patients undergoing procedures at high risk for bleeding complications. We have noticed an increase of bleeding complications in our vascular practice following administration of LMWH after major vascular reconstruction. Until larger studies are done, therapeutic anticoagulation with LMWH cannot be advised in patients undergoing surgical procedures at high risk for bleeding.

Alternative anticoagulants must be considered for patients unable to receive heparin because of heparin resistance or heparin antibodies. The direct thrombin inhibitors (eg, hirudin, lepirudin, argatroban, ximelagatran, and bilvalirudin) each have merits in specific clinical scenarios [26]. They inhibit thrombin without the necessity of antithrombin as a cofactor. Direct thrombin inhibition can overcome some of the limitations of standard heparin therapy, such as diminished efficacy in the face of an antithrombin deficiency. Direct thrombin inhibitors do not bind to platelet factor 4 and therefore are not susceptible to heparin-induced thrombocytopenia (HIT). In fact, both lepirudin and argatroban have been approved for this purpose. Finally, unlike heparin, they have the ability to inhibit clot-bound thrombin.

Thrombosis risk in specific states

Atrial fibrillation

The risk of arterial thromboembolism in patients with nonvalvular atrial fibrillation who are not anticoagulated is about 4.5% per year [27]. Patients with strokes caused by atrial fibrillation (AF) are more likely to die from the stroke than patients with strokes not associated with AF. Also, strokes caused by AF tend to be more disabling, and patients who have had such strokes have less chance of being discharged to home than their counterparts who have had strokes not associated with AF [28,29]. Furthermore, strokes caused by AF are more likely to recur than strokes from other causes [29]. The risk of an arterial thromboembolic complication for any single patient, however, varies depending on the clinical scenario. For example, patients with previous cerebral embolism may have a recurrent risk as high as 12% [26]. Anticoagulation reduces this risk by an estimated 66% [27,30]. The recommended INR for most effective therapy for atrial fibrillation is 2.0 to 3.0 [15]. This is the same recommendation found in the American College of Chest Physicians Guidelines for the Prevention and Management of Postoperative Atrial Fibrillation After Cardiac Surgery [31].

In patients with AF, anticoagulation is usually interrupted 4 days before surgery and resumed as soon as possible following surgery. Most procedures can safely be performed with an INR of 1.5. Therefore, a patient will likely have a subtherapeutic INR for about 2 days before surgery and 2 days following surgery [18]. While evidence suggests that surgery increases the risk of venous thromboembolism [32], no evidence shows that it increases the risk of arterial thromboembolism. Evidence indicates that only for compelling reasons is it necessary to bridge a patient chronically anticoagulated for atrial fibrillation with either unfractionated heparin or LMWH. Such a compelling circumstance might be a recent arterial thromboembolic complication.

Mechanical heart valves

Prosthetic valve thrombosis has a reported incidence of 0.1% to 5.7% per patient-year [33,34]. Inadequate anticoagulation and a mechanical valve placed in the mitral position are the most common reasons for valve thrombosis and arterial thromboembolism. These events have devastating clinical consequences and are fatal in 15% of cases [25]. The thrombogenicity of mechanical valves varies depending on the type of valve and the position in which it is placed. For example, a caged-ball valve placed in the mitral position has the highest potential for thrombogenicity, while a bileaflet-tilting disc in the aortic position has considerably less (Table 1) [35]. Homograft valves do not require anticoagulation [35,36]. The American College of Chest Physicians 2004 Guidelines recommend an INR of 2.5 to 3.5 for most patients with mechanical prosthetic valves and 2.0 to 3.0 for those with bioprosthetic valves and low-risk patients with bileaflet valves (such as the St. Jude Medical Device) in the aortic position [37]. In patients with a mechanical valve and additional risk factors, such as atrial fibrillation, myocardial infarction, left atrial enlargement, or low ejection fraction, a target INR of 3.0 (range 2.5–3.5) combined with low doses of aspirin (75–100 mg/day) is recommended.

In patients with mechanical heart valves, oral anticoagulation reduces the rate of thrombotic complications while increasing bleeding complications. The relative risk reduction of warfarin above antiplatelet therapy is 60% to 79% [38]. No consensus has been established for the management of anticoagulation in patients who have mechanical heart valves and who are about to undergo a procedure [39,40]. For minor procedures in which blood loss is expected to be minimal and easily managed, anticoagulant therapy can be continued without interruption. However, for major procedures with the potential for significant blood loss, discontinuation of warfarin therapy is recommended. Strategies of anticoagulation protection during warfarin cessation vary. At one extreme is the strategy of establishing a bridge with unfractionated or LMWH. At the other extreme is a minimalist strategy, such as discontinuation of warfarin use alone. A survey among members of the Canadian Society of Internal Medicine demonstrated that preoperative and postoperative IV unfractionated heparin was the most frequently selected anticoagulation option for patients undergoing elective noncardiac surgery. Of course, this is costly, requires hospital admission, is labor intensive, and has its own risks. This decision was primarily based on the risk of the inherent thrombosis with respect to the type of valve and its position and not on the risk of periprocedural bleeding [39]. In weighing

Table 1
Thrombogenicity of heart valves

Valve type	Thrombogenicity[a]	Recommended INR
Caged-ball	++++	4.0–4.9
Single-tilting disc	+++	3.0–3.9
Bileaflet-tilting disc	++	2.5–2.9
Heterograft bioprosthesis	++	2.0–3.0
Homograft bioprosthesis	+	Not indicated

[a] Relative thrombogenicity: + = least, ++++ = most.

risks, physicians probably considered thrombotic consequences likely to be more devastating than postoperative bleeding complications (eg, wound hematoma).

Patients with a history of deep vein thrombosis

Patients with a recent diagnosis of acute venous thromboembolism should avoid elective surgery for 1 month following the diagnosis. If this is not possible, the patient should receive IV unfractionated heparin therapy before and after the procedure while the INR is less than 2.0. The use of heparin should be discontinued 6 hours before the procedure and restarted 12 hours following the procedure. The use of heparin is generally restarted without a bolus at no more than the expected maintenance infusion rate [18].

A temporary inferior vena cava (IVC) filter should be considered for patients receiving anticoagulation for less than two weeks after a pulmonary embolism or proximal deep vein thrombosis (DVT). Any patient at unacceptable risk for bleeding with IV heparin should also undergo IVC filter placement.

Patients undergoing a procedure beyond three months of being diagnosed with an acute DVT may not need perioperative heparin if risk factors for DVT are no longer present. Members of this cohort should receive perioperative prophylaxis as if they were at high risk for postoperative venous thromboembolism [37,41]. Prophylaxis would include LMWH, if safe to do so, or IV unfractionated heparin until the INR is above 2.0.

Summary

The surgical management of the anticoagulated patient requires an understanding of blood thrombosis, the mechanisms behind common anticoagulants, and the indications for anticoagulation. As percutaneous cardiac and peripheral procedures become increasingly sophisticated, we can expect to encounter more patients on aspirin and clopidogrel. Management strategies will require continued appraisal of available literature for evidence-based surgical practice.

References

[1] Davie EW, Ratnoff OD. Waterfall sequence for intrinsic blood clotting. Science 1964;145: 1310–2.
[2] Monroe DM, Hoffman M, Roberts HR. Platelets and thrombin generation. Arterioscler Thromb Vasc Biol 2002;22(9):1381–9.
[3] Dahlback B. Blood coagulation. Lancet 2000;355(9215):1627–32.
[4] Mangano DT. Aspirin and mortality from coronary bypass surgery. N Engl J Med 2002; 347(17):1309–17.
[5] Dacey LJ, et al. Effect of preoperative aspirin use on mortality in coronary artery bypass grafting patients. Ann Thorac Surg 2000;70(6):1986–90.

[6] Neilipovitz DT, Bryson GL, Nichol G. The effect of perioperative aspirin therapy in peripheral vascular surgery: a decision analysis. Anesth Analg 2001;93(3):573–80.

[7] Stein PD, et al. Antithrombotic therapy in patients with saphenous vein and internal mammary artery bypass grafts: the Seventh ACCP Conference on Antithrombotic and Thrombolytic Therapy. Chest 2004;126(3 Suppl):600S–8S.

[8] Hollopeter G, et al. Identification of the platelet ADP receptor targeted by antithrombotic drugs. Nature 2001;409(6817):202–7.

[9] CAPRIE Steering Committee. A randomised, blinded, trial of clopidogrel versus aspirin in patients at risk of ischaemic events (CAPRIE). Lancet 1996;348(9038):1329–39.

[10] Fajadet J, et al. Maintenance of long-term clinical benefit with sirolimus-eluting coronary stents: three-year results of the RAVEL trial. Circulation 2005;111(8):1040–4.

[11] Antman EM, et al. ACC/AHA guidelines for the management of patients with ST-elevation myocardial infarction—executive summary: a report of the American College of Cardiology/ American Heart Association Task Force on Practice Guidelines (Writing Committee to Revise the 1999 Guidelines for the Management of Patients With Acute Myocardial Infarction). Circulation 2004;110(5):588–636.

[12] Hirsh J, et al. American Heart Association/American College of Cardiology Foundation guide to warfarin therapy. Circulation 2003;107(12):1692–711.

[13] Suzuki K, et al. Protein S is essential for the activated protein C-catalyzed inactivation of platelet-associated factor Va. J Biochem (Tokyo) 1984;96(2):455–60.

[14] Broekmans AW, et al. Protein C and the development of skin necrosis during anticoagulant therapy. Thromb Haemost 1983;49(3):251.

[15] Hirsh J, et al. Oral anticoagulants: mechanism of action, clinical effectiveness, and optimal therapeutic range. Chest 2001;119(1 Suppl):8S–21S.

[16] White RH, et al. Temporary discontinuation of warfarin therapy: changes in the international normalized ratio. Ann Intern Med 1995;122(1):40–2.

[17] Genewein U, et al. Rebound after cessation of oral anticoagulant therapy: the biochemical evidence. Br J Haematol 1996;92(2):479–85.

[18] Kearon C, Hirsh J. Management of anticoagulation before and after elective surgery. N Engl J Med 1997;336(21):1506–11.

[19] Sorensen B, et al. Reversal of the International Normalized Ratio with recombinant activated factor VII in central nervous system bleeding during warfarin thromboprophylaxis: clinical and biochemical aspects. Blood Coagul Fibrinolysis 2003;14(5):469–77.

[20] Ansell J, et al. The pharmacology and management of the vitamin K antagonists: the Seventh ACCP Conference on Antithrombotic and Thrombolytic Therapy. Chest 2004;126(3 Suppl): 204S–33S.

[21] Choay J, et al. Structure-activity relationship in heparin: a synthetic pentasaccharide with high affinity for antithrombin III and eliciting high anti-factor Xa activity. Biochem Biophys Res Commun 1983;116(2):492–9.

[22] Hirsh J, et al. Heparin and low-molecular-weight heparin: mechanisms of action, pharmacokinetics, dosing, monitoring, efficacy, and safety. Chest 2001;119(1 Suppl):64S–94S.

[23] Laposata M, et al. College of American Pathologists Conference XXXI on laboratory monitoring of anticoagulant therapy: the clinical use and laboratory monitoring of low-molecular-weight heparin, danaparoid, hirudin and related compounds, and argatroban. Arch Pathol Lab Med 1998;122(9):799–807.

[24] Nieuwenhuis HK, et al. Identification of risk factors for bleeding during treatment of acute venous thromboembolism with heparin or low molecular weight heparin. Blood 1991;78(9): 2337–43.

[25] Douketis JD, Johnson JA, Turpie AG. Low-molecular-weight heparin as bridging anticoagulation during interruption of warfarin: assessment of a standardized periprocedural anticoagulation regimen. Arch Intern Med 2004;164(12):1319–26.

[26] Di Nisio M, Middeldorp S, Büller H. Drug Therapy. Direct thrombin inhibitors. N Engl J Med 2005;353:1028–40.

[27] Risk factors for stroke and efficacy of antithrombotic therapy in atrial fibrillation. Analysis of pooled data from five randomized controlled trials. Arch Intern Med 1994;154(13): 1449–57.

[28] Lin HJ, et al. Stroke severity in atrial fibrillation. The Framingham Study. Stroke 1996; 27(10):1760–4.

[29] Jorgensen HS, et al. Acute stroke with atrial fibrillation. The Copenhagen Stroke Study. Stroke 1996;27(10):1765–9.

[30] EAFT (European Atrial Fibrillation Trial) Study Group. Secondary prevention in non-rheumatic atrial fibrillation after transient ischaemic attack or minor stroke. Lancet 1993; 342(8882):1255–62.

[31] The American College of Chest Physicians guidelines for the prevention and management of postoperative atrial fibrillation after cardiac surgery. Chest 2005;128(Suppl):1S–64S.

[32] Flanc C, Kakkar VV, Clarke MB. The detection of venous thrombosis of the legs using 125-I-labelled fibrinogen. Br J Surg 1968;55(10):742–7.

[33] Metzdorff MT, et al. Thrombosis of mechanical cardiac valves: a qualitative comparison of the silastic ball valve and the tilting disc valve. J Am Coll Cardiol 1984;4(1):50–3.

[34] Edmunds LH Jr. Thromboembolic complications of current cardiac valvular prostheses. Ann Thorac Surg 1982;34(1):96–106.

[35] Vongpatanasin W, Hillis LD, Lange RA. Prosthetic heart valves. N Engl J Med 1996;335(6): 407–16.

[36] Gherli T, et al. Comparing warfarin with aspirin after biological aortic valve replacement. A prospective study. Circulation 2004;110(5):496–500.

[37] The seventh ACCP conference on antithrombotic and thrombolytic therapy: evidence-based guidelines. Chest 2004;126(suppl):163S–696S.

[38] Mok CK, et al. Warfarin versus dipyridamole-aspirin and pentoxifylline-aspirin for the prevention of prosthetic heart valve thromboembolism: a prospective randomized clinical trial. Circulation 1985;72(5):1059–63.

[39] Douketis JD, et al. Physician preferences for perioperative anticoagulation in patients with a mechanical heart valve who are undergoing elective noncardiac surgery. Chest 1999;116(5): 1240–6.

[40] Salem DN, Stein PD, Al-Ahmad A, et al. Antithrombotic therapy in valvular heart disease—native and prosthetic: the seventh AACP conference on antithrombotic and thrombolytic therapy. Chest 2004;126:457S–82S.

[41] Geerts WH, Pineo GF, Heit JA, et al. Prevention of venous thromboembolism: the seventh ACCP conference on antithrombotic and thrombotic therapy. Chest 2004;126:338S–400S.

ELSEVIER
SAUNDERS

Surg Clin N Am 85 (2005) 1191–1213

SURGICAL
CLINICS OF
NORTH AMERICA

The Management of Postoperative Bleeding

T. Forcht Dagi, MD, MPH

Division of Health Sciences and Technology, The Harvard-MIT Program in Health Sciences and Technology, 423 Commonwealth Avenue, Newton Center, MA 02459, USA

This article addresses the management of postoperative bleeding. The problem is called postoperative bleeding rather than postoperative hemorrhage to emphasize the fact that perfect postoperative hemostasis rather than acceptable postoperative blood loss is the ideal. Postoperative bleeding is a risk of all surgical procedures. The best way to reduce the risk of hemorrhage is to identify and correct potential causes of coagulopathy preoperatively as well as postoperatively.

In the presence of bright red bleeding from any site, if the prothrombin time (PT), activated partial thromboplastin time ($_a$PTT), platelet count, and temperature are normal, urgent re-exploration is indicated unless other factors dictate a more thorough diagnostic workup. In the presence of life-threatening hemorrhage, control of bleeding takes priority. The hematologic workup is pursued in parallel.

Throughout this article, a distinction is made between technical causes of bleeding and coagulopathy, or disorders of hemostasis [1]. The term "technical causes of bleeding" refers to four broad categories of postoperative blood loss:

1. Inadequate repair of vessels or vascular structures that are knowingly opened or divided, whether purposefully or accidentally
2. Occult or undiagnosed and therefore unrepaired injury to the vascular system

---

In writing this article, the author has drawn liberally from the several authors cited, particularly references 1 and 14. In several instances the author has paraphrased and combined the authors and followed their outline closely, with only small changes in language and order of presentation of flow for purposes and to make the material more pertinent to the perioperative setting and to this publication.

E-mail address: tdagi@post.harvard.edu

3. Injury or damage during the course of surgery to organs or structures within the operative field, whether recognized at the time or not
4. Injury or damage during the course of surgery or in the immediate postoperative period to organs or structures remote from the surgical site

Except in the most general sense, this article does not cover the management of intraoperative or postoperative hemorrhage arising from technical causes, the management of anticoagulation in the perioperative period, the management of trauma, the management of transfusion, or the treatment of shock.

Few surgeons have the expertise in hematology or the time to manage the medical aspects of coagulopathy without consultation. This article provides the surgeon with a basis on which to engage, rather than to replace, the medical specialist. Early consultation may be prudent and useful.

Preoperative screening strategies

Routine preoperative screening

In terms of surgical complications, "an ounce of prevention is worth a pound of cure," and preoperative screening has evolved with the thought of preventing intra- and postoperative problems. What constitutes a reasonable stratagem for preoperative screening for hemostasis? The guidelines of the Joint Commission on Accreditation of Health care Organizations mandate a preoperative evaluation to assess a patient's readiness and risk for surgical intervention but leave the details up to each individual organization [2]. As increasingly sophisticated screening tests have entered the market, their cost and their aggregate effectiveness and utility for *routine use* have come into question. Unlike their quantifiable value in elucidating the cause of demonstrated coagulopathy, their screening value, as measured in terms of (1) preventing postoperative bleeding and (2) the costs of sorting out abnormalities of questionable significance, remains in question [3,4].

The significance of abnormal test results

Test results may be reported on a continuum (ie, a set of values between 0 and infinity, as in a patient's weight), on an ordinal scale with a small number of discrete and discontinuous values (ie, 1 +, 2 +, and so forth, as with dipstick examination of proteinuria), or categorically (eg. as normal or abnormal). Tests that report results on a continuum must provide cutoff points for abnormally high or low values. The intervening values, classically obtained by calculating the mean and allowing 2 standard deviation on either side, typically represent the range of results in 95% of a reference population. As a result, 5% of any population comparable to the reference population would be expected to have an abnormal result on any given test, and this probability increases when multiple tests are ordered. In a patient who has no disease, there is a 64% likelihood of an abnormality being found on a chemistry panel of 20 tests [4].

Nevertheless, for medico-legal reasons, to detect unsuspected and potentially correctable abnormalities that increase surgical risk, to establish a baseline value for laboratory values that might change postoperatively or need to be monitored because of perioperative medications (eg, anticoagulants), or because of the importance of diagnosing related conditions (such as carotid stenosis in the face of symptomatic coronary artery disease), routine preoperative screening is standard of care.

It has been noted that clinicians ignore between 30% and 60% of abnormalities elicited on routine screening [4–6]. Ignoring abnormalities without comment increases the risk of suit. Unless the chart contains good documentation reflecting the reasons for setting aside an abnormal screening result, the physician is at risk for a plaintiff's verdict in the event of legal action following a surgical complication or adverse result [4].

The term "screening" is properly reserved for patients who do not have signs and symptoms of underlying abnormality and who are free of any known conditions that increase the likelihood of abnormal results. Screening tests are useful when they

1. Cost little
2. Are consistent
3. Carry negligible risk
4. Demonstrate high sensitivity and selectivity
5. Offer high positive and negative predictive value
6. Accurately foreshadow surgical morbidity
7. Are appropriate to the population at hand (eg, there is questionable value to skin testing for tuberculosis in a population known to have been vaccinated with Bacille Calmette-Guérin [BCG])
8. Uncover common conditions contributing to surgical morbidity and for which effective intervention is available [4]

Thus, to be efficient and effective, screening stratagems must be useful and pertinent. The literature cautions that estimates of unsuspected abnormalities in healthy populations are probably exaggerated and that routine preoperative screening is of limited measurable value unless abnormal results are suspected, or abnormal results have been obtained previously [4,7,8].

Nevertheless, the risks accompanying surgical intervention, both to the patient and to the surgeon, justify judicious screening to detect and correct pertinent underlying abnormalities.

History and physical examination

Patients who do not have a personal or family history of bleeding difficulties or abnormal bleeding associated with dental extractions, previous surgery, routine childhood and adolescent trauma, or childbirth are unlikely to suffer from familial or congenital coagulopathy. Patients taking no medications and without history of bleeding disorders are also at very low risk. Many patients, however, do not recognize that over-the counter-medications—nonsteroidal anti-inflammatory drugs most notably—do count as medications and can interfere with normal coagulation. The history must specifically address the casual use of over-the-counter drugs as well as the routine and prescribed use of any medications.

The absence of bruising or other signs of bleeding on routine physical examination helps confirm that the patient is at low risk for surgical bleeding. This finding should be clearly listed in the physical examination.

Abnormalities in routine screening and their significance

The following statistics refer to only the results of tests performed for screening purposes in the context described previously.

Complete blood cell count

The overall incidence of hemoglobin abnormalities in a combined review of 9363 patients was 1.8%, but anemia occurs in 4% to 9% of patients 70 years of age and older (n = 526) and predicts the need for transfusion in patients at risk for blood loss [4,9–11]. The prevalence of an elevated white blood cell count in a combined review of 5359 patients was less than 1% and was unrelated to perioperative morbidity [4,11,12]. The prevalence of platelet abnormalities in a combined review of 8670 patients was calculated to be 0.9% [4,12]. The abnormality in the preponderance of cases was thrombocytopenia, but management was changed in only 0.02% of cases [4].

Coagulation

The yield for abnormal PT in a combined review of 3786 patients was 0.3%, but in no case was management influenced [4]. Evidence suggests that the PT alone is a poor screening test and neither predicts nor excludes clinically relevant perioperative bleeding abnormalities [10]. The yield for abnormalities in PTT was 6.5% in a combined review of 2955 patients [4].

These figures are summarized in Table 1.

Bleeding time

The use of bleeding time for screening is controversial [13]. On the one hand, there is good evidence to suggest the actual times are variable and depend on technique. It has been asserted that bleeding time offers no screening advantage in normal reference populations, and therefore it has no role to play [4,13,14].

On the other hand, bleeding time is a good way to detect abnormalities of platelet function. Disruption of platelet function is increasingly common in the aging population because of the regular use of aspirin (ASA) for primary

Table 1
Prevalence of hematological abnormalities in preoperative screening

Test	Number of Patients	Prevalence of Abnormality (%)
Hemoglobin	9363	1.8%
Leukocytes	5359	0.7%
Platelets	8670	0.9%
Prothrombin time	4786	0.3%
Partial thromboplastin time	2955	6.5%

and secondary prophylaxis in ischemic heart disease and cerebrovascular occlusive disease, the occasional and often unreported use of ASA for pain and inflammation, and the use of ticlopidine hydrochloride or clopidogrel bisulfate for platelet inhibition in cerebrovascular disease (where ASA has failed) or for stenting in coronary artery disease (clopidogrel and ASA in combination) [14]. Bleeding times normalize after these drugs have been discontinued, but the time required for normalization cannot be predicted with certainty [14].

Eptifibatide, abciximab, and tirofiban hydrochloride block the integrin $\alpha_{IIb}\beta_3$ receptor on the platelet membrane. Blocking this receptor paralyzes the platelet and prevents activation. Platelets fail to aggregate normally, and their endothelial attachments do not withstand high shear forces. Abciximab has additional effects as well [15].

Bleeding time typically returns to normal 6 hours after the discontinuation of eptifibatide but more than 24 hours after the discontinuation of abciximab.

Abciximab is also associated with thrombocytopenia, generally within the first 24 hours of use. Platelet counts drop below 100,000 in 6% of patients and below 50,000 in 1.5% [15]. The prevalence of thrombocytopenia is lower with tirofiban and apparently is nonexistent with eptifibatide [14]. Thrombocytopenia has also been associated with the use of clopidogrel [16].

Statistics for the prevalence of abnormalities of bleeding time in screening of a reference population are not available, perhaps because bleeding times are not routinely measured. Even so, the measurement of bleeding time is indicated in patients treated with platelet-inhibiting agents, irrespective of symptomatology or findings, and in patients who are likely to self-medicate with ASA, wittingly or not. (Many patients and some physicians are unaware that ASA may be found in combination with antihistamines and decongestants in cold and headache remedies, and, in some parts of the United States, packaged as a powder or as a branded pill without ASA in its name.)

Abnormalities of bleeding time do represent a coagulopathy and must be respected as such. They should not be ignored. In some cases it is easier to wait until platelet function returns to normal. In other cases, platelet transfusions are in order. Plasma exchange may be indicated for drug-induced thrombocytopenia purpura [16].

Surgery in higher-risk populations

Sometimes it is necessary to proceed with surgery urgently despite the likelihood of defective hemostasis and intra- or postoperative bleeding. In these cases, preoperative screening has three purposes: to identify defects in hemostasis that can be corrected preoperatively, to guide the management of hemostatic defects that cannot be corrected in the time remaining before surgery, and to help manage the bleeding that cannot be prevented.

A perspective on risk management and benefits of screening

Increasing emphasis on cost containment in medicine has resulted in attempts to distinguish "essential" from "nonessential" measures in patient care. This trend has been balanced, at least in part, by concerns for patient safety and fears of medical liability actions. Even the terms used create difficulty: where does "advisable" or "prudent" fit in the spectrum of "nonessential to essential"? The literature on preoperative screening reports a low prevalence of abnormal findings in study populations and an even lower likelihood that management would be altered by any single discovered abnormality. In populations at different and usually greater risk, such as patients treated with low-dose ASA after transient ischemic attack, the prevalence of abnormality will be greater if the appropriate test is performed. Bleeding time may not be indicated as a screening test in the population at large, but bleeding time may be very useful to screen for coagulopathy in patients whose platelet function is inhibited for therapeutic purposes or in patients likely to self-medicate unwittingly with platelet-inhibiting preparations.

What is the real significance of these observations? Given the large number of surgical procedures performed every day, a 0.01 prevalence of abnormality leading to even a 0.00001 likelihood of alteration in management affects a large aggregate number of patients and surgeons in the aggregate. The aggregate risk of surgical bleeding in a particular population is derived by combining the risk of bleeding in the study population with an estimate of the risk of technical causes of bleeding associated with the procedure. It is reasonable to attempt to identify situations in which both the population-based risk of bleeding and the technical risk are exceptionally low and to raise the threshold for screening accordingly. One thoroughly studied example is cataract surgery in patients who have absolutely no known or discoverable risk factors for bleeding, for whom routine screening really does seem to convey no measurable benefit [17].

In the broader perspective of cost-benefit analysis, it is prudent to think not only in terms of the technical risk of surgery but also of the consequences of bleeding. Because of the specific problems associated with intracranial pressure and vasospasm following intracranial hemorrhage, for example, the cost–benefit analysis of screening in intracranial surgery may shift in comparison to other operations with similar technical risk.

A classification of surgical risk that factors anticipated blood loss into the risk of surgery can serve as a useful guide. A good example is the Johns Hopkins Risk Classification System [3]. It can be used either alone or in combination with other classification systems. The Hopkins system associates category I (minimally invasive) with little or no blood loss, category II (minimally to moderately invasive) with blood loss less than 500 mL, category III (moderately to significantly invasive) with a blood loss potential of 500 to 1500 mL, and categories IV and V (both considered highly invasive) with blood loss in excess of 1500 mL [3].

Every classification system has inherent limits. Risk analysis is useful for predicting the events in a set (a defined population) but not the behavior of a statistic (a single member of the set) in the abstract. Thus, there is no way to know exactly what will transpire with a particular patient because there is no perfect way to combine the pertinent risks into a perfect prediction for an individual case.

For this reason alone, it is often appropriate to move beyond routine screening protocols when there is concern about factors that might jeopardize patient safety, even in category I or category II patients. In the face of such concerns, it may be advisable to move from screening protocols to diagnostic protocols such as those reviewed here and used to rule out technical causes of bleeding.

Diagnostic protocols

Overview

The first step in diagnosis is recognizing that the patient is bleeding. This recognition is neither as obvious nor as easy as it might seem.

Vital signs may remain remarkably stable, especially in the young, until shock ensues. Normal blood pressure may be preserved despite the loss of 1.5 to 2 L, or 40% of total blood volume. Falling hematocrits and hemoglobin levels are often dismissed as artifacts of dilution. Drains placed intraoperatively and intended to monitor and drain blood from a closed cavity may become blocked, kinked, or malpositioned, thereby providing a false sense of security. Finally, the bleeding may be remote from the site of surgery or it may accumulate in an undrained compartment.

The results of physical examination should be integrated with all other data sources. Tachycardia, diminished cardiac output, dropping central venous pressure, reductions in urine output, and abnormal capillary refill pattern are all suggestive of bleeding, as are flank bruises and swelling of the extremities with discoloration. The search for an occult technical cause of bleeding should continue, regularly and repeatedly, until the patient is stable and bleeding has stopped.

Technical causes of bleeding and coagulopathy may coexist and often do. It may be difficult to address the technical cause before stabilizing the coagulopathy. On the other hand, massive transfusion of blood products may induce or worsen coagulopathy. Both lines of management—control of technical causes of bleeding and reversal of coagulopathy—should be pursued simultaneously. The precise details of intervention and timing are often a matter of judgment and cannot be reduced effectively to protocol.

Intracranial bleeding may lead to neurogenic shock or neurogenic pulmonary edema, but the volume of hemorrhage does not *per se* reduce circulating blood volume enough to lead to shock except in infants, and even then very rarely.

The search for technical sources of hemorrhage includes repeated physical examination and appropriate imaging techniques (CT, MRI, MR angiography, ultrasound). Sometimes angiography is indicated. Angiography should be seen as an opportunity for endovascular repair, if possible and appropriate.

Screening protocols versus diagnostic protocols

The approach to preoperative screening differs from the approach to the diagnosis of coagulopathy. In the preoperative situation, the patient can be assumed to have normal hemostatic function unless history or findings dictate otherwise. In the setting of postoperative hemorrhage (and following the exclusion of technical causes of bleeding), the patient is assumed to have a coagulopathy. For preoperative purposes, normal test results up to 4 months old are generally deemed reliable if the patient is clinically unchanged [4,8]. In the postoperative setting, test results can change quickly, and serial studies may be required.

The diagnosis of coagulopathy is directed at assessing the function of the factors, cells, and other elements that contribute to normal coagulation. Technical causes of bleeding and coagulopathy may occur simultaneously or sequentially. Until the bleeding has come under control, until it has been shown not to recur, and until the patient is stable, neither the exclusion of one nor the confirmation of the other suffices.

Assessment of coagulopathy

The six initial steps in assessing coagulopathy are to

1. Perform complete blood cell count and coagulation studies
2. Check for and correct hypothermia
3. Review the history
4. Review medications
5. Obtain additional studies if indicated
6. Check serially for new or ongoing sources of bleed loss

One of the most cogent algorithms has been published by Owings and Gosselin in *ACS Surgery* [1]. The discussion that follows draws liberally on their work.

Complete blood cell count and coagulation studies. Blood is drawn and sent in two tubes, one containing ethylenediaminetetraacetic acid [EDTA] for a complete blood cell count, and the other citrated for coagulation analysis. The tubes must be carefully labeled for identification. It is easy for samples to be confused or mislabeled in the press of resuscitation. The samples should be sent stat.

It is the responsibility of the treating physician to follow up on the studies and make sure both the studies and their results are documented in the chart.

Hypothermia. A body temperature below 35°C (95°F) may inhibit clotting mechanisms. In pure hypothermic coagulopathy, coagulation mechanisms normalize when normal temperature is restored. Hypothermia may contribute to or be the sole source of coagulopathy. Hypothermic patients are actively rewarmed.

Differential diagnosis of coagulopathy. Most coagulopathies can be diagnosed, or at least separated into categories reflecting the most likely mechanism or mechanisms of coagulopathy, on the basis of the international normalized ratio (INR), the ₐPTT, platelet count, platelet function, and family history. Sometimes, the diagnosis cannot be further refined without assays for specific factors. The number of platelets in circulation and platelet function are independent variables. Bleeding time is the traditional test used to assess platelet function. Its limitations have been noted. Although a number of far more sophisticated tests have been introduced recently, the problem of adequate assessment of platelet dysfunction is beyond the scope of this article.

A summary of differential diagnosis is given in Table 2.

A discussion of the INR is given in Appendix 1.

The management of postoperative bleeding

Overview

In the presence of bright red bleeding from any site, if the PT, ₐPTT, platelet count, and temperature are normal, urgent re-exploration is indicated unless other factors dictate a more thorough diagnostic workup. In the presence of life-threatening arterial hemorrhage, control of bleeding takes priority. The hematologic workup is pursued in parallel.

The most basic principles of management are

1. Diagnose and treat shock and any other potentially life-threatening conditions
2. Rule out technical sources of bleeding
3. Restore clotting parameters to normal by means of medications, transfusion of blood products or clotting factors, restoration of normothermia, diagnosis and treatment of sepsis, or control of other precipitating or contributing factors (eg, retained products of conception, as discussed later)
4. Monitor for stability of clotting parameters

Table 2
Differential diagnosis of postoperative coagulopathies

Symptom	INR	aPTT	Platelet Number	Platelet Function[a]	Family or Personal History	Diagnosis	Differential Diagnosis	Comments
Persisting ooze, low-volume bleeding	Normal	Normal	Normal	Impaired	Negative	Impaired platelet function		Spontaneous bleeding with thrombocytopenia <50,000 is rare (some authorities cite 20,000 [1], but postoperative needs may be higher
Persisting ooze, low-volume bleeding	Normal	Normal	Low	Normal	Negative	Thrombocytopenia		
Persisting ooze, low-volume bleeding	Normal	Normal	Normal	Normal	Negative		Consider factor XIII deficiency, hypofibrinogenemia, dyfibrinogenemia, altered fibrinolysis	
Minor or major bleeding	Normal	Prolonged	Normal	Normal	Negative	Drug-induced coagulopathy, most likely unfractionated heparin in the US	Effects of direct thrombin inhibitors such as hirulog and lepirudin	
Minor or major bleeding	Normal	Prolonged slightly	Normal	Abnormal	Negative		von Willebrand's disease	Confirm by testing for circulating von Willebrand's factor levels
Major or minor bleeding, oozing	Normal	Normal	Normal	Normal	Positive for hemophilia	Hemophilia	Hemophilia A: factor VIII deficiency. Hemophilia B: factor IX deficiency. Hemophilia C: factor XI deficiency.	Rarely encountered without prior family or personal history. Specific factor analysis is indicated.

Clinical scenario							
Major or minor bleeding	Increased	Normal	Normal	n/a	Hepatitis, liver disease, ETOH, oral anticoagulation	Factor deficiency, vitamin K deficiency, warfarin effect	Undiagnosed liver disease, malabsorption, malnutrition, warfarin effect or superwarfarin (rat poison) toxicity, antibiotic effect	Reversal of anticoagulation with vitamin K accurately reflected in INR
Major bleeding	Prolonged	Prolonged	Normal	Normal		Multiple factor deficiencies	DIC, hemodilution, uremia and nephrotic syndrome Isolated, rare factor deficiencies of the common pathway include factors X, V, and prothrombin Autoimmune conditions resulting in acquired factor V deficiencies Factor X deficiency associated with amyloidosis Acquired hypoprothrombinemia associated in lupus Warfarin overdose Rodenticide toxicity Animal venoms	D-dimer level assay helps the diagnosis of DIC. If level < 1000 ng/mL, DIC unlikely; level > 2000 ng/mL without confounding explanation, DIC highly likely

5. Correct as needed
6. Monitor for new or ongoing sources of bleeding or blood loss
7. Monitor for treatable complications associated with new or ongoing sources of bleeding or blood loss (eg, intracranial hemorrhage)

Generally accepted criteria for transfusion are published widely and are not reviewed here. Table 3 provides a summary of current recommendations for replacement transfusion in acute blood loss [18].

Technical causes

The following discussion draws liberally from McKenna [14].

Postoperative bleeding can result from one cause or many, and the causes may be related or linked or not. By default, the surgeon must first consider a surgically remediable technical cause of bleeding. Technical causes are least likely to respond to nonsurgical intervention.

Principles of surgical hemostasis are reviewed in all standard general surgical and specialty textbooks and are not revisited here, except to note that the use of certain materials and techniques in surgery may cause coagulopathy in unexpected ways. For example, high levels of suction have been associated with diffuse intravascular coagulation (DIC) after surgery for scoliosis when a cell-saver has been deployed. The development of antibovine antibodies after the use of topical bovine thrombin in neurosurgery has been associated with coagulopathy [14].

Nontechnical causes

Hypothermia

The effects of hypothermia have already been noted. Hypothermia may be the sole cause of coagulopathy or may contribute to coagulopathy

Table 3
Transfusion Guidelines in Acute Blood Loss

Criterion	Significance
Ischemia	High risk of occurrence, impending and/or increased risk to patient because of underlying medical issues: transfusion usually indicated
Degree of blood loss	> 30% rapid blood loss: transfusion may be indicated (< 30% rapid blood loss in previously healthy patient: usually well tolerated)
Hemoglobin concentration	< 6 g/dL: transfusion generally required. 6–10 g/dL: dictated by clinical circumstances. > 6 g/dL: transfusion rarely required
Vital signs	Tachycardia and hypotension refractory to volume expansion with hemoglobin concentration in 6–10 g/dL range and extent of blood loss unknown: transfusion usually required
O_2 extraction ratio	O_2 extraction ratio > 50% with VO_2 decrease: transfusion usually required

From Simon TL, Alverson DC, AuBuchon J, et al. Practice parameters for the use of red blood cell transfusions: developed by the Red Blood Cell Administration Practice Guideline Development Task Force of the College of American Pathologists. Arch Pathol Lab Med 1998;122:130–8; with permission.

from other root causes. Laboratories warm samples to 37°C. In pure hypothermic coagulopathy, normal coagulation parameters will be documented.

If the patient exhibits normal coagulation parameters and is normothermic, attention should revert to the diagnosis of occult technical causes of bleeding [1].

In instances of induced hypothermia for therapeutic purposes, a thorough risk–benefit analysis comparing the risks of coagulopathy with the risks of normothermia should be conducted.

Drugs

Aspirin. ASA is the most common platelet-inhibiting drug. The effect is dose related and affects bleeding times. ASA effects may last up to 10 days and cannot be completely reversed directly, unlike those of other nonsteroidal anti-inflammatory drugs such as ibuprofen [1]. The effects are potentiated when ASA is given in conjunction with other platelet-function inhibitors or to patients who have other causes of coagulopathy, such as type I von Willebrand's disease or hepatic or renal dysfunction. The bleeding time may become very prolonged. The first line of treatment is platelet transfusion. Desmopressin acetate may be helpful, particularly in patients who have renal failure [19]. Desmopressin acetate may cause water retention, hyponatremia, and, more rarely, arterial thrombotic complications.

Platelet inhibitors. The effects of ticlopidine, clopidogrel, eptifibatide, abciximab and tirofiban have been noted. Prolonged bleeding time may be reversed with platelet transfusions, which are indicated specifically when an accompanying thrombocytopenia ensues after the use of abciximab or tirofiban.

Anticoagulants. Unfractionated heparin (UFH) is commonly administered in large doses to provide systemic anticoagulation in the management of venous thrombosis, hypercoagulability, arterial dissection, and arterial embolic states such as transient ischemic attack or stroke-in-evolution. UFH prolongs the $_a$PTT. In low, prophylactic doses, heparin is used to prevent deep venous thrombosis or for catheter flushing. Even low doses of UFH may cause clinically significant anticoagulation in the setting of hepatic or renal dysfunction.

When the consequences of bleeding or hematoma are not critical, it may be possible to manage UFH-mediated anticoagulation by modifying the dose of UFH. When the consequences are critical (eg, intracranial surgery), the effects must be reversed. The effects of UFH last 24 to 72 hours after administration. If more urgent reversal is required, prolonged $_a$PTT may be reversed by protamine sulfate infusion.

Rapid reversal, however, may precipitate unwanted thrombosis. Protamine administration may also lead to allergic reactions and anaphylaxis, and in excess, protamine may actually prolong the $_a$PTT. Sensitivity to protamine may be related to sensitization to insulin [1].

The $_a$PTT may be artifactually prolonged when blood is drawn from a heparin-flushed catheter. Confirmation may be obtained by comparison with an $_a$PTT drawn by venipuncture.

UFH administration may also induce the formation of heparin platelet antibodies and result in heparin-induced thrombocytopenia (HIT), or, even more rarely and paradoxically, in a life-threatening heparin-induced thrombocytopenia thrombosis syndrome (HITTS). These syndromes develop in approximately 1% to 5% of patients within 3 to 5 days of starting treatment with heparin, and approximately 30% to 40% of patients who have HIT progress to HITTS. The mortality and morbidity associated with HITTS reaches 40% to 55% [20]. The heparin–platelet antibody interactions may explain only one part of HIT. It is a complex phenomenon that remains to be elucidated fully [14].

The importance of HIT and HITTS derives in part from the prevalence of heparin administration. These conditions also exemplify a complex coagulopathy with both hemorrhagic and thrombotic features. The diagnosis may elude the surgeon unless specifically pursued.

The diagnosis of HIT is made on the basis of a 50% drop in baseline platelet count or thrombocytopenia below 100,000. A 30% drop serves as an indication to assay heparin-platelet antibodies using a combination of the three tests currently available: ^{14}C-serotonin release assay which measures the presence of functionally active heparin-platelet antibody; the platelet factor 4 ELISA, a more sensitive but less specific for identifying heparin-platelet antibodies; the platelet aggregation assay, which helps confirm the diagnosis when abnormal. Other methods to identify heparin-platelet antibodies are in development.

Low molecular weight heparins (LMWH) such as enoxaparin sodium, tinzaparin sodium, and dalteparin sodium have greater than a 90% cross-reactivity with heparin–platelet antibodies and must not be used as substitutes, even when the immediate threat of postoperative bleeding has past. A full discussion of the management of HIT and HITTS goes beyond the purview of this article, but, very broadly, the recommendation is to treat with warfarin supplemented by recombinant hirudin or argatroban until the dose is stabilized and satisfactory anticoagulation achieved.

The anticoagulant effects of LMWHs are best assayed by an anti-factor X_a assay. Levels exceeding 1.3 to 2.0 IU/mL may be deemed abnormally high. The $_a$PTT does not effectively measure the anticoagulant effect of LMWHs. A normal $_a$PTT may still be associated with a bleeding diathesis [14]. In contrast to the effectiveness of protamine administration in reversing anticoagulation with UFH, protamine does not reliably reverse the anticoagulant effect after LMWH administration.

Fresh-frozen plasma (FFP) contains antithrombin. Antithrombin is potentiated by both UFH and LMWHs. FFP will not correct the anticoagulant effect of either UFH or LMWH and may, in fact, worsen the problem.

FFP may be used to correct $_a$PTT prolongations caused by direct thrombin inhibitors such as hirulog and lepirudin, with one important caveat. Circulating, unbound inhibitor binds the prothrombin in the FFP. For this reason, the effective dose is diminished. The amount of FFP needed to normalize $_a$PTT will be greater than might otherwise be estimated to correct a simple factor deficiency, for example [1].

Chronic illness, malignancy, malnutrition, or treatment with broad-spectrum antibiotics may result in the rapid onset of vitamin K deficiency through reduction in the vitamin K–dependent coagulation factors VII, IX, X, and II. Vitamin K deficiency prolongs both the PT and the $_a$PTT. This problem is prevented by the routine administration of vitamin K weekly or biweekly to vulnerable patients.

Warfarin sodium has an effect that parallels to vitamin K deficiency. Prolongation of PT is used to monitor adequacy of treatment. An INR of 1.5 or less generally allows satisfactory hemostasis during and after surgery, except for intracranial procedures and other critical situations in which *any* increased risk is problematic.

PT prolongations are corrected by the oral administration of vitamin K in doses of 1 to 5 mg. Sometimes multiple doses must be given over time [14] because of warfarin's long half-life (about 40 hours), during which the reversal wears off. Complicating factors in warfarin use include malabsorption, hepatic disease, and the simultaneous administration of other anticoagulants.

Principles in the management of the patient who has increased INR are as follows [1]:

1. For prolonged INR less than 5.0 without bleeding, hold the next dose
2. For INR between 5.0 and 9.0 without significant bleeding either
   a. Withhold next 1 or 2 doses if clinically reasonable or
   b. Withhold next dose and administer vitamin K, 1.0 to 2 mg orally
3. For INR between 5.0 and 9.0 when rapid normalization is required, administer vitamin K, 2.0 to 4.0 mg, for reduction of INR within 24 hours
4. For INR above 9.0
   a. Without significant bleeding, administer vitamin K, 3.0 to 5.0 mg
   b. With serious bleeding, administer vitamin K, 10 mg intravenously, and FFP; monitor INR at 12-hour intervals because additional vitamin K supplementation may be required
   c. With life-threatening hemorrhage, consider prothrombin complexes in addition to measures in (b)
5. For INR above 20.0
   a. Whether or not serious bleeding is present, administer vitamin K, 10 mg intravenously, and FFP to reduce INR to therapeutic levels; monitor INR at 12-hour intervals because additional vitamin K supplementation may be required
   b. With life-threatening hemorrhage, consider administration of prothrombin complexes in addition to measures in (a)

Thrombolytic agents. Acute vascular thrombosis in the perioperative setting may be treated with thrombolytic agents such as streptokinase or urokinase that act as plasminogen activators, or with tissue plasminogen activators such as Alteplase, recombinant and Reteplase. Free plasmin degrades both pathologic and physiologic fibrin clots of recent origin, as well as lysing fibrinogen and factors V and VIII. These drugs generate large amounts of plasmin [21]. Plasmin has other effects on hemostasis as well, the sum total of which is described broadly as "chaotic" [14].

The effects of these thrombolytic agents are reversed with anti-fibrinolytics such as ϵ-aminocaproic acid and tranexamic acid, or by aprotinin, a protease inhibitor. FFP increases levels of factor V and of α_2-antiplasmin, a physiologic plasmin inhibitor. Cryoprecipitate increases fibrinogen and factor VIII levels and is indicated for use in the presence of active bleeding, reduction of thrombin-clottable fibrinogen below 70 mg/dL, of factor V below 35%, and of factor VIII below 30%. Conversely, assessments of these factors help sort out the diagnosis.

Diffuse intravascular coagulation

DIC is a complex condition with both thrombotic and hemorrhagic features. It may occur whenever the coagulation system is activated and the level of thrombin increases. Thrombin promotes coagulation, also activates anticoagulant pathways and modulates fibrinolysis. The severity of the coagulopathy depends on fibrinogen levels and reflects the balance between fibrinogen production and physiological antithrombotic mechanisms.

The imbalance between thrombosis and fibrinolysis creates a complex hemostatic disorder with both thrombotic and thrombolytic features. The thrombolytic features are responsible for bleeding diatheses.

In mild forms of DIC, microthrombi are formed in the vascular system and are cleared. The condition may remain subclinical. In moderate forms, microthrombi occlude the circulation and may be associated with acute respiratory distress syndrome or hepatorenal failure. The severe form more familiar to surgeons occurs when massive fibrinolysis intervenes to clear the thrombi. Bleeding follows at sites of endothelial damage when the clots are lysed. Tissue factor release induces factor VII activation with heightened coagulation. Additional microthrombi form. The cycle continues and eventually depletes or consumes the store of coagulation factors. Hence, DIC is categorized as a consumption coagulopathy [1].

Acute DIC results from an overwhelming and sudden clotting stimulus, such as a massive crush injury, or from a more moderate clotting stimulus accompanied by shock, as in sepsis or abruptio placentae. A slower, chronic, low-level DIC may occur in other circumstances such as fetal death with retained products of conception, cancer, or large aortic aneurysm [1,14,20].

The mechanisms by which septic shock induces DIC are well described in standard textbooks and are not repeated here.

DIC may result from acute hepatic insult, such as shock liver, massive hypotension-induced hepatic necrosis, massive hepatic trauma, acute massive hepatitis, or transplantation. It may also result from events in the setting of chronic liver failure ranging from sepsis to peritoneovenous shunt placement. Hepatic disease induces coagulopathy through reduction and abnormality of coagulation factors, prolonged circulating plasmin levels, reduced fibrinolysis, disordered platelet function, and sometimes through an associated thrombocytopenia.

DIC in the obstetric population is associated with abruptio placentae, amniotic fluid embolism, septic abortion, and, less commonly, with second-trimester saline-induced abortions. The low-grade DIC associated with retained products of conception may not manifest until 4 to 5 weeks after death of the fetus.

Malignancies, particularly slower-growing adenocarcinomas, are associated with a low-grade and chronic DIC. Chemotherapy, radiotherapy, and other modalities that induce tumor necrosis may accelerate the process. This problem may become more common as tumor angiogenesis inhibitors come to market.

A coagulopathy with mixed thrombotic/hemorrhagic features may result in bleeding from acute promyelocytic leukemia. It is accompanied by hypofibrinogenemia, increased fibrin degradation, and thrombocytopenia, possibly ascribable to platelet consumption. Blood products to correct the coagulopathy should be given before surgical intervention.

In trauma, DIC is common, particularly in the settings of head injury, multiple fractures with fat embolism, extensive soft tissue damage, and burns over large areas. Potential comorbidities that should be anticipated include shock, hypothermia, acidosis, sepsis, adult respiratory distress syndrome, adrenal failure, massive occult hemorrhage, and sepsis.

DIC has been reported after volume expansion with hydroxyethyl starch (hetastarch). The likelihood of bleeding correlates with age, duration of treatment, and dose (>5 mL/kg). The likelihood increases in the presence of renal failure and other underlying hemostatic defects [14,22,23].

DIC is associated with the administration of specific blood products under particular circumstances. These include the rapid transfusion of prothrombin complex concentrates to correct coagulopathy in patients who have liver disease, after warfarin administration, or after the administration of factor VII to correct deficiencies. The problem has been avoided by the addition of small concentrations of heparin to the mixture and slower administration. DIC has also been associated with recombinant factor VII administration. A dose–response effect has been reported [14].

Finally, the chronic low-grade DIC associated with vascular malformations and slowly expanding aortic aneurysms can transform into an acute DIC.

Principles of management in acute diffuse intravascular coagulation

The following principles guide the management of acute DIC [14]:

1. Diagnosis and treatment of the underlying precipitating factors responsible for the clotting stimulus (may require débridement and amputation of devitalized tissue, drainage of abscesses, or other, similar measures)
2. Cryoprecipitate infusion when fibrinogen levels are below 70 mg/dL and factor VIII-C is below 40%
3. FFP plasma when factor V levels are below 40%
4. Platelet transfusion to raise platelet count above 50,000 or 100,000, depending on the underlying clinical situation and the type of surgery performed (eg, above 100,000 after intracranial surgery)
5. Low doses of heparin if thrombin activation persists
6. Continuing to work toward normalization of the INR, replacement of blood volume, and restoration of hematocrit

In chronic DIC associated with malignancy, patients generally respond to low levels of heparin while undergoing chemotherapy.

In patients who have liver disease, FFP provides replacement of coagulation factors. If volume becomes a problem, diuresis or even plasmapharesis may be indicated. In the face of demonstrated excessive fibrinolysis *without DIC*, fibrinolysis inhibitors are recommended.

In patients undergoing repair of abdominal aneurysm, factor replacement usually suffices, although other stratagems are used as well [14].

After trauma, the emphasis is on volume replacement, treatment of sepsis, and blood product replacement as called for by assessment of clinical status and circulating coagulation factors.

Renal dysfunction and uremia

Renal failure induces platelet dysfunction. Some antibiotics and anti-inflammatory agents exacerbate this situation. The simplest diagnostic clinical assay is the bleeding time, which should be reserved, however, for patients who have adequate platelet counts ($>60,000$).

For prolonged bleeding times in the presence of abnormal bleeding, the treatment options include [14]

1. Desmopressin acetate at 0.3 µg/kg given intravenously over 20 to 30 minutes (second or third doses may be given, but tachyphylaxis is to be expected if the interval between doses is less than 3 to 5 days)
2. Transfusion of fresh platelets after dialysis
3. Conjugated estrogens at 0.6 mg/kg intravenously each day for 5 days (effect lasts about 2 weeks)
4. Correction of anemia (hematocrit $> 26\%$) with erythropoietin

The use of cryoprecipitate is controversial [14].

Uterine bleeding

Excessive uterine bleeding has been reported after minor surgical interventions, such as the placement of an intrauterine device or cone biopsy of the cervix, and after other uterine surgery in which no reason for hemorrhage could be found. Uterine bleeding of this nature has been ascribed to localized hyperfibrinolysis and to high uterine plasminogen activator activity. It has been linked statistically to the secretory phase of the menstrual cycle and to menstrual bleeding at the time of surgery.

The bleeding responds readily to antifibrinolytic agents including intravenous or oral ε-aminocaproic acid [14].

Postprostatectomy hemorrhage

Urinary urokinase that seeps into the surgical bed after prostatectomy may lead to increased local plasmin production and an anticoagulant effect attributable to local hyperfibrinolysis. The mechanism is similar to that ascribed to unanticipated uterine bleeding.

Antifibrinolytic agents successfully reduce bleeding in this setting as well. Bleeding responds to the administration of intravenous or oral ε-aminocaproic acid [14].

Posttransfusion coagulopathy

Coagulopathy may follow after the rapid replacement of two thirds of the body's blood volume. This level of transfusion is generally required only after massive trauma, although it may be called for in the course of vascular and oncologic surgery.

The roots of this problem lie in the changes that occur when whole blood is stored. After several days, the concentration of two thermolabile coagulation factors, V and VIII-C, is reduced by 15% to 50%. After 2 or 3 days, platelet function is lost.

Once transfused, platelets that do not function well are rapidly removed from circulation. As a result, bleeding time may be prolonged irrespective of the platelet count. A consumptive coagulopathy ensues frequently resulting in thrombocytopenia.

The scenario often includes massive tissue injury, hypotension, acidosis, hypoxia, some level of hepatorenal dysfunction, and hypothermia, all of which contribute to hemostatic defects and may result in DIC. McKenna [14], however, asserts that overtly decompensated DIC is uncommon in this setting [1].

Whole blood has the advantage of availability and volume. For the reasons outlined previously, however, transfusion with components of whole blood is theoretically preferable to whole blood transfusion. One protocol recommends transfusing one unit of FFP for every three to four units of

RBC when patients are expected to lose more than one unit of blood volume rapidly [14]. Platelet concentrates are used to correct bleeding time and treat thrombocytopenia.

The details of and controversies surrounding resuscitation theory are beyond the scope of this article, but the principle of choosing blood components over whole blood when possible and of anticipating a multifactorial coagulopathy in the setting of massive transfusion is broadly accepted [1]. Treatment should involve replacement of diluted factors by FFP, cryoprecipitate, calcium, and platelets. Replacement is continued until coagulation parameters normalize. Bleeding from non-technical causes should then cease.

Posttransfusion purpura syndrome

Posttransfusion purpura syndrome refers to the sudden onset of severe thrombocytopenia 7 to 10 days after transfusion of RBC, FFP, or platelets. The thrombocytopenia is accompanied by sudden and dramatic hemorrhage. Mortality from intracranial hemorrhage is high. The differential diagnosis includes sepsis and drug-induced thrombocytopenia. The population at greatest risk seems to be multiparous women. Sensitization is generally attributed to pregnancy or, less commonly, to previous transfusions of blood products.

The syndrome is a form of transfusion reaction. It occurs when the human platelet antigen (HPA-1a) antigen in blood products elicits an anti-HPA-1a antibody in the 2.5% of whites and 0.5% of African Americans who lack the antigen. The precise mechanisms that lead to platelet destruction are not understood.

The management of posttransfusion purpura syndrome involves urgent platelet transfusion after the documentation of posttransfusion purpura syndrome antibodies in a serum sample. This treatment may seem counterintuitive, but the intention is to deplete the store of available anti-HPA-1a platelet antibodies through the destruction of newly supplied HPA-1a-positive platelets while simultaneously depending on the non-antigenic platelets and on platelet fragments to assist in hemostasis and control the bleeding.

Plasmapharesis scrubs the antibodies in 80% of the cases, and intravenous IgG blocks further antigen–antibody reactions. Steroids may be useful in nonspecific indications such as vascular support and treatment of overall stress [14].

Hemophilia

Hemophilia rarely enters the differential diagnosis in the absence of a personal or family history of bleeding. There are three common forms. Type A involves a deficiency of factor VIII, type B involves a deficiency of factor IX, and type C involves a deficiency of factor XI.

The diagnosis is made through specific factor analysis. Treatment involves replacement of the factor or factors that are deficient. After extensive transfusions, hemophiliac patients may develop antibodies to blood products or to bioengineered factors of recombinant origin, such as recombinant activated factor VII.

There are approximately 20 approved products on the market providing some combination of factor VIII replacement, factor IX replacement, or von Willebrand's factor replacement. Approximately 20% are recombinant, 5% are porcine derived, and the rest are plasma derived. Each of the six products supplying von Willebrand's factor also provides factor VIII replacement. Most surgeons will want to seek consultation to oversee the treatment of congenital or familial blood dyscrasias and provide long-term follow-up.

Summary

The risks and complications associated with postoperative bleeding can be substantially reduced through measures such as adequate preoperative assessment; the identification and correction of deficiencies in circulating clotting factors, in platelet number and function, in hematocrit and blood volume, and body temperature; and the treatment of infection. It is important to optimize the condition of the patient before surgery.

A risk–benefit calculus is always at play. If surgery can be delayed until all pertinent problems are identified and addressed, so much the better. If not, the patient's risk may be reduced by choosing a less invasive or less radical procedure, by appropriate preoperative consultations, by staging the operation, by judicious choice of anesthetic technique, by operating on an inpatient rather than an outpatient basis, and by arranging in advance for adequate postoperative monitoring and the appropriate intensity of care.

This article has addressed the prevention and management of postoperative hemorrhage. For reasons of focus and space, it has not addressed two important and related subjects: the management of chronic anticoagulation and the problem of prophylaxis for deep vein thrombosis in the perioperative period. Whenever possible, the patient should go to surgery with normal coagulation parameters. The decision to proceed despite abnormal coagulation parameters (within therapeutic range or not) is equivalent to deciding either that the risk of intraoperative and postoperative hemorrhage is of lesser consequence to the patient's overall welfare than a delay, or that no marginal benefit will accrue from normalizing coagulation. This decision may well be in the patient's best interests. The consent obtained for surgery ought to reflect in detail the thinking and discussion that surrounded the decision.

Acknowledgments

Dr. Rodney Falk provided important insights and perspective.

Appendix 1

Prothrombin time and international normalized ratio

The traditional method of determining the efficacy of anticoagulation therapy is the prothrombin time (PT). A blood sample is collected in a tube containing citrated sodium. After centrifugation, a specific volume of thromboplastin reagent is added. The interval until a fibrin clot forms, measured in seconds, is reported as the PT. The thromboplastin reagent can be either an extract of mammalian tissue (lungs heart or brain of animals) rich in tissue factor or a recombinant proportion of human tissue factor in combination with phospholipids. The sensitivity of individual thromboplastin reagents is variable. Higher sensitivity results in prolonged PT. Sensitivity is also affected by shelf life.

The international normalized ratio (INR) corrects for potential variability by calibrating results against a standardized measure of the sensitivity of the thromboplastin reagents used. It has become a standard for monitoring oral anticoagulant therapy and serves the same purpose as the PT. The prothrombin time ratio relates the observed PT (in seconds) to each laboratory's calculated mean normal PT (in seconds).

Target anticoagulation ranges are commonly expressed in terms of INRs: while a range of 2.0 to 3.0 is recommended for most indications, a range of 2.5 to 3.5 is recommended for patients at higher risk (eg, those with mechanical prosthetic heart valves). The INR alone is insufficient to assess coagulopathy.

Hirsh and Poller [24] provide a fuller discussion.

References

[1] Owings JT, Gosselin RC. Bleeding and transfusion. In: Wilmore WW, Cheung LY, Harken AH, et al, editors. American College of Surgeons surgery principles and practice. Chicago: American College of Surgeons; 2001. p. 77–90.

[2] Comprehensive accreditation manual for hospitals: the official handbook. Oakbrook Terrace (IL): Joint Commission on the Accreditation of Healthcare Organizations; 1998.

[3] Litaker D. Preoperative screening. Med Clin North Am 1999;83:1565–81.

[4] Smetana GW, Macpherson DS. The case against routine preoperative laboratory testing. Med Clin North Am 2003;87:7–40.

[5] Turnbull JM, Buck C. The value of pre-operative screening investigations in otherwise healthy individuals. Arch Intern Med 1987;147:1101–5.

[6] Roizen MF. More preoperative assessment by physicians and less by laboratory tests. N Engl J Med 2000;342:204–5.

[7] Charpak Y, Blery C, Chastang C, et al. Usefulness of selectively ordered preoperative tests. Med Care 1988;26:95–104.

[8] Macpherson DS, Snow R, Lofren RP. Preoperative screening; value of previous tests. Ann Intern Med 1990;113:969–73.

[9] Dzankic S, Pastor D, Gonzales C, et al. The prevalence and predictive value of abnormal preoperative laboratory tests in elderly surgical patients. Anesth Analg 2001;93:301–8.

[10] Sanders DP, McKinney FW, Harris WH. Clinical evaluation and cost effectiveness of pre-operative laboratory assessment on patients undergoing total hip arthroplasty. Orthopedics 1989;12:1449–53.

[11] Faris PM, Spence RK, Larhol KM, et al. The predictive power of baseline hemoglobin for transfusion risk in surgery patients. Orthopedics 1999;22(Suppl):S135–40.

[12] Rohrer M, Mechelotti M, Nahrwold D. A prospective evaluation of the efficacy of preoper-ative coagulation testing. Ann Surg 1988;208:554–7.

[13] Cobas M. Preoperative assessment of coagulation disorders. Int Anesthesiol Clin 2001;39: 1–15.

[14] McKenna R. Abnormal coagulation in the postoperative period contributing to excessive bleeding. Med Clin North Am 2001;85:1277–310.

[15] Kereiakis DJ, Berkowitz SD, Lincoff AM, et al. Clinical correlates and course of thrombo-cytopenia during percutaneous coronary intervention in the era of abciximab platelet glyco-protein IIb/IIIa blockade. Am Heart J 2000;14:74–80.

[16] Bennet CL, Connors JM, Carwille JM, et al. Thrombotic thrombocytopenic purpura asso-ciated with clopidogrel. N Engl J Med 2000;342:1773–7.

[17] Bellan L. Preoperative testing for cataract surgery. Can J Ophthalmol 1994;29:111–4.

[18] Simon TL, Alverson DC, AuBuchon J, et al. Practice parameters for the use of red blood cell transfusions: developed by the Red Blood Cell Administration Practice Guideline Develop-ment Task Force of the College of American Pathologists. Arch Pathol Lab Med 1998;122: 130–8.

[19] Despotis GJ, Levine V, Saleem R, et al. Use of point-of-care test in identification of patients who can benefit from desmopressin during cardiac surgery: a randomized controlled trial. Lancet 1999;354:106–10.

[20] Warkentin TE, Levine MN, Hirsch J, et al. Heparin-induced thrombocytopenia in patients treated with low-molecular-weight heparin or unfractionated heparin. N Engl J Med 1995; 332:1330–5.

[21] McKenna R, Walenga JM. Alpha 2-plasma inhibitor (a2-PI) deficiency. E Medicine Journal (serial online) 2001. Available from: http://www.emedicine.com/medicine,obstetrics and gynecology, psychiatry and surgery/109.htm. Accessed September 2, 2005.

[22] Strauss RG, Stump DC, Henriksen RA. Hydroxyethyl starch accentuates von Willebrand's disease. Transfusion 1985;25:234–7.

[23] Symington BE. Hetastarch and bleeding complications. Ann Intern Med 1986;105:627–8.

[24] Hirsh J, Poller L. International normalized ratio: a guide to understanding and correcting its problems. Arch Int Med 1994;154:282–8.

SURGICAL
CLINICS OF
NORTH AMERICA

Surg Clin N Am 85 (2005) 1215–1227

Perioperative Anemia

Lena M. Napolitano, MD[a,b,]*

[a]*University of Michigan School of Medicine, Ann Arbor, MI, USA*
[b]*Department of Surgery, University of Michigan Medical Center,*
1500 East Medical Center Drive, 1C340 University Hospital,
Box 0033, Ann Arbor, MI 48109-0033, USA

Anemia refers to red blood cell (RBC) mass, amount of hemoglobin (Hb), or volume of RBCs less than normal, determined either as an hematocrit or Hb concentration more than 2 standard deviation below the normal mean for age in children or below the lower limit of normal values in adults. The World Health Organization chose 12.5 g/dL as the normative value for both adult men and women. In the United States, limits of 13.5 g/dL for men and 12.5 g/dL for women are more realistic. Using these values, approximately 4% of men and 8% of women in the United States have anemia.

Perioperative anemia is a common occurrence and is associated with increased need for blood transfusion in the perioperative period. Perioperative anemia has also been linked to increased morbidity and mortality in surgical patients [1]. Some studies suggest that higher Hb concentrations are associated with better early functional recovery [2]. Anemia may impede a patient's ability to recover fully and participate in postoperative rehabilitation [3].

Pre- and postoperative anemia and the resultant increased need for blood transfusion are independent risk factors for postoperative infection, longer hospital stay, and death in noncardiac surgical patients. In the United States, 55% of RBC transfusions (6.6 million units annually) are administered to elective surgical patients.

Treatment of perioperative anemia has been shown to decrease the need for RBC transfusion and improve patient outcome. A rational approach, therefore, is to establish the diagnosis of anemia early enough preoperatively to be able to proceed with a diagnostic workup and initiation of appropriate treatment.

---

* Correspondence. Department of Surgery, University of Michigan Health System, Room 1C340, University Hospital, 1500 East Medical Center Drive, Ann Arbor, MI 48109.
E-mail address: lenan@umich.edu

doi:10.1016/j.suc.2005.10.012   *surgical.theclinics.com*

Prevalence and epidemiology

One third to one half of surgical patients may be anemic preoperatively because of the conditions for which they require surgery (ie, cancer, gastrointestinal bleeding) or underlying medical conditions associated with anemia. Perioperative anemia prevalence varies because of three factors: (1) differences in definition of anemia, (2) differences in surgical procedures and associated blood loss, and (3) differences in patients and comorbidities.

A large study examining the incidence of perioperative anemia used prospective data from the National Surgical Quality Improvement Program, an ongoing observational study based at Veterans Affairs Medical Centers, and included 6301 noncardiac surgical patients [4]. Anemia (defined as an hematocrit less than 36%) was present preoperatively in 39% of the patients. During the perioperative period the subgroup that had preoperative anemia required five times more blood than nonanemic patients. This study also documented that transfusion of more than four units of blood increased the risk of death by a factor of 2.84 and increased the risk of perioperative infection by a factor of 9.28 by logistic regression analysis.

Anemia was present postoperatively in 84.1% of patients. The incidence of postoperative infection increased from 2.6% to 5% with increasing degrees of anemia, and 92% of all infections occurred in patients who had anemia. Postoperative anemia, intraoperative transfusion, and transfusion of more than four units of blood were also significant predictors of increased length of hospital stay ($P < .001$).

Multiple logistic regression analysis documented that low preoperative hematocrit, low postoperative hematocrit, and increased blood transfusion rates were associated with increased mortality ($P < .01$), increased postoperative pneumonia ($P \leq .05$), and increased length of hospital stay ($P < .05$). The mean age of patients in this study was 61 years. Anemia is more prevalent with increasing age.

Anemia is common in patients who have cancer and is associated with reduced survival. The incidence of preoperative anemia (defined as a Hb level < 12.0 g/dL) was assessed in 1688 patients who underwent curative resection for gastric cancer. Preoperative anemia was present in 39.9% of the patients. The 10-year overall survival rate in anemic patients was 48.2%, versus 62.6% in nonanemic patients ($P < .001$). Multivariate analysis confirmed that anemia was an independent prognostic predictor in patients who had stage I and stage II disease ($P = .007$; relative risk, 1.466; 95% CI, 1.109–1.937) [5].

The high incidence of preoperative anemia (46.1%) in patients who have colorectal cancer (n = 311) was identified in a single-institution cohort study [6]. Preoperative anemia was most common in patients who had right colon cancer (incidence 57.6%), followed by left colon cancer (42.2%) and rectal cancer (29.8%). Patients who had right colon cancer had significantly lower

preoperative hematocrits than patients who had left colon cancer (33 ±
8.5 versus 36 ± 7.4; *P* < .01) or rectal cancer (33 ± 8.5 versus 38 ± 6.0;
P < .0001). Age was not a significant risk factor for preoperative anemia in
colorectal cancer.

To understand the prevalence of anemia in surgical patients (with a primary focus on preoperative anemia) and the impact that pre-existing anemia
has on transfusion rates as well as on clinical and functional outcomes, a systematic review was performed of articles published between January 1966
and February 2003 [7]. The estimates of anemia prevalence in the literature
ranged widely, from 5% in geriatric women who had hip fracture to 75.8%
in patients who had Duke's stage D colon cancer. Diagnosis of anemia was
most strongly associated with an increased risk of receiving an allogeneic
blood transfusion.

Preoperative anemia and outcome

Preoperative Hb levels were inversely related to operative mortality in
surgical patients. A preoperative Hb concentration of less than 8 g/dL
was associated with a 16.2-fold increased mortality rate compared with patients who did not have anemia preoperatively [8]. Preoperative anemia has
also been associated with a decreased overall survival in patients who have
lung cancer [9].

Previous studies have also documented that patients who have preoperative anemia and cardiovascular disease have a higher mortality rate than patients who have preoperative anemia alone (Fig. 1) [10]. Blood transfusion is
commonly used for the treatment of anemia in the perioperative period, and
blood transfusion is also an independent risk factor for adverse outcome in
surgery. It has been difficult to separate anemia and blood transfusion as independent risk factors in these clinical studies.

The impact of preoperative anemia and blood transfusion on survival in
patients who have resected non–small cell lung cancer (n = 439) was recently

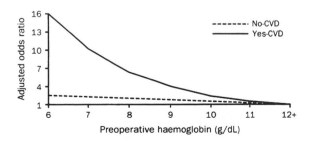

Fig. 1. The association between preoperative anemia, cardiovascular disease, and mortality in
surgical patients. CVD, cardiovascular disease. (*From* Carson JL, Duff A, Poses RM, et al. Effect of anaemia and cardiovascular disease on surgical mortality and morbidity. Lancet
1996;348(9034):1057; with permission.)

examined. Survival was lower in patients who had Hb concentrations equal to or less than 10 g/dL than in those who had Hb concentrations higher than 10 g/dL ($P = .012$) and survival was lower in the transfused population ($P = .046$). At multivariate analysis, independent prognostic indicators included patient age, pathologic stage, and preoperative Hb concentration. This study suggests that anemia could represent an important prognostic factor in resected lung cancer, and correction of anemia before surgical intervention may be an effective strategy for improving outcome [11].

Anemia is common in patients who have cancer; a recent systematic literature search (1966–2003) identified the prevalence of anemia in specific cancers and assessed the impact of anemia on survival and quality of life [12]. Anemia prevalence varied widely; most studies found that between 30% and 90% of patients who had cancer had anemia. Prevalence was affected strongly by the definition of anemia: 7% of patients who had Hodgkin disease had anemia when the condition was defined as a Hb concentration lower than 9 g/dL; as many as 86% of patients had anemia when it was defined as a Hb concentration lower than 11 g/dL. Prevalence varied by cancer type and disease stage: 40% of patients who had early-stage colon tumors and nearly 80% of patients who had advanced disease had anemia. Patients who had anemia had poorer survival and local tumor control than did their nonanemic counterparts in 15 of 18 studies. In 8 of 12 studies, patients who did not have anemia (most treated with epoetin) needed fewer transfusions. Quality of life was positively correlated with Hb concentration in 15 of 16 studies. There was no significant difference in treatment toxicity between patients who did and did not have anemia. Tumor hypoxia, which has been associated with resistance to radiation therapy and chemotherapy, may stimulate angiogenesis, leading to poor local control of tumors and increased morbidity and mortality. Treatment of anemia may have a significant effect on patient survival and quality of life. Given these findings, consideration should be given to establishing preoperative protocols for early diagnosis and correction of anemia in all patients who have cancer and who are scheduled for surgical intervention.

Pathophysiology

Perioperative anemia has many potential causes (Box 1), including chronic blood loss (hemorrhoids, gastrointestinal tumors, peptic ulcer disease, bleeding disorders), nutritional deficiencies (iron, vitamin B_{12}, folate deficiency), hematologic abnormalities (sickle-cell anemia, hemolytic anemia) and chronic diseases (renal or hepatic insufficiency).

A large number of patients who require surgery manifest the anemia of chronic disease (ACD). ACD is the second most prevalent anemia after anemia caused by iron deficiency and occurs in patients who have acute or chronic immune activation [13]. ACD is driven by the immune system. Cytokines and cells of the reticuloendothelial system induce changes in iron homeostasis

Box 1. Potential causes of anemia in surgical patients

Genetic
 Hemoglobinopathies
 Thalassemias
 Enzyme abnormalities of the glycolytic pathways
 Defects of the RBC cytoskeleton
 Congenital dyserythropoietic anemia
 Rh-null disease
 Hereditary xerocytosis
 Abetalipoproteinemia
 Fanconi anemia
Nutritional
 Iron deficiency
 Vitamin B_{12} deficiency
 Folate deficiency
 Starvation and generalized malnutrition
Hemorrhage
Immunologic- or antibody-mediated abnormalities
Physical effects
 Trauma
 Burns
 Frostbite
 Prosthetic valves and surfaces
Drugs and chemicals
 Aplastic anemia
 Megaloblastic anemia
Chronic diseases and malignancies
 Renal disease
 Hepatic disease
 Chronic infections
 Neoplasia
 Collagen vascular diseases
Infections
 Viral: hepatitis, infectious mononucleosis, cytomegalovirus
 Bacterial: clostridia, gram-negative sepsis
 Protozoal: malaria, leishmaniasis, toxoplasmosis
Thrombotic thrombocytopenic purpura and hemolytic uremic
 syndrome

(diversion of iron from the circulation into the reticuloendothelial system resulting in iron-restricted erythropoiesis), reduced proliferation of erythroid progenitor cells, reduced production of erythropoietin, and reduced life span of RBCs, all of which contribute to the pathogenesis of anemia.

Diagnosis

Preoperative anemia is easily diagnosed and treated. All patients should be carefully evaluated for anemia during the preoperative evaluation [14]. A detailed history and physical examination constitute the most important elements of the perioperative evaluation of patients for anemia. A complete blood cell count is commonly obtained before surgery simply to ensure that the patient has an adequate hematocrit. This value should be reviewed; if it is abnormal, additional diagnostic testing is usually required.

If a surgical patient is anemic preoperatively, a diagnostic workup a month or two before surgery is recommended to provide adequate time for initiation of appropriate treatment after diagnosis is established. It is important to differentiate between the two most common anemia diagnoses, iron-deficiency anemia and ACD (Fig. 2). The mainstays of therapy for ACD are erythropoietic agents and supplemental iron therapy.

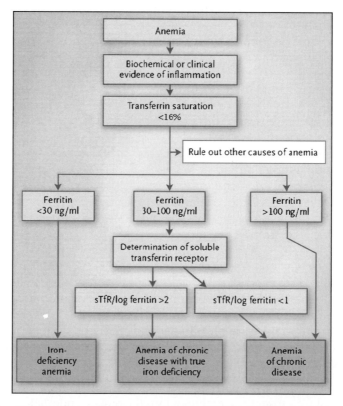

Fig. 2. Algorithm for differential diagnosis of anemia. STfR/log ferritin, ratio of the concentration of soluble transferrin receptor to the log of the serum ferritin level in conventional units. (*From* Weiss G, Goodnough LT. Anemia of chronic disease. N Engl J Med 2005;352:1020; with permission.)

Treatment of anemia

The evaluation and treatment of anemia play an important role in the perioperative period. It is important to define the cause of anemia and to institute appropriate corrective therapy. Correction of anemia preoperatively can minimize the amount of blood the patient will be exposed to in the operating room and in the postoperative period.

Anemia treatment strategies include iron, vitamin B_{12}, or folate supplementation, administration of recombinant human erythropoietin (rHuEpo), and blood transfusion.

Iron, folate, or vitamin B_{12} deficiency

For patients who have diagnosed vitamin (vitamin B_{12}, folate) or iron deficiency, initiation of appropriate replacement therapy is easily accomplished preoperatively. For patients who have anemia of chronic disease (renal insufficiency or failure, cancer), the mainstay of treatment is recombinant rHuEpo and concomitant iron supplementation.

Recombinant human erythropoietin

The availability of rHuEpo for the treatment of anemia offers an option in selected patients to reduce or eliminate the need for RBC transfusion. A number of studies have documented that the use of rHuEpo preoperatively is associated with a significant reduction in the number of blood transfusions in the perioperative period.

A double-blind, placebo-controlled trial in 30 patients who had colorectal cancer and anemia randomly assigned patients to receive rHuEpo, 150 IU/kg body weight subcutaneously every 2 days from 10 days before surgery to 2 days after surgery [15]. Twenty patients were randomly assigned to receive rHuEpo, and 10 were assigned to placebo treatment. No supplemental iron was administered. rHuEpo therapy was associated with increased Hb ($P = .069$) and increased reticulocyte count ($P = .0004$) but with no difference in blood transfusion rates. Low ferritin was associated with a decreased Hb response in the rHuEpo group. The authors concluded that hematopoiesis in anemic patients can be stimulated by rHuEpo, but clinical efficacy is limited in patients who have decreased iron availability. A significant deficiency of this trial was the lack of use of iron supplementation to achieve maximal erythropoietin efficacy.

Another double-blind, placebo-controlled trial enrolled 100 patients who had preoperative anemia (Hb < 8.5 g/dL) and randomly assigned patients to receive rHuEpo, 300 IU/kg body weight on day 4 before surgery and 150 IU/kg body weight for the following 7 days. All patients received oral iron (200 mg daily × 4). The use of rHuEpo was associated with a significant reduction in RBC transfusion (0.3 versus 1.6 units transfused, $P < .05$) and no difference in discharge Hb (7.8 versus 7.2, respectively) [16].

A small double-blind, placebo-controlled study (n = 58) in anemic patients who had head and neck cancer (prestudy Hb ≥ 10.0 g/dL and ≤ 13.5 g/dL) administered rHuEpo, 600 IU/kg body weight for a total of three doses pre-operatively. All patients received oral iron (150 mg iron sulfate two times/d). The rHuEpo patients manifested increased mean Hb on day of surgery ($P = .016$), increased hematocrit ($P = .015$), increased reticulocyte count ($P < .001$), and resultant transfusion avoidance in 34.5% of patients [17].

The efficacy of rHuEpo in patients undergoing surgery for gastrointestinal tract malignancies was investigated in a double-blind, placebo-controlled trial (n = 63) with rHuEpo dosing of 300 IU/kg body weight. All patients received 100 mg iron intravenously. Medications were administered for at least 7 days before and 7 days after the operation. Patients who received rHuEpo received significantly fewer blood transfusions intraoperatively and postoperatively, had significantly higher hematocrit, Hb, and reticulocyte count, had reduced postoperative complications, and had improved 1-year survival [18].

The European Epoetin Alfa Surgery Trial enrolled patients undergoing orthopedic surgery with preoperative Hb concentrations between 10 and 13 g/dL (epoetin n = 460; control n = 235) in an open, randomized, controlled multicenter trial [19]. Epoetin-treated patients had higher Hb values from the day of surgery until discharge ($P < .001$) and lower transfusion rates (12% versus 46%, $P < .001$). Epoetin treatment had no significant effect on postoperative recovery, but the time to ambulation and the time to discharge was longer in transfused patients than in nontransfused patients.

Epoetin efficacy has also been investigated in anemic patients who have colorectal cancer (n = 223) scheduled for surgery [20]. Patients were randomly assigned to receive epoetin alfa, 150 or 300 IU/kg/d subcutaneously for 12 days (from day 10 before surgery to day 1 after surgery) or to a control group. All received iron (200 mg/d by mouth) for 10 days before surgery. Mean Hb levels were significantly higher in the 300 IU/kg group than in the control group, both 1 day before surgery ($P = .008$) and 1 day after surgery ($P = .011$). Blood loss during and after surgery was similar in all groups. Patients who received epoetin alfa 300 IU/kg required significantly fewer perioperative transfusion units than control patients (0.81 versus 1.32; $P = .016$) and significantly fewer postoperative units (0.87 versus 1.33; $P = .023$). This study documented that preoperative epoetin alfa (300 IU/d) increased Hb in patients undergoing colorectal surgery and was associated with a reduced need for perioperative and postoperative transfusions.

Daily or every-other-day dosing of rHuEpo is cumbersome, and clinical studies have documented similar efficacy with rHuEpo daily and weekly dosing in the preoperative period [21].

The strategy of preoperative weekly dosing of rHuEpo recommends initiating the first dose 21 days preoperatively, continuing weekly dosing of 40,000 units subcutaneously for a total of four doses before surgery, and administering an additional dose postoperatively. Iron supplementation is recommended in all patients because rHuEpo stimulates bone marrow production of RBCs and requires increased iron for maximal efficacy.

Blood transfusion

A recent review of 62 studies (observational or interventional) examined variables and patient characteristics associated with allogeneic RBC transfusion in surgical patients. Preoperative anemia was documented as a significant risk factor for blood transfusion in 46 studies. Advancing age and female gender, both associated with a higher rate of preoperative anemia, were also associated with increased risk for perioperative blood transfusion [22]. An observational study in 307 patients examined predictors of blood transfusion in patients undergoing cardiac surgery and confirmed preoperative anemia as a significant risk factor by multivariate analysis [23].

The "10/30" (Hb/hematocrit) rule has long been recognized in the medical community as the threshold for transfusion in the perioperative setting, but this rule has recently been challenged [24]. An increasing number of publications suggest there is no absolute threshold for blood transfusion for anemia and that this decision should be based solely on a physiologic assessment of each patient. Blood transfusion should be reserved for patients manifesting physiologic indications for transfusion, including tachycardia and hypotension.

Transfusion of RBCs is useful in restoring oxygen-carrying capacity in patients who have symptomatic anemia. In general, physicians should avoid transfusing blood based on the criterion of Hb concentration alone. Instead, they should focus on the impact of anemia on the patient's symptoms and level of activity. The concern for HIV infection and viral hepatitis has served to highlight the potential risks associated with homologous transfusion therapy [25]. These concerns, along with possible alternatives, should be considered carefully before a decision is made to transfuse.

A recent meta-analysis reported the relationship of allogeneic blood transfusion to postoperative bacterial infection in surgical patients and included 20 peer-reviewed articles published from 1986 to 2000 [26]. The total number of subjects included in this meta-analysis was 13,152 (5215 in the transfused group and 7937 in the nontransfused group). The common odds ratio for all articles included in this meta-analysis evaluating the association of allogeneic blood transfusion to the incidence of postoperative bacterial infection was 3.45 (range, 1.43–15.15), with 17 of the 20 studies demonstrating a value of $P \leq .05$. These results provide overwhelming evidence that allogeneic blood transfusion is associated with a significantly increased risk of postoperative bacterial infection in the surgical patient. The common odds ratio of the subgroup of trauma patients was 5.263 (range, 5.03–5.43), with all studies showing a value of $P < .05$ (0.005–0.0001). These results demonstrate that allogeneic blood transfusion is an associated and apparently significant and frequently overlooked risk factor for the development of postoperative bacterial infection in the surgical patient. Allogeneic blood transfusion is a greater risk factor for the development of postoperative bacterial infection in traumatically injured patients than in patients undergoing elective surgery.

Guidelines for blood transfusion have been issued by several organizations, including a consensus conference of the National Institutes of Health [27], the American College of Physicians [28], the American Society of Anesthesiology [29], and the Canadian Medical Association [30]. The guidelines recommend that in patients without known risk factors, the threshold for transfusion should be a Hb level in the range of 6.0 to 8.0 g/dL. They also indicate that patients who have Hb levels higher than 10 g/dL are unlikely to benefit from blood transfusion.

Possible indications for RBC transfusion include

- Otherwise stable patients, if the Hb level is below 7 g/d
- Patients who have cardiovascular disease, if the Hb level is below 9 to 10 g/dL
- Bleeding patients, if anticipated blood loss will result in the Hb level falling below the transfusion thresholds listed previously
- Patients who have symptomatic anemia

Despite the guideline recommendations, it has been documented that transfusion rates for standard surgical procedures vary significantly among institutions [31]. This recent study documented variation in transfusion practice following repair of hip fracture or cardiac surgery and in patients requiring intensive care following a surgical intervention or multiple trauma (high-risk patients). Rates of allogeneic RBC transfusion were reported in 41,568 patients admitted to 11 hospitals across Canada between August 1998 and August 2000 as part of a retrospective observational cohort study. In the subgroup of 7552 patients receiving RBCs, the author and colleagues also compared mean nadir Hb concentrations from center to center. The overall rate of RBC transfusion was 38.7% and ranged from 23.8% to 51.9% across centers. Women were more likely to be transfused than men (43.7% versus 35.3%, $P < .0001$), with higher rates of transfusion in 8 of 11 centers. Compared with a chosen reference hospital that had a crude transfusion rate near the median, the adjusted odds of transfusion ranged from 0.44 to 1.53 overall, from 0.42 to 1.22 in patients undergoing a hip fracture repair, from 0.72 to 3.17 in patients undergoing cardiac surgery, and from 0.27 to 1.11 in critically ill and trauma patients. In the 7552 transfused patients, the mean adjusted nadir Hb was 7.4 ± 4.8 g/dL overall and ranged from 6.7 to 8.5 g/dL across centers.

Preventive strategies for perioperative anemia

A number of strategies are available for the prevention of anemia in the perioperative period, including attempts to minimize diagnostic blood testing and the use of low-volume adult or pediatric sampling tubes, surgical techniques to minimize blood loss intraoperatively, perioperative cell salvage and autotransfusion, acute normovolemic hemodilution, and the prompt evaluation and correction of any bleeding disorders or complications.

Perioperative cell salvage and autotransfusion have been documented to decrease blood usage significantly following surgery [32,33]. In a randomized clinical trial of intraoperative autotransfusion in patients undergoing surgery for abdominal aortic aneurysm, the use of autotransfusion effectively reduced the need for blood transfusion and also was associated with a reduced incidence of postoperative systemic inflammatory response syndrome and infectious complications [34].

It has been documented that transfusion-free surgery can be accomplished successfully, even in the conduct of complex surgical procedures such as cardiac surgery and hepatic transplantation [35]. In these cases, however, special attention is paid to the preoperative treatment of anemia to increase Hb concentration preoperatively and to the intraoperative use of acute normovolemic hemodilution and intraoperative cell salvage.

Summary

Perioperative anemia is common and is associated with increased need for blood transfusion. Preoperative assessment of patients for the presence of anemia is necessary with subsequent diagnostic workup to evaluate the potential cause of anemia. Preoperative treatment of anemia based on the diagnostic cause is associated with a reduction in the need for blood transfusion in the perioperative period. Additional advances in surgical technology that reduce blood loss intraoperatively are associated with a reduction in postoperative anemia and should be used whenever possible. All strategies to prevent anemia in the perioperative period should be considered in an effort to minimize exposure of surgical patients to blood transfusion.

References

[1] Kuriyan M, Carson JL. Anemia and clinical outcomes. Anesthesiol Clin North America 2005;23(2):315–25 [vii.].
[2] Lawrence VA, Silverstein JH, Cornell JE, et al. Higher Hb level is associated with better early functional recovery after hip fracture repair. Transfusion 2003;43(12):1717–22.
[3] Carson JL, Terrin ML, Jay M. Anemia and postoperative rehabilitation. Can J Anaesth 2003;50(6 Suppl):S60–4.
[4] Dunne J, Malone D, Tracy JK, et al. Perioperative anemia: an independent risk factor for infection, mortality and resource utilization in surgery. J Surg Res 2002;102(2):237–44.
[5] Shen JG, Cheong JH, Huyng WJ, et al. Pretreatment anemia is associated with poorer survival in patients with stage I and II gastric cancer. J Surg Oncol 2005;91(2):126–30.
[6] Dunne JR, Gannon CJ, Osborn TM, et al. Preoperative anemia in colon cancer: assessment of risk factors. Am Surg 2002;68(6):582–7.
[7] Shander A, Knight K, Thurer R, et al. Prevalence and outcomes of anemia in surgery: a systematic review of the literature. Am J Med 2004;116(7A):58S–69S.

[8] Carson JL, Poses RM, Spence RK, et al. Severity of anaemia and operative mortality and morbidity. Lancet 1988;1(8588):727–9.

[9] Jazieh AR, Hussain M, Howington JA, et al. Prognostic factors in patients with surgically resected stages I and II non-small cell lung cancer. Ann Thorac Surg 2000;70:1168–71.

[10] Carson JL, Duff A, Poses RM, et al. Effect of anaemia and cardiovascular disease on surgical mortality and morbidity. Lancet 1996;348(9034):1055–60.

[11] Berardi R, Brunelli A, Tamburrano T, et al. Perioperative anemia and blood transfusions as prognostic factors in patients undergoing resection for non-small cell lung cancers. Lung Cancer 2005;49(3):371–6.

[12] Knight K, Wade S, Balducci L. Prevalence and outcomes of anemia in cancer: a systematic review of the literature. Am J Med 2004;116(Suppl 7A):11S–26S.

[13] Weiss G, Goodnough LT. Anemia of chronic disease. N Engl J Med 2005;352:1011–23.

[14] Armas-Loughran B, Kalra R, Carson JL. Evaluation and management of anemia and bleeding disorders in surgical patients. Med Clin North Am 2003;87(1):229–42.

[15] Heiss MM, Tarabichi A, Delanoff C, et al. Perisurgical erythropoietin application in anemic patients with colorectal cancer: a double-blind randomized study. Surgery 1996;119(5):523–7.

[16] Qvist N, Boesby S, Wolff B, et al. Recombinant human erythropoietin and hemoglobin concentration at operation and during the postoperative period: reduced need for blood transfusions in patients undergoing colorectal surgery—prospective double-blind placebo-controlled study. World J Surg 1999;23(1):30–5.

[17] Scott SN, Boeve TJ, McCulloch TM, et al. The effects of epoetin alfa on transfusion requirements in head and neck cancer patients: a prospective, randomized, placebo-controlled study. Laryngoscopy 2002;112(7 Pt 1):1221–9.

[18] Kosmadakis N, Messaris E, Maris A, et al. Perioperative erythropoietin administration in patients with gastrointestinal tract cancer: prospective randomized double-blind study. Ann Surg 2003;237(3):417–21.

[19] Weber EW, Slappendel R, Hemon Y, et al. Effects of epoetin alfa on blood transfusions and postoperative recovery in orthopaedic surgery: the European Epoetin Alfa Surgery Trial (EEST). Eur J Anaesthesiol 2005;22(4):249–57.

[20] Christodoulakis M, Tsiftsis DD. Preoperative epoetin alfa in colorectal surgery: a randomized, controlled study. Ann Surg Oncol 2005;12(9):718–25.

[21] Goldberg MA, McCutchen JW, Jove M, et al. A safety and efficacy comparison study of two dosing regimens of epoetin alfa in patients undergoing major orthopedic surgery. Am J Orthop 1996;25(8):544–52.

[22] Khanna MP, Hebert PC, Fergusson DA. Review of the clinical practice literature on patient characteristics associated with perioperative allogeneic red blood cell transfusion. Transfus Med Rev 2003;17(2):110–9.

[23] Moskowitz DM, Klein JJ, Shander A, et al. Predictors of transfusion requirements for cardiac surgical procedures at a blood conservation center. Ann Thorac Surg 2004;77(2):626–34.

[24] Carson JL, Willett LR. Is a hemoglobin of 10 g/dL required for surgery? Med Clin North Am 1993;77(2):335–47.

[25] Jain R. Use of blood transfusion in management of anemia. Med Clin North Am 1992;76(3):727–44.

[26] Hill GE, Frawley WH, Griffith KE, et al. Allogeneic blood transfusion increases the risk of postoperative bacterial infection: a meta-analysis. J Trauma 2003;54(5):908–14.

[27] Consensus conference. Perioperative red blood cell transfusion. JAMA 1988;260:2700–3.

[28] American College of Physicians. Practice strategies for elective red blood cell transfusion. Ann Intern Med 1992;116:403–6.

[29] American Society of Anesthesiologists Task Force on Blood Component Therapy. Practice guidelines for blood component therapy: a report by the American Society of Anesthesiologists Task Force on Blood Component Therapy. Anesthesiology 1996;84:732–47.

[30] Expert Working Group. Guidelines for red blood cell and plasma transfusions for adults and children. Can Med Assoc J 1997;156(Suppl 11):S1–25.

[31] Hutton B, Fergusson D, Tinmouth A, et al. Transfusion rates vary significantly amongst Canadian medical centres. Can J Anaesth 2005;52(6):581–90.

[32] Dalrymple-Hay MJ, Dawkins S, Pack L, et al. Autotransfusion decreases blood usage following cardiac surgery—a prospective randomized trial. Cardiovasc Surg 2001;9(2):184–7.

[33] Murphy GJ, Allen SM, Unsworth-White J, et al. Safety and efficacy of perioperative cell salvage and autotransfusion after coronary artery bypass grafting: a randomized trial. Ann Thorac Surg 2004;77(5):1553–9.

[34] Mercer KG, Spark JI, Berridge DC, et al. Randomized clinical trial of intraoperative autotransfusion in surgery for abdominal aortic aneurysm. Br J Surg 2004;91(11):1443–8.

[35] Jabbour N, Gagandeep S, Mateo R, et al. Transfusion free surgery: single institution experience of 27 consecutive liver transplants in Jehovah's Witnesses. J Am Coll Surg 2005; 201(3):412–7.

ELSEVIER
SAUNDERS

SURGICAL
CLINICS OF
NORTH AMERICA

Surg Clin N Am 85 (2005) 1229–1241

Postoperative Nausea and Vomiting

Karen Stanley Williams, MD

*Department of Anesthesiology and Critical Care, George Washington
University Medical Center, 900 23rd Street, N.W., Washington DC 20037, USA*

Despite advances in our understanding of postoperative nausea and vomiting (PONV), the overall incidence of emetic sequelae after a balanced anesthetic remains between 20% and 30% [1], approaching 70% in patients in certain high-risk categories [2]. PONV may lead to dehydration, electrolyte imbalance, venous hypertension, bleeding, hematoma formation, suture dehiscence, esophageal rupture, hematoma formation, aspiration pneumonitis, delayed discharge from the hospital or ambulatory surgery center, prolonged nursing care, and unanticipated hospital admission, leading to increased health care costs.

Patients report that their concerns associated with PONV are more worrisome than postoperative pain [3] and are willing to spend up to $100 of their own money to avoid this discomfort and inconvenience [4]. Furthermore, the likelihood of nausea and vomiting occurring in the postanesthesia care unit (PACU) may not correspond to the likelihood of nausea and vomiting after discharge from the medical care facility. Approximately 36% of patients who experience postdischarge nausea and vomiting (PDNV) do not experience any nausea and vomiting before discharge [5], with the overall incidence of PDNV approaching 50% [6,7].

Anatomy

The neuroanatomical site controlling nausea and vomiting is an ill-defined region called the "vomiting center" within the lateral reticular formation in the brainstem [8]. The vomiting center receives afferent inputs from higher cortical centers, the cerebellum, the vestibular apparatus, and vagal and glossopharyngeal nerves [9]. Further interactions occur with the nucleus tractus solitarius and the chemoreceptor trigger zone (CTZ), which is located in the floor of the fourth ventricle [10]. The CTZ is outside the

E-mail address: santorinibound@aol.com

blood–brain barrier and in contact with cerebrospinal fluid (CSF). The CTZ enables substances in the blood and CSF to interact. Direct stimulation of the CTZ does not result in vomiting. Immunochemical studies of these anatomical sites show that these areas contain histamine, serotonin, cholinergic, neurokinin-1 and D2 dopamine receptors [11].

Literature review

In 2003, a multidisciplinary panel of experts published Consensus Guidelines for Managing Postoperative Nausea and Vomiting, which was based on a review of the medical literature through February 2002. The level of the medical evidence was rated I-V based on study size and design as well as the strength of the recommendation of expert opinion. The panel agreed that universal prophylaxis of patients for PONV is not cost-effective and may place patients at undue risk from the potential side effects of antiemetics. Patients at moderate risk of PONV should receive either monotherapy or combination prophylactic therapy (Fig. 1). Patients at high risk for PONV should receive multimodal prophylactic therapy of antiemetic agents from two or three different classes [12].

Apfel reported four independent predictors, enabling health care practitioners to identify adults at risk for PONV. Risks were greater for females, patients with a history of motion sickness or PONV, nonsmokers, and patients taking postoperative opioids. The rate of PONV was 10% when no risk factor was present, 23% when one factor was present, 39% when two factors were present, 61% when three factors were present, and 79% when all four factors were present [2]. These findings were supported in recent reports about inpatients [13,14]. Meanwhile, issues involving PONV among young adults remain controversial [15]. Also, the influence of postoperative pain on the incidence and management of PONV is unclear. The use of opioids may provoke nausea, but opioids are also used to relieve pain, resulting overall in a decreased incidence of PONV [16,17].

While the panel was unable to reach full consensus regarding the association between the type of surgery and risk of PONV, it noted that the bulk of data reviewed and reported was related to cases where variations in the duration of the operations and the types of anesthetic made it difficult to pinpoint how specific surgical procedures may relate to PONV. However, Sinclair also conducted a study on 17,638 ambulatory surgical patients, reporting an overall incidence of PONV of 4.6% in the PACU and 9.1% during a 24-hour follow-up [18]. In addition to confirming Apfel's four risk factors, Sinclair's study suggested that the use of general anesthesia resulted in an 11-fold increased risk of PONV compared with regional anesthesia. Also, each 30-minute increase in duration of anesthesia resulted in a 59% increase in the incidence of PONV. Patients undergoing plastic, ophthalmologic and orthopedic surgery were six times more likely to experience PONV than patients in a control group. Meanwhile, patients undergoing ear-nose-

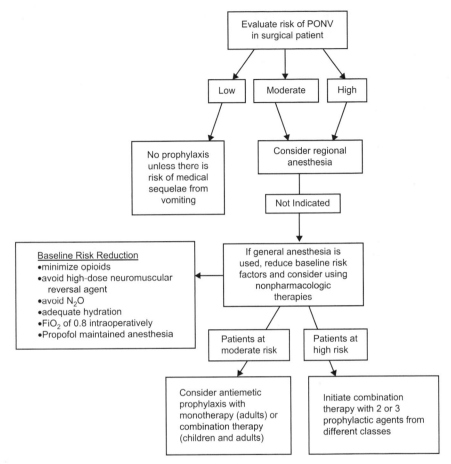

Fig. 1. Algorithm for management of postoperative nausea and vomiting. (*From* Gan TJ, Meyer T, Apfel C, et al. Consensus guidelines for managing postoperative nausea and vomiting. Anesth Analg 2003;97:62–71; with permission.)

throat, dental, general orthopedic, and gynecologic procedures were twice as likely to experience PONV than patients in the control group. Laparoscopic, breast, strabismus, laparotomy and plastic surgical procedures have also been reported as increasing the risk of PONV [18–20].

Postoperative vomiting is rare in children under 2 years old. However the incidence of postoperative vomiting (POV) increases to approximately 40% between ages 3 years and puberty, when the incidence gradually decreases [21]. Puberty also marks the onset of gender differences in the incidence of POV [22]. Adenotonsillectomy, strabismus repair, hernia repair, orchiopexy and penile surgery are specific operative procedures associated with an increased risk of POV in children [21]. Postoperative nausea is excluded from these studies in children because of the difficulty diagnosing nausea in young children. Box 1 summarizes strategies that may reduce the baseline risk of PONV.

Regional anesthesia

Patient factors linked to an increased risk of PONV following regional anesthetic, as opposed to general anesthesia, require further clarification. Most reported research does not distinguish between the two anesthetic techniques in their case mix or patient populations. Intraoperative sedation is also often used to relieve anxiety and improve patient perioperative satisfaction and comfort when a regional anesthetic is chosen. Current sedatives most commonly chosen are midazolam or propofol. Both sedatives have been effective in reducing nausea and vomiting [23].

Several mechanisms may play roles in the incidence of PONV in patients undergoing a regional anesthetic. Crocker and Vandam reported that a systolic blood pressure of less than 80 mmHg, a block higher than the fifth thoracic segment and the addition of vasoconstrictors to the local anesthetic, increased the incidence of nausea and vomiting during spinal anesthesia [16]. Low blood pressure may lead to brain stem ischemia, which may concurrently activate the circulatory, respiratory, and vomiting centers in the

---

Box 1. Risk factors for PONV in adults

Patient-specific risk factors
- Female sex
- Nonsmoking status
- History of PONV or motion sickness

Anesthetic risk factors
- Use of volatile anesthetics within 0–2 hrs
- Use of nitrous oxide
- Use of intraoperative and postoperative opioids

Surgical risk factors
- Duration of surgery (each 30-min increase in duration increases PONV risk by 60% so that a baseline risk of 10% is increased by 16% after 30 min)
- Type of surgery (risks higher for laparoscopy, ear-nose-throat, neurosurgery, breast, strabismus, laparotomy, plastic surgery, orthopedic surgery and gynecologic procedures)

From Gan TJ, et al. Consensus guidelines for managing postoperative nausea and vomiting. Anesth Analg 2003;97:62–71; with permission.

medulla [17], and may be relieved by oxygen [24]. There is also speculation that hypotension leads to gastrointestinal ischemia, releasing emetogenic substances, such as serotonin, from the intestines [25].

Table 1 summarizes the effect of varying admixtures to spinal and epidural anesthetics and their subsequent effect on PONV [26]. The addition of epinephrine to spinal anesthetics may increase the risk of PONV, regardless of the rate of hypotension [27]. The mechanism of action is unclear, but may be related to serotonin release [25] and the alpha-adrenergic effects on the CTZ [28]. Hydrophilic narcotics, such as morphine, are frequently added to supplement spinal anesthetics. They tend to remain in the cerebrospinal fluid for prolonged periods, moving rostrally by diffusion or bulk spread, reaching the CTZ within 5 to 6 hours, coinciding with the peak onset of nausea [29,30]. However, patients undergoing extensive surgical procedures, such as major orthopedic surgery, or transabdominal hysterectomy where postoperative analgesia is warranted, may not experience increased PONV, depending on the dose of intrathecal morphine used, particularly if a dose of less than 0.1 mg is chosen. By contrast, highly lipophilic opioids, such as fentanyl, administered intrathecally produce intense analgesia with infrequent nausea and vomiting.

Table 2 summarizes the effect of various medication admixtures on extremity and truncal nerve blocks [26]. The use of upper- and lower-extremity blocks for short procedures remains popular because of short operating times, limited surgery, and quick recovery after tourniquet release, all contributing to low PONV with reported incidence ranging from none to 10% regardless of the type of local anesthetic [31,32]. However, the addition of opioids to the local anesthetics may [33,34] be associated with increased nausea after tourniquet deflation following Bier blocks, but not with other upper-extremity blocks, such as interscalene, supraclavicular, infraclavicular or axillary [35–39]. Intercostal and paravertebral nerve blocks are also alternatives to general anesthesia for breast surgery, a documented risk factor for PONV. However, the techniques may be time-consuming and the failure rates are high.

Lower-extremity blocks such as femoral-sciatic or saphenous-popliteal report very low rates of PONV [40–43]. However, they may be time-consuming and cumbersome to perform if the medical facility does not have experienced staff and the appropriate physical space to provide the blocks without schedule delays.

Management of PONV

In managing PONV, medical professionals should consider the four major receptor systems that have been identified in the etiology of PONV. Antiemetic therapy may act at the muscarinic/cholinergic, dopaminergic (D2), histaminergic (H1), or serotonergic (5-HT3) receptors with NK-1 receptors

Table 1
Effect of intrathecal or epidural additives on PONV

Anesthetics	Epinephrine	Local anesthetic	Morphine	Fentanyl	Sufentanil	Meperidine	Clonidine	Neostigmine
Intrathecal	Increased	No change if avoid hypotension	Dose-dependent increase; modified by extent of surgery	Negligible, no change	Negligible, no change	Increased	No change if avoid hypotension	Increased; poorly treated with antiemetics
Epidural	Controversial	No change if avoid hypotension	No change up to 5 mg	No change	No change	No change	No change	No change up to 4 mcg/kg

Table 2
Effect of additives to local anesthetics on PONV during peripheral nerve blocks

Nerve blocks	Epinephrine	Local anesthetic	Morphine	Fentanyl	Sufentanil	Meperdine	Clonidine	Neostigmine
Upper extremity blocks		Very low (depending upon choice of IV sedatives)	No change if no prolonged plexus catheter used	No change if no prolonged plexus catheter used	Dose-dependent increase; mild, short duration	Increased	None if avoid bradycardia/hypotension	Increased
Truncal blocks		Low depending upon IV sedatives						
Lower extremity blocks		Low depending upon IV sedatives		No change			No change	

being investigated. Current pharmacotherapies available for the management of PONV are summarized in Table 3 [12].

Other interventions with potential antiemetic effects

Benzodiazepines are effective in the prophylaxis and treatment of PONV, particularly in persistent cases where other antiemetics failed to control symptoms [44–48]. Propofol used for the induction and maintenance of anesthesia is as effective as 4mg ondansetron in preventing PONV [49] and has a lower incidence of PONV than inhalation agents [5,50,51]. Its effects are most pronounced in the early postoperative period and are effective in subhypnotic dosages [52]. Intramuscular ephedrine (0.5 mg/kg) is also an effective prophylaxis in the early postoperative period (0–3 hr) [53–55]. Alpha 2 adrenergic agonists significantly reduce the incidence of PONV in adults and children [56,57]. Supplemental oxygen (80%) intraoperatively and for 2 hours postoperatively reportedly provides effective relief of PONV compared with 30% oxygen [58,59]. However, this finding was not confirmed in a subsequent study of females undergoing ambulatory gynecologic surgery [60]. Finally, adequate hydration significantly reduces the incidence of PONV [61].

Nonpharmacologic techniques

Twenty-four randomized trials by Lee and Done involving acupuncture, electroacupuncture, transcutaneous electrical nerve stimulation, acupoint stimulation and acupressure found a significant reduction in early PONV (0–6 hr) in adults treated with acupuncture compared with placebo, and

Table 3
Antiemetic doses and timing for administration in adults

Drug	Dose	Timing
Ondansetron	4–8 mg IV	At end of surgery
Dolasetron	12.5 mg IV	At end of surgery
Granisetron	0.35–1 mg IV	At end of surgery
Tropisetron	5 mg IV	At end of surgery
Dexamethasone	5–10 mg IV	Before induction
Droperidol	0.625–1.25 mg IV	At end of surgery
Dimenhydrinate	1–2 mg/kg IV	
Ephedrine	0.5 mg/kg IM	
Prochlorperazine	5–10 mg IV	At end of surgery
Promethazine	12.5–25 mg IV	At end of surgery
Scopolamine	Transdermal patch	Applied prior evening or 4 h before end of surgery

From Gan TJ, et al. Consensus guidelines for managing postoperative nausea and vomiting. Anesth Analg 2003;97:62–71; with permission.

that antiemetics (metoclopramide, cyclizine, droperidol, prochlorperazine) versus acupuncture were comparable in preventing early and late (0–48 hr) PONV in adults [23]. Although this study reported no beneficial effects in children, subsequent reports have documented prophylactic effectiveness in children [62–65]. Electoacupuncture at the P6 point provided similar efficacy to control PONV as compared with prophylactic ondansetron, including the added benefit of less pain. Combination therapy of acupoint electrical stimulation with ondansetron is associated with a lower incidence of PONV, less need for rescue medications, and improved patient satisfaction than with ondansetron alone [66,67]. Hypnosis has also been found to be more effective than placebo [68], but gingerroot has not been found to have a beneficial effect [69].

Future research

Neurokinin-1 (NK-1) receptor antagonists have been studied in humans and were found to be effective in the prophylaxis and treatment of PONV. Further, these in combination with ondansetron significantly prolonged the time to administration of rescue antiemetics compared with either drug alone [70].

All 5HT-3 antagonists are metabolized in various degrees by cytrochrome P-450. Dolasetron is predominantly metabolized by CYP2D6. Granisetron is metabolized predominantly by CYP3A4 and, to a lesser extent, by CYP2D6. In 2004, Candiotti and colleagues reported that results from a group of 250 healthy adult females undergoing general anesthesia were similar to results involving some chemotherapy patients showing decreased effectiveness of ondansetron when three or more alleles of the CYP2D6 genetic pathway of cytochrome P450 were present. Patients possessing three copies of the gene were statistically more likely than patients possessing one or two copies to have vomiting despite administration of ondansetron [71]. Janicki also investigated individual drug responses based on variations in drug biotransformation by genetically polymorphic enzymes. Patients classified as extensive metabolizers and ultrarapid metabolizers experienced more frequent vomiting following surgery conducted with general anesthesia. The difference was more pronounced with dolasetron than granisetron. Further genomic research and testing is anticipated. However, its use for the general surgical population is currently expensive and of limited feasibility [72].

Acknowledgments

Appreciation and gratitude is sincerely expressed to Dr. Michael Berrigan, Dr. Paul Dangerfield, and Cassandra King for their diligent assistance in the preparation of this manuscript.

References

[1] Cohen M, Duncan P, DeBoer D, et al. The postoperative interview: assessing risk factors for nausea and vomiting. Anesth Analg 1994;78:7–16.

[2] Apfel CC, Laara E, Koivuranta M, et al. A simplified risk score for predicting postoperative nausea and vomiting. Anesthesiology 1999;91:693–700.

[3] Marcario A, Weinger M, Carney S, et al. Which clinical anesthesia outcomes are important to avoid? Anesth Analg 1999;89:652–8.

[4] Gan T, Sloan F, Dear G, et al. How much are patients willing to pay to avoid postoperative nausea and vomiting? Anesth Analg 2001;92:393–400.

[5] Price M, Walmsley A, Swaine C, et al. Comparison of a total intravenous anaesthetic technique using a propofol infusion, with an inhalational technique using enflurane for day case surgery. Anaesthesia 1988;43:84–7.

[6] Carroll NV, Miederhoff P, Cox FM, et al. Postoperative nausea and vomiting after discharge from outpatient surgery centers. Anesth Analg 1995;80:903–9.

[7] Gan TJ. Postoperative nausea and vomiting: can it be eliminated? JAMA 2002;287(10): 1233–6.

[8] Wang SC, Borison HL. The vomiting center. Arch Neurol Psychiatry 1950;63:928–41.

[9] Watcha MF, White PF. Postoperative nausea and vomiting: its aetiology, treatment and prevention. Anesthesiology 1992;77:162–84.

[10] Leslie RA. Neuroactive substances in the dorsal vagal complex of the medulla oblongata: nucleus of the tractus solitarius, area postrema, and dorsal motor nucleus of the vagus. Neurochem Int 1985;7:191–211.

[11] Leslie RA, Shah Y, Thejomayen M, et al. The neuropharmacology of emesis: the role of receptors in neuromodulation of nausea and vomiting. Can J Physiol Pharmacol 1990;68: 279–88.

[12] Gan TJ, Meyer T, Apfel C, et al. Consensus guidelines for managing postoperative nausea and vomiting. Anesth Analg 2003;97:62–71.

[13] Apfel CC, Kranke P, Eberhart LH, et al. Comparison of predictive models for postoperative nausea and vomiting. Br J Anesth 2002;88:234–40.

[14] Pierre S, Benais H, Pouymayou J. Apfel's simplified score may favorably predict the risk of postoperative nausea and vomiting. Can J Anaesth 2002;49:237–42.

[15] Lee A, Done ML. The use of nonpharmacologic techniques to prevent postoperative nausea and vomiting: a meta-analysis. Anesth Analg 1999;88:1362–9.

[16] Crocker JS, Vandam LD. Concerning nausea and vomiting during spinal anesthesia. Anesthesiology 1959;20:587–92.

[17] Data S, Alper MH, Ostheimer GW, et al. Method of ephedrine administration and nausea and hypotension during spinal anesthesia for cesarean section. Anesthesiology 1982;56: 68–70.

[18] Sinclair DR, Chung F, Mezei G. Can postoperative nausea and vomiting be predicted? Anesthesiology 1999;91:109–18.

[19] Fabling JM, Gan TJ, El-Moalem HE, et al. A randomized, double-blinded comparison of ondansetron, droperidol and placebo for prevention of postoperative nausea and vomiting after supratentorial craniotomy. Anesth Analg 2000;91:358–61.

[20] Gan TJ, Ginsberg B, Grant AP, et al. Double blind, randomized comparison of ondansetron and intraoperative propofol to prevent postoperative nausea and vomiting. Anesthesiology 1996;85:1036–42.

[21] Lerman J. Surgical and patient factors involved in postoperative nausea and vomiting. Br J Anaesth 1992;69(Suppl 1):S24–32.

[22] Rowley MP, Brown TCK. Postoperative vomiting in children. Anaesth Intensive Care 1982; 10:309–13.

[23] Borgear A, Ekatodramis G, Schenker C. Postoperative nausea and vomiting in regional anesthesia. Anesthesiology 2003;98:530–47.

[24] Ratra CK, Badola RP, Bhargava KP. A study of factors concerned in emesis during spinal anaesthesia. Br J Anaesth 1972;44:1208–11.

[25] Racke K, Schworer H. Regulation of serotonin release from the intestinal mucosa. Pharmacol Res 1991;23:13–25.

[26] Borgeat A, Ekatodramis G, Schenker C. Postoperative nausea and vomiting in regional anesthesia, a review. Anesthesiology 2003;98:530–47.

[27] Carpenter RL, Caplan RA, Brown DL, et al. Incidence and risk factors for side effects of spinal anesthesia. Anesthesiology 1992;76:909–16.

[28] Jenkins L, Lakay D. Central mechanism of vomiting related to catecholamine response: anaesthetic implication. Can Anaesth Soc J 1971;18:434–41.

[29] Angst MS, Ramaswamy B, Riley ET, et al. Lumbar epidural morphine in humans and supraspinal analgesia to experimental heat pain. Anesthesiology 2000;92:312–24.

[30] Gjessing J, Tomlin PJ. Postoperative pain control with intrathecal morphine. Anaesthesia 1981;36:268–76.

[31] Bone HG, Van Aken H, Booke M, et al. Enhancement of axillary brachial plexus block anesthesia by co-administration of neostigmine. Reg Anesth Pain Med 1999;24:405–10.

[32] Simon MAM, Gielen MJM, Alberink N, et al. Intravenous regional anesthesia with 0.5% articaine, 0.5% lidocaine, or 0.5% prilocaine. Reg Anesth 1997;22:29–34.

[33] Lavin PA, Henderson CL, Vaghadia H. Non-alkalinized and alkalinized 2-chloroprocaine vs. lidocaine for intravenous regional anesthesia during outpatient hand surgery. Can J Anesth 1999;46·939–45.

[34] Arthur JM, Heavner JE, Mian T, et al. Fentanyl and lidocaine versus lidocaine for Bier block. Reg Anesth 1992;17:223–7.

[35] Racz H, Gunning K, Dellasanta D, et al. Evaluation of the effect of perineuronal morphine on the quality of postoperative analgesia after axillary plexus block: a randomized double-blind study. Anesth Analg 1991;72:769–72.

[36] Gormley WP, Murray JM, Ree JPJ, et al. Effect of the addition of alfentanil to lignocaine during axillary brachial plexus anaesthesia. Br J Anaesth 1996;76:802–5.

[37] Bouaziz H, Kinirons BP, Macalou D, et al. Sufentanil does not prolong the duration of analgesia in a mepivacaine brachial plexus block: a dose response study. Anesth Analg 2000;90: 383–7.

[38] Erlacher W, Schuschnig C, Orlicek F, et al. The effects of clonidine on ropivacaine 0.75% in axillary perivascular brachial plexus block. Acta Anaesthesiol Scand 2000;44:53–7.

[39] Bouaziz H, Paqueron X, Bur ML, et al. No enhancement of sensory and motor blockade by neostigmine added to mepivacaine axillary plexus block. Anesthesiology 1999;91:78–83.

[40] Vloka JD, Hadzie A, Mulcare R, et al. Femoral and genitofemoral nerve blocks versus spinal anesthesia for outpatients undergoing long saphenous vein stripping surgery. Anesth Analg 1997;84:749–52.

[41] Mansour NY, Bennetts FE. An observational study of combined continuous lumbar plexus and single-shot sciatic nerve blocks for post-knee surgery analgesia. Reg Anesth 1996;21: 287–91.

[42] Casati A, Cappelleri G, Fanelli G, et al. Regional anaesthesia for outpatient knee arthroscopy: a randomized clinical comparison of two different anesthetic techniques. Acta Anaesthesiol Scand 2000;44:543–7.

[43] Singelyn FJ, Aye F, Gouverneur JM. Continuous popliteal sciatic nerve block: an original technique to provide postoperative analgesia after foot surgery. Anesth Analg 1997;84: 383–6.

[44] Splinter W, Noel LP, Roberts D, et al. Antiemetic prophylaxis for strabismus surgery. Can J Ophthalmol 1994;29:224–6.

[45] Splinter W, MacNeill H, Menard E, et al. Midazolam reduces vomiting after tonsillectomy in children. Can J Anaesth 1995;42:201–3.

[46] Khalil S, Berry J, Howard G, et al. The antiemetic effect of lorazepam after outpatient strabismus surgery in children. Anesthesiology 1992;77:915–9.

[47] Di Florio T. The use of midazolam for persistent postoperative nausea and vomiting. Anaesth Intensive Care 1992;20:383–6.

[48] Di Florio T, Goucke C. The effect of midazolam on persistent postoperative nausea and vomiting. Anaesth Intensive Care 1999;27:38–40.

[49] Gan TJ, Ginsberg B, Grant A, et al. Double blind, randomized comparison of ondansetron and intraoperative propofol to prevent postoperative nausea and vomiting. Anesthesiology 1996;85:1036–42.

[50] Doze V, Shafer A, White P. Propofol-nitrous oxide versus thiopental-isoflurane-nitrous oxide for general anesthesia. Anesthesiology 1988;69:63–71.

[51] Lebenbom-Mansour M, Pandit S, Kothary S, et al. Desflurane versus propofol anesthesia: a comparative analysis in outpatients. Anesth Analg 1993;76:936–41.

[52] Tramer M, Moore A, McQuay H. Propofol anaesthesia and postoperative nausea and vomiting: quantitative systematic review of randomized controlled studies. Br J Anaesth 1997;78:247–55.

[53] Rothenberg D, Parnass S, Litwack K, et al. Efficacy of ephedrine in the prevention of postoperative nausea and vomiting. Anesth Analg 1991;72:58–61.

[54] Naguib K, Osman H, Al-Khayat H, et al. Prevention of post-operative nausea and vomiting following laparoscopic surgery. Ephedrine vs. propofol. Middle East J Anesthesiol 1998;14:219–30.

[55] Hagemann E, Halvorsen A, Holgersen O, et al. Intramuscular ephedrine reduces emesis during the first three hours after abdominal hysterectomy. Acta Anaesthesiol Scand 2000;44:107–11.

[56] Mikawa K, Nishina K, Maekawa N, et al. Oral clonidine premedication reduces vomiting in children after strabismus surgery. Can J Anaesth 1995;42:977–81.

[57] Oddby-Muhrbeck E, Eksborg S, Bergendahl H, et al. Effects of clonidine on postoperative nausea and vomiting in breast cancer surgery. Anesthesiology 2002;96:1109–14.

[58] Goll V, Akca O, Greif R, et al. Ondansetron is no more effective than supplemental intraoperative oxygen for prevention of postoperative nausea and vomiting. Anesth Analg 2001;92:112–7.

[59] Grief R, Laciny S, Rapf B, et al. Supplemental oxygen reduces the incidence of postoperative nausea and vomiting. Anesthesiology 1999;91:1246–52.

[60] Purhonen S, Turunen M, Ruohoaho U, et al. Supplemental oxygen does not reduce the incidence of postoperative nausea and vomiting after ambulatory gynecologic laparoscopy. Anesth Analg 2003;96:91–6.

[61] Yogendrean S, Asokumar B, Cheng D, et al. A prospective randomized double-blinded study of the effect of intravenous fluid therapy on adverse outcomes on outpatient surgery. Anesth Analg 1995;80:682–6.

[62] Boehler M, Mitterschiffthaler G, Schlager A. Korean hand acupressure reduces postoperative nausea and vomiting after gynecological laparoscopic surgery. Anesth Analg 2002;94:872–5.

[63] Schlager A, Offer T, Baldissera I. Laser stimulation of acupuncture point P6 reduces postoperative vomiting in children undergoing strabismus surgery. Br J Anaesth 1998;81:529–32.

[64] Rusy L, Hoffman G, Weisman S. Electro acupuncture prophylaxis of postoperative nausea and vomiting following pediatric tonsillectomy with or without adenoidectomy. Anesthesiology 2002;96:300–5.

[65] Somri M, Vaida S, Sabo E, et al. Acupuncture versus ondansetron in the prevention of postoperative vomiting. A study of children undergoing dental surgery. Anaesthesia 2001;56:927–32.

[66] Coloma M, White P, Ogunnaike B, et al. Comparison of acustimulation and ondansetron for the treatment of established postoperative nausea and vomiting. Anesthesiology 2002;97:1387–92.

[67] White P, Issioui T, Hu J, et al. Comparative efficacy of acustimulation versus ondansetron in combination with droperidol for preventing nausea and vomiting. Anesthesiology 2002;97: 1075–81.

[68] Enqvist B, Bjorklunmd C, Engman M, et al. Preoperative hypnosis reduces postoperative vomiting after surgery of the breasts. A prospective, randomized and blinded study. Acta Anaesthesiol Scan 1997;41:1028–32.

[69] Ernst E, Pittler M. Efficacy of ginger for nausea and vomiting: a systematic review of randomized clinical trials. Br J Anaesth 2000;84:367–71.

[70] Gesztesi Z, Scuderi P, White P, et al. Substance P (Neurokinin-1) antagonist prevents postoperative vomiting after abdominal hysterectomy procedures. Anesthesiology 2000;93: 931–7.

[71] Candiotti K, Nhuch F, Kamat A, et al. Pharmacogenomics affects postoperative nausea and vomiting: the effects of CYP2D6 allelc frequency on ondansetron prophlaxis failure. Anesthesiology 2004;101:A1611.

[72] Janicki P. Efficacy of antiemetic prophylaxix with granisetron and dolasetron depends on cytochrome P-450 2D6 genotypes. Anesthesiology 2004;101:A1606.

ELSEVIER
SAUNDERS

SURGICAL
CLINICS OF
NORTH AMERICA

Surg Clin N Am 85 (2005) 1243–1257

Perioperative Pain Control: A Strategy for Management

Mitchell Jay Cohen, MD,
William P. Schecter, MD, FACS*

*University of California, San Francisco, San Francisco General Hospital,
1001 Potrero Avenue, San Francisco, CA 94110, USA*

A thorough understanding of the anatomy and neurophysiology of the pain response is necessary for the effective treatment of perioperative pain. Pain begins with stimulation of specialized nerve endings called nociceptors. Nociceptors exist throughout the body and serve as the proximal end of the sensory nerves. Most prevalent in highly sensate areas, such as the fingertips, extremities, and face, these receptors are most often stimulated directly by injury and surgical incision. In addition to responding to direct stimulation, these receptors also respond to mediators released during surgical trauma, inflammation and stress, leading to impulse formation and pain [1–4]. These mediators, which include prostaglandins, bradykinins, histamine, and serotonin, act by two mechanisms to cause pain [1,5,6]. First, they act on nerve endings to cause pain impulse formation. Second, they amplify other pain signals caused by direct stimulation. These mediators have also been implicated in prolonged up-regulation of nociceptors, which leads to chronic pain, phantom pain, and hypersensitization [1,4].

Nociceptor stimulation causes depolarization of the nerve, creating an all-or-nothing response. The nerve impulse travels from the periphery to the dorsal horn of the spinal cord via Lissauer's tract. Myelinated A-δ nerve fibers conduct nerve impulses rapidly. Relatively slow conduction takes place in unmyelinated C fibers in the viscera, which join autonomic nerves as they travel to join somatic nerves entering the central nervous system. This union of visceral and somatic nerves is responsible for the phenomena of referred pain. Because the visceral nerves enter the cord at the level of the somatic nerves with which they travel, the pain is perceived to be originating from the area innervated by the somatic nerves.

---

* Corresponding author. 1001 Potrero Avenue, Ward 3A33, San Francisco, CA 94110.
E-mail address: bschecter@sfghsurg.ucsf.edu (W.P. Schecter).

The sensory fiber nerves enter the dorsal horn. Pain and temperature fibers cross the midline and ascend to the brain in the lateral spinothalamic tract. Substance P is the primary neurotransmitter at the synapse between the afferent peripheral and ascending spinothalamic tract nerves. Interestingly, substance P has also been well described as a primary mediator in the neuroinflammatory cascade providing a connection between inflammation and chronic pain. The ascending fibers in the spinothalamic tract terminate primarily in the brain stem and thalamus, which then relay the information to the perceptive cerebral cortex. Signal transmission to and within the cerebral cortex causes perception and localization of pain. Other signals are sent to the limbic system, further processed in the emotional centers, and are thereby responsible for the emotional response to pain.

Inflammation and pain

Inflammation is itself painful. Often this simple fact is not recognized and patients are undertreated. Inflammation causes pain through the up-regulation of stimulated nociceptors and the recruitment of nonstimulated or dormant receptors [1,3,4]. Proinflammatory mediators, including TNF-α, IL-1, IL-6, and the interferons, decrease the threshold for impulse generation, and raise the intensity of the nociceptic impulse. Additionally, the basal rate of discharge of peripheral nociceptors increases in a proinflammatory state [7]. These mechanisms make pain control in the patient with inflammatory conditions both complicated and difficult. These mediators explain why the pro-inflammatory state is itself painful. Patients with inflammation generally require analgesia at levels equal to or greater than levels required by patients with more direct and obvious sources of pain [7].

Inflammation can generate pain, but pain in turn also generates inflammation. As described above, nociceptor stimulation and the resultant generation of the nerve impulse take place in an all-or-nothing fashion. Several factors modulate pain intensity. These factors include the number of receptors stimulated, the duration of stimulation, and how efficiently the central nervous system processes the impulses. When the pain response is sufficiently intense or prolonged, the pain impulse is further amplified by neurogenic inflammation [6]. Neurogenic inflammation is mediated by the release of substance P, which is also the primary central neurotransmitter at the presynaptic nerve ending. During intense or prolonged pain, substance P acts peripherally to induce inflammation, vascular permeability, and other tissue injury, causing both nociceptor stimulation and amplification of nerve impulses [5].

Pain and subsequent neurogenic inflammation have the same physiologic effects as direct tissue injury or surgical stress. These effects include elevation of the heart rate, higher blood pressure, increased O_2 consumption, myocardial ischemia, lung injury, and release of adrenocorticotropic hormone (ACTH), antidiuretic hormone (ADH), cortisol and proinflammatory mediators, including IL-1, Il-6 and TNF-α [6,8,9]. Intense pain leads to changes that can reorganize the dorsal horn ultra structure. Dorsal horn changes result in new feedback loops, causing central sensitization and precipitating the onset of chronic pain [5,7].

Along with the inflammatory and structural changes, which are responsible for sensitization and chronic pain, a change in gene expression takes place with intense painful stimuli. Previous pain and ongoing chronic pain modulate the pain experienced with each new painful stimulus. Painful stimuli have been shown in animal studies to produce gene expression changes that precipitate changes in pain perception and impulse formation in as little as 1 hour [5]. Posttranslational modification causes inflammatory amplification of painful stimuli and pain perception. Preemptive analgesia and balanced analgesia become especially important in patients who have been previously sensitized [5,6,10,11].

Certain receptors may be especially important for the transformation from acute to chronic pain. N-nitrosodimethylamine (NDMA) is the primary receptor involved in chronic pain and sensitization, but substance P and protein kinase C have been implicated as well [12,13]. Acute pain leads to sensitization of these receptors, decreasing the threshold for future impulse as well as increasing the baseline impulse level in much the same manner as described above for neurogenic inflammation [5].

Descending modulation of pain

Descending pain fibers from the cerebral cortex and midbrain modulate the afferent nerve stimuli that transmit nociceptive impulses to the central nervous system. Other molecular neurotransmitters, including enkephalin, noradrenaline, serotonin, and gamma aminobutyric acid (GABA), also modulate and inhibit the frequency and degree of nociceptive impulses, thereby attenuating the pain response [11]. These substances, including the endogenous opioids and endorphins, are released from the central nervous system, bind to opioid receptors, and prevent presynaptic release of neurotransmitters, including substance P, thereby inhibiting the perception and response to painful stimuli [11].

Nerve anatomy

Peripheral nerves are made of millions of axons bundled into fascicles. At the end of each of these nerves are the nociceptors. Multiple fascicles are then bundled into nerves. This bundling is brought about by the Schwann cell, which is also responsible for myelination.

Myelin provides some structure for the nerve and increases the speed of conduction of the nerve impulse. A protective sheath, called the endoneurium, surrounds each axon. Each fascicle is in turn surrounded and protected by the perineurium and each nerve by epineurium. Each of these layers serves to protect the nerve from trauma and allows the nerve to flex and move without injury. Pharmacologically, the layers are important because they inhibit the penetration, slow the diffusion, and prolong the duration of local anesthetic.

At the cellular level, each nerve cell membrane is made of a phospholipid bilayer, which separates the nerve into hydrophobic and hydrophilic domains. Bridging these domains are transmembrane channels, including the sodium channels necessary for depolarization and conduction. In the nerve cell, the principle extracellular cation is sodium, while potassium is the principle intracellular cation. Active transport of sodium and potassium maintains a transmembrane gradient of -70 to -90 mV thereby creating a polarized, charged electrical potential for nerve signaling.

Peripheral nerves are further classified into myelinated and unmyelinated fibers. Myelin is a lipid-based substance made by Schwann cells. It is found on larger sensory and motor nerves. Myelin serves to increase the speed of impulse conduction by salutary conduction. In unmyelinated nerve fibers, conduction proceeds by sequential opening of closely spaced sodium channels. In all myelinated nerves, however, transmembrane sodium channels are found only intermittently along the nerve axon at specialized nodes called the nodes of Ranvier. In a myelinated axon, transmembrane sodium channels are widely spaced at the nodes of Ranvier, allowing electric potential to "jump" from node to node, thereby increasing the velocity of impulse conduction.

Pharmacology of nonopioid analgesia

Nonopioid analgesics can be separated into two categories: nonsteroidal anti-inflammatory drugs (NSAIDs) and acetaminophen. Acetaminophen has long been the gold standard for mild to moderate pain control and is often used for its antipyretic effects. It has an excellent safety profile at standard dosing of 325 to 1000 mg every 4 to 6 hours. Unlike most opioids, dose escalation does not provide greater drug effect. Acetaminophen's only major side effect is hepatotoxicity. Although hepatotoxicity has been reported at the recommended dose of 325 to 1000 mg every 6 hours, hepatotoxicity at doses less than 4 g over 24 hours is unlikely [10].

Acetaminophen is a metabolic product of phenacetin, an analgesic that has a significant risk of nephrotoxicity and, as a result, is no longer available for prescription. Prolonged use of large doses of acetaminophen is associated with an increased risk of renal insufficiency, although this event is considered unlikely at normal doses. Unlike many NSAIDs, acetaminophen is not associated with platelet dysfunction and, as a result, does not increase bleeding risk [10,14].

Making up the class of NSAIDs are the salicylates, proprionic acids, acetic acids, oxylates, and fenamates, all of which act through the blockage of cyclooxygenase (COX). COX is an enzyme that converts arachidonic acid to prostaglandin, which is necessary for neurosensitization to painful stimuli and subsequent hyperalgesia. Cellular injury leads to release of phospholipids, which are an important component of the cell membrane. Phospholipids are then metabolized to arachidonic acid in the presence of the enzyme phospholipase. Arachidonic acid is metabolized in the presence of COX, resulting in the formation of prostaglandin. Prostaglandins are molecular signals that stimulate nociceptive nerve impulse transmission from the site of injury. By blocking prostaglandin synthesis, NSAIDs block transduction of the physical stimulus to the nociceptors [3,10,14].

The alternative pathway for COX metabolism is the production of leukotrienes. Inhibition of COX can theoretically increase leukotriene production, accounting for rare asthmatic and anaphylactic reactions to NSAIDs [14].

COX exists in two isoforms, which have markedly different physiologic effects. COX-1 influences platelet function, gastric mucosal protection, and hemostasis, while the COX-2 isozyme affects the inflammatory cascade and pain [14]. Aspirin and most of the NSAIDs are nonselective and block both isoforms, resulting in analgesia along with varying degrees of side effects, including injury to the gastric mucosal barrier, coagulopathy, and platelet dysfunction [15,16]. The inhibition of prostaglandin synthesis is the prime cause of the side effects of COX inhibitors. Prostaglandins influence the creation and maintenance of the gastric mucosal barrier and NSAIDs have long been implicated in the destruction of this barrier and subsequent ulceration. NSAIDs also act directly on the gastric mucosa, causing direct mucosal injury and ulceration [5,10,14]. Although the risk of bleeding from NSAID use is small, the risk increases with older patients, higher drug dosages, and longer periods of therapy.

COX-1 is present in the stomach, intestines, kidneys, and platelets, and helps produce prostaglandins, which have a role in regulating gastrointestinal function and platelet aggregation. COX-2 is produced during inflammatory states and serves as an enzyme for production of prostaglandins that mediate inflammation pain and fever. Theoretically, a drug that inhibits only COX-2 would, as a result, be primarily anti-inflammatory, without incurring the adverse risks of gastrointestinal ulceration and bleeding [16].

Despite great hope that the selective COX-2 inhibitors would provide analgesia without gastrointestinal side effects, little evidence supports that claim. Additionally, recent evidence shows the COX-2 inhibitors to be associated with adverse cardiovascular events, including myocardial infarction and cerebrovascular accident (CVA). A study testing the efficacy of rofecoxib in preventing colonic polyps showed that patients treated with rofecoxib had a higher rate of cardiovascular events. As a result of this data, Merck withdrew rofecoxib from the market in September 2004. Similarly, a National Institutes of Health trial examining celecoxib was ended because of the unexpected finding of cardiovascular toxicity. At the time of this writing, celecoxib and valdecoxib have also been withdrawn [17–23].

NSAIDs alone are useful for mild to moderate pain. For perioperative pain they are useful adjuncts to opioids and local anesthetics [10,24]. NSAIDs can reduce perioperative opioid dose requirements by up to 50% [25]. NSAIDs help modulate and treat the inflammatory milieu and attenuating the pain caused and heightened by inflammation. NSAIDs are most often given orally. Ketorolac is a nonselective COX inhibitor that can be given intramuscularly or intravenously in the perioperative period [14,26,27].

Pharmacology of opioid analgesia

Because of its potency, opioid analgesia is the gold standard for perioperative pain control. Opioid receptors exist in the periphery, spinal cord, and central nervous system. Recently, opioid receptors have also been identified on inflammatory and immunologic cells. Opioids act by binding to presynaptic receptors and preventing the release of substance P at the presynaptic vesicle, thereby preventing impulse transmission. The three opioid receptors are μ, κ, and δ. Each receptor is in a different location and produces different effects. The μ receptor is responsible for spinal and supraspinal analgesia and also mediates undesirable opioid side effects, such as respiratory depression, bowel dysmotility, urinary retention, and pruritus. The κ receptor also provides spinal and supraspinal analgesia while mediating miosis, sedation, and dysphasia. The δ receptor mediates spinal and supraspinal analgesia.

While some opioid receptors exist in the periphery, most are located centrally. To function, the opioids must cross the blood-brain barrier. The opioids have differing partition coefficients and lipid solubilities, which determine distribution, onset, and duration of action. Opioids with greater lipid solubility have a faster onset of action because of their rapid distribution and ability to cross the blood-brain barrier. Fentanyl is an example of a lipid-soluble drug with a high potency and a rapid onset of action.

Unlike acetaminophen and the NSAIDs, opiates do not have a ceiling effect and escalating doses will stop pain once enough drug is given. Often, as doses escalate, respiratory depression and other less serious side effects make it imprudent to further escalate doses [28]. Careful monitoring of opioid administration in the opioid naïve and elderly patient is essential.

Opioids are divided into two categories. In one category are the μ agonists, which include morphine, hydromorphone, fentanyl, oxycodone, codeine, methadone, and meperidine. In the other category are the agonist/antagonists. The agonist/antagonists are further divided into the mixed agonist/antagonists, because they bind at both the μ and κ receptors, and partial agonists, so called because of their limited efficacy.

Morphine is the model opioid to which all others are compared. Intravenous morphine is most commonly used in the perioperative period, although it is also available for oral, rectal, intrathecal, and epidural use. Subcutaneous or intramuscular morphine administration is an option but inconsistent uptake and distribution of the drug from these sites make intravenous use a better choice in the perioperative period. Intravenous morphine has an onset of action at approximately 5 minutes, a peak effect within 20 minutes, and duration of action of 3 to 4 hours. Unfortunately, morphine has a relatively high incidence of associated nausea and vomiting, which can delay discharge from the recovery room or same-day surgery unit [10,29].

Fentanyl is a highly potent lipophilic drug with an onset of action of approximately 30 seconds after intravenous administration and a short duration of action because of rapid redistribution from fat stores. The short duration of action of fentanyl is ideally suited to outpatient surgery and makes for easy rapid titration in the inpatient setting. Fentanyl remains an ideal drug for drip titration in the ICU. In addition to offering the benefits of rapid titration, fentanyl has a lower incidence of nausea and vomiting compared with morphine, making fentanyl a better choice for analgesia in outpatient surgery.

Meperidine is another opiate available for perioperative use. Meperidine has a similar time-to-onset but only one tenth the potency of morphine. In addition, it has atropine-like side effects, including tachycardia and ampullary dilatation. Meperidine has a toxic metabolite (normeperidine), which is excreted in the urine. Normeperidine causes anxiety, tremor, and seizures. While meperidine should be avoided in patients with renal insufficiency, the drug is effective in the treatment of postoperative shivering when given in small doses.

Oxycodone and hydrocodone are opiates available orally and often used in conjunction with acetaminophen. These drugs are effective for mild to moderate pain and the dose can be increased if the pain is more severe. Oxycodone is also available in sustained release form, which can provide analgesia for up to 12 hours.

Codeine is a weak opioid that is also often combined with acetaminophen. The maximum recommended analgesic dose of codeine is 60 mg every 6 hours. Codeine is not very effective for severe pain but can be a useful adjunct to reduce other opioid requirements. Once the patient is ready to transition from the ICU to the floor or hospital to home, codeine usually provides well-tolerated analgesia [10,14].

Tramadol is a relatively new analgesic drug. Both tramadol and meperidine have a similar efficacy [30–32]. Tramadol works through two mechanisms. First, as a weak opioid agonist, the drug acts on μ receptors [30–32]. Second, tramadol inhibits monoamine neurotransmitter re-uptake, which weakly hinders norepinephrine and serotonin re-uptake in a manner similar to an antidepressant. Tramadol has two enantiomers, which lead to better efficacy. Safety and efficacy are similar to other opioids and meperidine. Tramadol may be given in doses of 50 to 100 mg orally every 4 to 6 hours in adult patients. Concomitant use of antiemetics may be necessary in outpatient surgery when tramadol is used because of the increased risk of nausea and vomiting [33].

Over the past 5 years, ketamine has seen increasing use as an analgesic/sedative drug outside the operating room. Ketamine owes its increased use to its opioid-sparing effect. Ketamine works through NDMA modulation and has been effective in preemptive analgesia and reduction of narcotic requirements [34–36].

Pharmacology of local anesthesia

While local anesthetics vary widely in their applicability, onset, and duration, they all eliminate conduction of nociceptive impulses along the nerve axon. Local anesthetics bind to receptors in the sodium channel, blocking sodium influx, arresting depolarization, and interrupting conduction. All local anesthetics are made up of a lipophilic aromatic ring linked by either an amide or ester group to a hydrophilic amino group. This tertiary amine structure allows the anesthetic to penetrate the nerve and diffuse into its lipid-rich environment. All local anesthetics are weak bases with Pkas that range from 7.6 to 8.9 [33].

Ester-linked local anesthetics are metabolized by cholinesterase produced in the synaptic nerve endings. The anesthetics are then broken down into para-aminobenzoic acid (PABA), a common ingredient in many healthcare products, lotions, and creams. Because most patients are already sensitized to PABA, cross-reaction and allergy can take place [33].

The potency of local anesthetics depends on their lipid solubility, which is measured by the oil-water partition coefficient. The more lipid soluble an anesthetic is, the more binding takes place, resulting in increased potency. The potency additionally depends on vasodilatation and redistribution in the particular tissue bed. Potency is not based on the characteristics of the anesthetic alone but also on the distribution and washout of the drug. Duration of action is based on the degree of binding of the drug. Duration of action can be prolonged by adding epinephrine to the anesthetic, thereby causing vasoconstriction and slowing washout of the drug [33].

There are six major adverse reactions to local anesthetics: cardiac arrhythmias, hypertension, direct tissue toxicity, central nervous system toxicity, methemoglobinemia, and allergic reactions. Of all local anesthetics, bupivacaine is associated with the most serious cardiac arrhythmias. Bupivacaine depresses conduction of cardiac tissue, which can result in reentrant arrhythmias. These arrhythmias can in turn rapidly degenerate into ventricular fibrillation [37,38]. Great care must be taken to avoid intravascular injection of bupivacaine. In addition, recommended doses of bupivacaine should not be exceeded.

All local anesthetics have central nervous side effects, which include dizziness, lightheadedness, paresthesias, nervousness, and disorientation. Severe toxicity can result in seizures, coma, and even respiratory arrest. For this reason, care must be taken to avoid intravascular injection when doing a field block or nerve block. Intraneural injection can result in neurotoxicity.

All local anesthetics in high concentrations are neurotoxins. Injection of a drug into a nerve can result in nerve injury because of the needle. Finally, the direct injection of a drug into a nerve sheath can result in a compartment syndrome occurring within the epineurium, resulting in nerve injury from increased pressure.

An unusual but potentially fatal complication of local anesthesia is methemoglobinemia. Prilocaine is the drug most commonly associated with methemoglobinemia. Methemoglobinemia occurs as a result of oxidation of the iron in hemoglobin from the ferrous to the ferric form. This oxidation can take place as a result of exposure to prilocaine, resulting in increased affinity of oxygen to the hemoglobin molecule. Because of this affinity, oxygen does not dissociate from the hemoglobin molecule in peripheral tissues, thereby causing decreased oxygen delivery. Tachypnea, cyanosis and spuriously increased hemoglobin oxygen saturation are the clinical signs of methemoglobenemia. Supplemental oxygen will not increase oxygen saturation. A high index of suspicion is essential to make the diagnosis. Methemoglobinemia is easily treated by the administration of methylene blue intravenously in doses of 1 to 2 mg/kg [39]. Methylene blue reduces the ferric ion to the ferrous form, thereby allowing hemoglobin molecules to release oxygen to the peripheral tissues. Methemoglobinemia usually results when prilocaine is used as either a topical anesthetic in the oral pharynx or in the eutectic mixture local anesthetic (EMLA) cream [39,40]. Methemoglobinemia is most commonly associated with this form of prilocaine administration because of the difficulty in controlling the amount of drug administered in a spray or in a topical cream.

Assessment of pain

Assessment of pain depends on level of consciousness and degree of cooperation. In patients who are awake and able to communicate, pain and sedation are best assessed by a good history and physical examination [41]. Multiple objective scales have been developed to measure the severity and nature of pain. These scales can be further broken down into unidimensional and multidimensional scales. Unidimensional scales are the simplest and most widely used. They measure only the intensity of pain. The two most common scales are the visual analog scale (VAS) and the numeric rating scale (NRS). The VAS consists of a straight line with the words "no pain at all" written on one end and the words "the worst pain" written at the other end. Patients indicate their level of pain by placing a mark along the scale. Measurement improves when a standard 10 cm line is used. The VAS is most useful when it tracks the changing pattern of a patient's pain, and less useful for comparing the level of pain between different patients [10].

The NRS is a numerical scale to evaluate the level of pain. The most commonly used scale is between zero and 100. Zero represents no pain and 100 represents the worst pain imaginable. With all these scales, patient self-reporting is the most reliable indication of the existence and the intensity of pain [42].

There are a variety of multidimensional scales. However, these scales are most useful in evaluating chronic pain and have limited use in the management of perioperative pain [43–45].

Balanced perioperative analgesia

The concept of balanced analgesia implies that pain is treated with the least amount of the most specific drug necessary. Balanced analgesia treats all aspects of the pain axis, including stimulation, modulation, inflammation, and psychology with a combination of drugs and therapies each aimed at creating a synergistic pain-control regimen.

Balanced analgesia begins before the onset of stimuli with the preoperative interview. This interview is critical to the notion of balanced analgesia and effective pain control. Careful interrogation regarding baseline pain, previous painful stimuli, and treatment methods, both effective and failed, guides both the choice and application of analgesia while also comforting the patient. This preoperative interview can rate discomfort and separate pain from anxiety while providing careful assessment of the emotional lability of the patient. In the preoperative setting, a careful explanation of the details of the anesthetic and pain-control strategy combined with medication before the beginning of surgery reduces anxiety and modulates pain perception. The interview sets the stage for attenuation of pain and identifies emotionally labile individuals who may benefit from modifications in the anesthetic technique and perioperative pain-treatment regimen.

After the preoperative interview, preemptive medication also is essential to attenuate the pain response. Preoperative sedation helps to achieve a state of conscious sedation and amnesia. The sedation allows the patient to cooperate without fear or anxiety. Short-acting drugs with anxiolytic and amnesic properties, such as midazolam, can be used because they have proven benefits with limited hemodynamic effects and a good safety profile. Preoperative opiates and anxiolytics can reduce intraoperative anesthesia and postoperative analgesia requirements. Attention to preemptive pain control reduces central sensitization, hyperexcitability, and inflammation [46]. Effective preoperative analgesia with a combination of agents reduces perioperative morbidity, shortens hospital stays, and improves patient satisfaction [17,47–49].

Continuous epidural catheters are another useful adjunct to traditional pain control. They are most appropriate in orthopedic, abdominal, and thoracic procedures and in the treatment of blunt chest injury. When placed before induction of anesthesia, continuous epidural analgesia reduces intraoperative and postoperative anesthetic requirements [50–54]. In addition, epidural analgesia reduces ileus and postoperative nausea and vomiting. In appropriate circumstances, continuous epidural analgesia with local anesthetic, opioids, or clonidine will attenuate the perioperative neuro-endocrine response. Single-dose neuraxial anesthetics will reduce the incidence of postoperative pulmonary complications, myocardial infarction, and thromboembolism [51,52,54,55].

Early and continuous attention to analgesia incorporating a combination of techniques and drugs is essential. Insufficient analgesia at any point in the perioperative period, even for a short time, will predispose the patient to sensitization, inflammation, and chronic pain at levels similar to those seen with long-term untreated pain [6,56].

Pain assessment is mandatory. While assessment is relatively easy in the patient who is awake, oriented, and able to communicate, many postoperative patients are unable to accurately assess and communicate their level of pain. Careful monitoring of vital signs, levels of agitation, and other clues allows proper titration of analgesia. Patients who are in pain may show objective signs such as tachypnea, tachycardia, and sweating similar to the signs of hypovolemia. A careful assessment should allow appropriate management of both pain and volume status [5,6,27,41].

A balanced analgesia approach should continue into the postoperative period. Sedation does not provide proper analgesia and should not be used as a substitute for adequate analgesia. This rule is sometimes forgotten in the ICU where sedated patients in pain are often undertreated behind the cover of sedation. Aberrant vital signs, increased oxygen consumption, tissue injury, and a perpetuation of the pro-stress, pro-inflammatory milieu are all consequences of pain when undertreated, even if it is masked by sedation [4,11,48,54,55,57].

Opiates are the mainstay of a postoperative analgesic program. As a general rule, the intravenous route is the most accurate method of opiate administration. Whenever possible, we prefer to administer opioids using patient-controlled analgesia. This improves patient satisfaction, reduces patient anxiety, and provides more effective analgesia when compared with standard nurse-provided intravenous administration [58–62]. However, no evidence shows that postoperative cardiac pulmonary or thromboembolic complications are reduced with patient-controlled anesthesia compared with intermittent opioid administration. NSAIDs should be used with the opioids if possible. The concomitant use of NSAIDs with opioids provides moderate analgesia and has an opioid-sparing effect.

A recent development in perioperative pain control is the use of continuous regional infusions of local anesthetic. These infusions are administered through small catheters, which are placed directly into the surgical wound at the time of surgery. Small infusion pumps are filled with local anesthetic (usually bupivacaine), which is infused at a continuous rate directly into the wound site. At the end of the acute pain period the catheter is removed by the patient or in the doctor's office.

A number of studies have shown the efficacy and safety of these new devices. One study conducted on 80 patients who underwent inguinal hernia repair showed that use of a continuous bupivacaine pump was closely associated with reduced time in the recovery room, reduced worst-pain score on postoperative day 1, and higher patient satisfaction. No differences in pain score were seen from days 2 to 5. Additionally, there was no difference in narcotic analgesia use between the group that used the pumps and the group that did not. Another recent double-blind study of 52 patients undergoing open hernia repair showed a statistically significant decrease in VAS-scored pain and daily narcotic use for patients using the continuous bupivacaine pump. One additional study of patients undergoing median sternotomy for cardiac surgery showed a significant decrease in VAS pain score and higher patient satisfaction among pump users. This study showed no difference in patient-controlled morphine use between the group that used the pump and the group that did not [63,64]. Meanwhile, patients using the pump required less time before ambulation and experienced shorter hospital stays than patients not equipped with the pump [65]. None of the studies reported catheter related complications. The use of direct-wound anesthetic infusion seems to provide a useful adjunct to opioid and nonopioid analgesia in the postoperative setting.

The most recent Practice Guidelines for Acute Pain Management in the Perioperative Setting were published in 2004 and provide additional evidence-based recommendations from the American Society of Anesthesiologists Task Force on Acute Pain Management [66]. The US Department of Veterans Affairs offers Clinical Practice Guidelines for the Management of Postoperative Pain [67]. These guidelines include useful and practical treatment algorithms.

Summary

Balanced analgesia employs different drugs in a complementary fashion to target different points in the afferent and efferent pain pathway. Effective perioperative analgesia is an important responsibility of the surgical team, which includes the surgeon, anesthesiologist, nursing staff, patient, and the family. Careful attention to perioperative analgesia improves the patient experience, resulting in a higher quality of care.

References

[1] Caterina MJ, Julius D. The vanilloid receptor: a molecular gateway to the pain pathway. Annu Rev Neurosci 2001;24:487–517.

[2] Mantyh PW, et al. Molecular mechanisms of cancer pain. Nat Rev Cancer 2002;2(3):201–9.

[3] Schaible HG, Richter F. Pathophysiology of pain. Langenbecks Arch Surg 2004;389(4): 237–43.

[4] Winkelstein BA. Mechanisms of central sensitization, neuroimmunology & injury biomechanics in persistent pain: implications for musculoskeletal disorders. J Electromyogr Kinesiol 2004;14(1):87–93.

[5] Carr DB, Goudas LC. Acute pain. Lancet 1999;353(9169):2051–8.

[6] Desborough JP. The stress response to trauma and surgery. Br J Anaesth 2000;85(1):109–17.

[7] Besson JM. The neurobiology of pain. Lancet 1999;353(9164):1610–5.

[8] Kehlet H. Modification of responses to surgery by neural blocade. In: Cousins MJ, editor. Neural blockade in clinical anesthesia and management of pain. Philadelphia: Lippencott-Raven; 1999.

[9] Kehlet H, Holte K. Effect of postoperative analgesia on surgical outcome. Br J Anaesth 2001;87(1):62–72.

[10] Schecter WP, et al. Pain control in outpatient surgery. J Am Coll Surg 2002;195(1):95–104.

[11] Wallace KG. The pathophysiology of pain. Crit Care Nurs Q 1992;15(2):1–13.

[12] Wu CL, et al. Gene therapy for the management of pain: part I: methods and strategies. Anesthesiology 2001;94(6):1119–32.

[13] Basbaum AI. Spinal mechanisms of acute and persistent pain. Reg Anesth Pain Med 1999; 24(1):59–67.

[14] Zuckerman LF. Nonopioid and opioid analgesics. In: Ashburn MRL, editor. The management of pain. New York: Churchill Livingstone; 1998. p. 111–140.

[15] Kwong MF. Have Cox2 inhibitors lived up to expectations? Best Pract Res Clin Gastroenterol 2004;18(Suppl):13–6.

[16] Lefkowith JB. Cyclooxygenase-2 specificity and its clinical implications. Am J Med 1999; 106(5B):43S–50S.

[17] Barratt SM, et al. Multimodal analgesia and intravenous nutrition preserves total body protein following major upper gastrointestinal surgery. Reg Anesth Pain Med 2002;27(1): 15–22.

[18] Bresalier RS, et al. Cardiovascular events associated with rofecoxib in a colorectal adenoma chemoprevention trial. N Engl J Med 2005;352(11):1092–102.

[19] Drazen JM. COX-2 inhibitors—a lesson in unexpected problems. N Engl J Med 2005; 352(11):1131–2.

[20] Nussmeier NA, et al. Complications of the COX-2 inhibitors parecoxib and valdecoxib after cardiac surgery. N Engl J Med 2005;352(11):1081–91.

[21] Seibert K, et al. COX-2 inhibitors—is there cause for concern? Nat Med 1999;5(6):621–2.

[22] Solomon DH, et al. Relationship between selective cyclooxygenase-2 inhibitors and acute myocardial infarction in older adults. Circulation 2004;109(17):2068–73.

[23] Solomon SD, et al. Cardiovascular risk associated with celecoxib in a clinical trial for colorectal adenoma prevention. N Engl J Med 2005;352(11):1071–80.

[24] Rawal N. Analgesia for day-case surgery. Br J Anaesth 2001;87(1):73–87.

[25] Souter AJ, Fredman B, White PF. Controversies in the perioperative use of nonsterodial antiinflammatory drugs. Anesth Analg 1994;79(6):1178–90.

[26] Chen JY, et al. Effect of adding ketorolac to intravenous morphine patient-controlled analgesia on bowel function in colorectal surgery patients a prospective, randomized, double-blind study. Acta Anaesthesiol Scand 2005;49(4):546–51.

[27] Rawal N. Treating postoperative pain improves outcome. Minerva Anestesiol 2001; 67(9, Suppl 1):200–5.

[28] Taylor DA, Fleming WW. Unifying perspectives of the mechanisms underlying the development of tolerance and physical dependence to opioids. J Pharmacol Exp Ther 2001;297(1): 11–8.

[29] Claxton AR, et al. Evaluation of morphine versus fentanyl for postoperative analgesia after ambulatory surgical procedures. Anesth Analg 1997;84(3):509–14.

[30] Putland AJ, McCluskey A. The analgesic efficacy of tramadol versus ketorolac in day-case laparoscopic sterilisation. Anaesthesia 1999;54(4):382–5.

[31] Rawal N, et al. Postoperative analgesia at home after ambulatory hand surgery: a controlled comparison of tramadol, metamizol, and paracetamol. Anesth Analg 2001;92(2):347–51.

[32] Roelofse JA, Payne KA. Oral tramadol: analgesic efficacy in children following multiple dental extractions. Eur J Anaesthesiol 1999;16(7):441–7.

[33] Schecter WP, Swisher JL. Local anesthesia in surgical practice. Curr Probl Surg 2000;37(1): 10–67.

[34] Tverskoy M, Oren M, Vaskovich M, et al. Ketamine enhances local anesthetic an danalgesic effects of bupivicatine by peripheral mechanism: a study in postoperative patients. Neurosci Lett 1996;215(1):5–8.

[35] Suzuki M, Tsueda K, Lansing PS, et al. Small dose ketamine enhances morphine induced analgesia after outpatient surgery. Anesth Analg 1999;89(1):98–103.

[36] Schmid RL, Sander AN, Katz J. Use and efficacy of low-dose ketamine in the management of acute postopertive pain: A review of current techniques and outcomes. Pain 1999;82(111): 111–25.

[37] Tanz RD, et al. Comparative cardiotoxicity of bupivacaine and lidocaine in the isolated perfused mammalian heart. Anesth Analg 1984;63(6):549–56.

[38] Timour Q, et al. Cardiac accidents of locoregional anesthesia: experimental study of risk factors with bupivacaine. Bull Acad Natl Med 1998;182(2):217–32.

[39] Rodriguez LF, Smolik LM, Zbehlik AJ. Benzocaine-induced methemoglobinemia: report of a severe reaction and review of the literature. Ann Pharmacother 1994;28(5):643–9.

[40] Elsner P. Signs of methaemoglobinemia after topical application of EMLA cream in an infant with haemangioma. Dermatology 1997;195:153–4.

[41] Panel APMG. Acute pain management: operative or medical procedures and trauma: clinical practice guideline. Rockland (MD): 1992. Agency for Health Policy and Research, Public Health Service, US Department of Health and Human Services, AHCPR Publication 92–0032.

[42] McCormack HM, Horne DJ. Clinical applications of visual analogue scales: a critical review. Psychol Med, 1988;18:1007–19.

[43] Gracely RH. Evaluation of multi-dimensional pain scales. Pain 1992;48(3):297–300.

[44] Hasegawa M, et al. The McGill Pain Questionnaire, Japanese version, reconsidered: confirming the theoretical structure. Pain Res Manag 2001;6(4):173–80.

[45] Lowe NK, Walker SN, MacCallum RC. Confirming the theoretical structure of the McGill Pain Questionnaire in acute clinical pain. Pain 1991;46(1):53–60.

[46] Perkins FM, Kehlet H. Chronic pain as an outcome of surgery. A review of predictive factors. Anesthesiology 2000;93:1123–33.

[47] Basse L, et al. Accelerated postoperative recovery programme after colonic resection improves physical performance, pulmonary function and body composition. Br J Surg 2002; 89(4):446–53.

[48] Brodner G, et al. Acute pain management: analysis, implications and consequences after prospective experience with 6349 surgical patients. Eur J Anaesthesiol 2000;17(9):566–75.

[49] Brodner G, et al. Multimodal perioperative management—combining thoracic epidural analgesia, forced mobilization, and oral nutrition—reduces hormonal and metabolic stress and improves convalescence after major urologic surgery. Anesth Analg 2001;92(6): 1594–600.

[50] Fernandez MI, et al. Does a thoracic epidural confer any additional benefit following video-assisted thoracoscopic pleurectomy for primary spontaneous pneumothorax? Eur J Cardiothorac Surg 2005;27(4):671–4.

[51] Holte K, Kehlet H. Epidural analgesia and risk of anastomotic leakage. Reg Anesth Pain Med 2001;26(2):111–7.

[52] Holte K, Kehlet H. Effect of postoperative epidural analgesia on surgical outcome. Minerva Anestesiol 2002;68(4):157–61.

[53] Subramaniam B, Pawar DK, Kashyap L. Pre-emptive analgesia with epidural morphine or morphine and bupivacaine. Anaesth Intensive Care 2000;28(4):392–8.

[54] Wu CT, et al. Pre-incisional epidural ketamine, morphine and bupivacaine combined with epidural and general anaesthesia provides pre-emptive analgesia for upper abdominal surgery. Acta Anaesthesiol Scand 2000;44(1):63–8.

[55] Woolf CJ. Phenotypic modification of primary sensory neurons: the role of nerve growth factor in the production of persistent pain. Philos Trans R Soc Lond B Biol Sci 1996;351(1338): 441–8.

[56] Katz J, et al. Acute pain after thoracic surgery predicts long-term post-thoracotomy pain. Clin J Pain 1996;12(1):50–5.

[57] Kehlet H. Effect of postoperative pain treatment on outcome current status and future strategies. Langenbecks Arch Surg 2004;389(4):244–9.

[58] Kanjhan R. Opioids and pain. Clin Exp Pharmacol Physiol 1995;22(6–7):397–403.

[59] Korpela R, Korvenoja P, Meretoja OA. Morphine-sparing effect of acetaminophen in pediatric day-case surgery. Anesthesiology 1999;91(2):442–7.

[60] McCaffery M, Pasero C. Pain: clinical manual. 2nd ed. St. Louis (MO): Mosby; 1999.

[61] Stein C, Machelska H, Schafer M. Peripheral analgesic and antiinflammatory effects of opioids. Z Rheumatol 2001;60(6):416–24.

[62] Stein C, Yassouridis A. Peripheral morphine analgesia. Pain 1997;71(2):119–21.

[63] Schurr MJ, et al. Continuous local anesthetic infusion for pain management after outpatient inguinal herniorrhaphy. Surgery 2004;136(4):761–9.

[64] Vintar N, et al. Incisional self-administration of bupivacaine or ropivacaine provides effective analgesia after inguinal hernia repair. Can J Anaesth 2002;49(5):481–6.

[65] White PF, et al. Use of a continuous local anesthetic infusion for pain management after median sternotomy. Anesthesiology 2003;99(4):918–23.

[66] American Society of Anesthesiologists Task Force on Acute Pain Management. Practice guidelines for acute pain management in the perioperative setting. Anesthesiology 2004; 100:1573–81.

[67] Department of Veterans Affairs, Veterans Health Administration, Office of Quality & Performance. Post operative pain: clinical practice guidelines. Available at: http://www.oqp. med.va.gov/cpg/pain/pain_base.htm. Accessed September 16, 2005.

SURGICAL
CLINICS OF
NORTH AMERICA

Surg Clin N Am 85 (2005) 1259–1266

Perioperative Management of Special Populations: The Geriatric Patient

David B. Loran, MD, Brannon R. Hyde, MD,
Joseph B. Zwischenberger, MD*

*Department of Surgery, The University of Texas Medical Branch,
301 University Boulevard, Galveston, TX 77555, USA*

Americans over age 65 represent the fastest growing segment of the United States population [1]. As a result, the demographic landscape of America is changing. Knowledge of aged physiology is necessary to construct a risk–benefit analysis tailored for each patient to improve perioperative outcomes and lower the morbidity and mortality rates among the elderly. Benefit estimates should account for a patient's life expectancy and quality of life before and after surgery. Pain control, postoperative cognitive dysfunction, end-of-life issues, and realistic expectations after surgery are paramount issues throughout the perioperative period.

Preoperative assessment

With aging, baseline functions of almost every organ system undergo progressive decline resulting in a decreased physiologic reserve and ability to compensate for stress. Coexisting disease has more impact on morbidity and mortality than age alone in the geriatric population [2]. An elderly patient has increased risk of morbidity and mortality if the patient:

- has severe systemic disease (American Society of Anethesiologists (ASA) Class III or IV);
- requires an emergency procedure;
- suffers from renal failure;
- has chronic obstructive pulmonary disease;
- has had a recent myocardial infarction or unstable angina;
- has albumin level of <3.5 g/dL;

* Corresponding author.
E-mail address: jzwische@utmb.edu (J.B. Zwischenberger).

0039-6109/05/$ - see front matter © 2005 Elsevier Inc. All rights reserved.
doi:10.1016/j.suc.2005.09.004
surgical.theclinics.com

- is anemic (Hb <8.0 g/dL);
- has been bedridden; or
- has before the operation required assistance with activities of daily living.

Preoperative workup should begin with basic laboratory screening based on an individual's identified comorbidities.

Cardiovascular physiology

Cardiac disease is the most common comorbid condition in the elderly [3] as 80% of patients over 80 have identifiable cardiovascular disease. Starting in the third decade, cardiac output and the maximum rate of oxygen use (VO_2max) steadily decline. Congestive heart failure (CHF) is present in 10% of individuals over 65 years of age and is the leading cause of postoperative morbidity and mortality following surgical procedures. Patients with CHF have an increased rate of stroke, myocardial infarction, and postoperative renal failure. Pre-existing CHF can lead to a twofold to fourfold increase in postoperative cardiovascular complications, including myocardial infarction, supraventricular tachycardia, hypotension or hypertension, and cardiac arrest [4].

Age-related changes to the cardiovascular system include stiffening of the vascular wall and increased peripheral vascular resistance. With prolonged exposure to high afterload, myocyte turnover through apoptosis is accelerated with subsequent hypertrophy of the ventricular myocardium and impaired diastolic filling. The ventricle remains stiff during passive diastolic filling, thus reducing left ventricular end diastolic volume (LVEDV) and cardiac output. The aged heart is less responsive to sympathetic stimulation and, therefore, relies on increased preload with atrial enlargement to compensate for diastolic dysfunction. A patient who develops atrial fibrillation loses atrial kick, leading to further reduced LVEDV and cardiac output. Fatty infiltration and fibrosis of the myocardium increases the incidence of conduction abnormalities [5]. These changes underscore the importance of maintaining the cardiovascular system in a nonstressed, normotensive sinus rhythm during surgical procedures in elderly patients.

Estimation of cardiac reserve can be difficult because most elderly patients with cardiac dysfunction are compensated and will only show signs of disease when stressed [4]. Cardiac assessment usually begins with an ECG. However, 75% of patients over 70 years of age have some abnormality on their baseline ECG, which ironically has not been shown to predict outcomes. Arrhythmias, however, have been shown to increase postoperative cardiac morbidity in elderly patients. Atrial fibrillation is the most common arrhythmia (10% over 80 years) and accounts for 75,000 thromboembolic events per year [6]. Provocative testing with thallium scans, dobutamine stress tests, or echocardiography should follow guidelines of the American College of Cardiologists/American Heart Association [7].

Pulmonary physiology

Evidence of age-related changes in the pulmonary system include a loss of elastic recoil of the lung and impaired chest wall movement caused by muscle atrophy, joint stiffening, and skeletal changes. Impaired elasticity causes air trapping and ventilation-perfusion (V/Q) mismatching leading to decreased oxygen transfer [8]. Oxygenation is further impaired by the closure of an increasing number of small airways and decreased surface area for gas exchange. Vital capacity decreases with age, reflecting an increase in dead space ventilation. The forced expiratory volume in 1 second (FEV1) also progressively declines. The respiratory changes associated with aging cumulatively limit the maximal breathing capacity by age 70% to 50% of that at age 30 [9]. Ciliary function and cough are also reduced, decreasing the clearance of secretions postoperatively and leading to an increased risk for aspiration and pneumonia [10].

Preoperative pulmonary assessment in the elderly should focus on identifying patients with limited pulmonary reserve and maximizing performance status. Smoking cessation can reduce surgical risk in as little as 6 weeks [11]. In patients over 70 years of age, the number of stairs a patient can climb before the operation is inversely proportional to cardiopulmonary complication rates after the operation [12]. Achieving an exercise capacity of just 2 minutes with a heart rate of 99 beats per minute can lower an elderly patient's complication rate from 42% to 9% and mortality rate from 7% to 1% [13]. A structured pulmonary rehabilitation program can improve 6-minute walk distances, dyspnea, and patient perceived pulmonary function. Improvement from pulmonary rehabilitation allows a quicker and more persistent return to activity.

Splinting from inadequate pain control restricts lung expansion, limits cough to clear secretions, and leads to an increased risk for atelectasis, pneumonia, and hypoxia. The functional residual capacity (FRC) can be suppressed up to 70% from baseline and remain severely suppressed for as long as 7 days postoperatively [14]. To reduce the likelihood of pulmonary complications, an aggressive pulmonary toilet regimen of coughing, deep breathing, and early ambulation should be implemented immediately after surgery. Preoperative education regarding the need for pulmonary toilet and incentive spirometry is of paramount importance in elderly patients.

Renal physiology

Age-related changes in the renal system are characterized by a progressive reduction in renal mass and creatinine clearance. Glomerulosclerosis results in a decline in renal plasma flow (RPF) and in glomerular filtration rate (GFR) [9]. Additionally, age-related decline in cardiac output also causes the RPF and the GFR to decline. Patients with an impaired GFR are more susceptible to volume overload in the perioperative period as well as accumulation of metabolic substances and drugs that rely on renal clearance for excretion [3]. Slowed drug elimination can lead to prolonged sedative effects of anesthetic and narcotic medication and drug-induced acute renal dysfunction following administration of nonsteroidal anti-inflammatory medications, diuretics, and antibiotics [9]. Impaired renal sodium conservation can lead to electrolyte imbalances, which could affect cardiac conduction and lead to arrhythmias. The plasma creatinine may measure low because of reduced skeletal muscle mass. However, the calculated creatinine clearance remains the most sensitive marker of renal function in the elderly.

Nutrition

Risk factors associated with nutritional deficiency among elderly patients have been documented [15]. Low weight is the most significant factor. Other factors include:

- poverty
- alcohol abuse
- deterioration in physical and cognitive function
- change in the number or type of medications
- recent hospitalization or surgery
- micturition dysfunction

Although history and physical examination are as effective as any biochemical marker in assessing nutrition [16], low preoperative albumin correlates directly with mortality. Mortality was <1% for albumin levels above 46 g/L and rose to 29% for levels <21 g/L in one large study [17]. The Mini Nutritional Assessment and Subjective Global Assessment also predicts mortality in geriatric patients [18].

Anesthesia

The physiologic changes seen in the elderly and their effects on drug bioavailability and side effect profiles can define the type and dose of agent used for anesthesia in the elderly patient. A decrease in total body water seen with aging leads to higher peak drug concentrations following bolus or rapid infusion. A relative reduction in perfusion to organs such as the liver and kidneys can prolong a drug's duration of action by slowing metabolism and excretion [19]. Most anesthetic drugs have some degree of cardiac depressant activity, necessitating a reduced dose in the elderly. In a patient with congestive heart failure, using benzodiazepines or opioids that have minimal effects on cardiac contractility and heart rate can reduce the likelihood of hypotension or arrhythmia at induction [20,21]. For patients with minimal cardiac functional reserve, tachycardia has deleterious effects. Avoiding such drugs as pancuronium, which induce tachycardia, can help avoid cardiac ischemia [22]. Epidural anesthesia decreases perioperative cardiac stress and decreases tachycardia-induced cardiac ischemia [23].

Pain control

Better analgesic techniques for the elderly need to be discovered [24]. Elderly often communicate less pain because of cognitive impairment or fear of being a "bad patient." Physicians may perceive this as evidence that elderly feel less pain than younger patients. In fact, up to 45% of patients may feel their pain is undertreated while hospitalized [25]. Scheduled dosing invariably leads to inadequate pain control or overdosing.

Inadequate pain control can increase morbidity and mortality in the elderly, perhaps because of the increased incidence of ischemic heart disease, decreased ventilatory reserve, and altered drug metabolism, response, and excretion [24]. For acute postoperative pain, intravenous morphine titration using the same protocol for elderly (>70 years) and younger patients appears safe [26]. Two milligrams (weight <60 kg) or 3 mg (weight >60 kg) of intravenous morphine every 5 minutes for a visual analog score of greater than 30 has been shown to provide adequate pain control in the immediate postoperative period. No difference appears in morphine-related adverse effects (nausea, vomiting, respiratory depression, urinary retention, pruritus, and allergy) or sedation incidence [26].

Several days after a major operation, however, elderly patients require less opioid than do younger cohorts. In a prospective patient-controlled analgesia (PCA) study of patients undergoing elective major surgery, 44 older patients (67 $\pm$ 8 years) self-administered less opioid than 45 younger (39 $\pm$ 9 years) patients [27]. In patients with a declining mental status, however, PCA use is not recommended. Compared with PCA involving intravenous opioids, patient-controlled epidural analgesia (PCEA) may be more effective in relieving pain at rest or after coughing in the elderly. The epidural route is also associated with earlier improved mental status and bowel activity [28].

Postoperative delirium and cognitive assessment

Postoperative cognitive impairment can be classified as postoperative delirium (PD) or postoperative neurocognitive disorder (POCD). PD is characterized by fluctuating levels of consciousness and temporary abnormalities in memory and perception. POCD is a condition with a variable time course characterized by impaired concentration, language comprehension, and social integration. These characteristics can become evident days to weeks after surgery.

The incidence of PD in the elderly varies widely from 3% to 61%, depending on the type of surgery [29]. Risk factors for PD include age, chronic impaired cognitive functioning, physical debilitation, and dementia.

Independent precipitating factors for delirium include use of physical restraints, malnutrition, addition of more than three medications, and use of a bladder catheter [30]. Perioperative factors associated with PD include intraoperative blood loss, postoperative hematocrit <30%, electrolyte abnormalities, and sepsis [31]. Perioperative hypoxemia, hypotension, and general anesthesia itself have not been shown to increase PD [32]. Treatment of PD should focus on identifying organic causes, including electrolyte abnormalities, hypoxemia, pain, sepsis, dehydration, and malnutrition. Protocols that provide cognitive stimulation, facilitate adequate sleep, promote early mobilization, and reduce sensory deficit lower the incidence of PD [33].

POCD differs from PD in that the memory loss, slower central processing time, and changes resulting in decreased ability to learn new information do not fluctuate and may last months to years. The incidence of POCD in elderly patients is difficult to determine because methods for diagnosis are unreliable. Factors that increase the risk for POCD include advanced age, extended duration of anesthesia, lack of education, a second operation, postoperative infection, and respiratory complications. Hypoxemia and hypotension are not associated with cognitive decline [32].

Quality-of-life and end-of-life issues

Most patients would rather maintain an independent lifestyle rather than gain a few months of life in a debilitated state. When weighing the risks and benefits for an elderly patient, a surgeon must consider the predicted life expectancy of the patient and quality of life after intervention. Unfortunately, literature concerning surgery in the elderly is often based on cases with an inherent selection bias for the healthiest patients.

The patient should be aware of the specific risks involved based on age and comorbidities, and the potential need for rehabilitation services or nursing home care after the operation. The average hospital stay for patients over 70 years old is from 7 to 12 days. Although 90% to 95% of elderly patients return to their preoperative lifestyle, 5% to 7% of patients need some form of long-term care assistance [34].

Death and dying discussions facilitate the transition from life-saving treatment to palliative care. Patients should be encouraged to take control of end-of-life decisions by outlining their care. Physicians, on the other hand, must resist proceeding with invasive and heroic measures late in the disease course. Candid discussions preoperatively between patient, physician, and family can help preserve patient autonomy in medical decisions.

References

[1] US Department of Census. 65+ in the United States. Washington, DC: US Bureau of the Census; 1996.

[2] Schneider JR, Droste JS, Schindler N, et al. Carotid endarterectomy in octogenarians: comparison with patient characteristics and outcomes in younger patients. J Vasc Surg 2000; 31(5):927–35.

[3] Rosenthal RA, Kavic SM. Assessment and management of the geriatric patient. Crit Care Med 2004;32(4 Suppl):S92–105.

[4] Leung JM, Dzankic S. Relative importance of preoperative health status versus intraoperative factors in predicting postoperative adverse outcomes in geriatric surgical patients. J Am Geriatr Soc 2001;49(8):1080–5.

[5] Lakatta EG. Cardiovascular regulatory mechanisms in advanced age. Physiol Rev 1993; 73(2):413–67.

[6] Liu LL, Dzankic S, Leung JM. Preoperative electrocardiogram abnormalities do not predict postoperative cardiac complications in geriatric surgical patients. J Am Geriatr Soc 2002; 50(7):1186–91.

[7] Eagle KA, Berger PB, Calkins H, et al. ACC/AHA guideline update for perioperative cardiovascular evaluation for noncardiac surgery—executive summary. A report of the American College of Cardiology/American Heart Association Task Force on Practice Guidelines (Committee to Update the 1996 Guidelines on Perioperative Cardiovascular Evaluation for Noncardiac Surgery). Anesth Analg 2002;94(5):1052–64.

[8] Erskine RJ, Murphy PJ, Langton JA, et al. Effect of age on the sensitivity of upper airway reflexes. Br J Anaesth 1993;70(5):574–5.

[9] Tonner PH, Kampen J, Scholz J. Pathophysiological changes in the elderly. Best Pract Res Clin Anaesthesiol 2003;17(2):163–77.

[10] Zaugg M, Lucchinetti E. Respiratory function in the elderly. Anesthesiol Clin North America 2000;18(1):47–58 [vi.].

[11] Warner MA, Offord KP, Warner ME, et al. Role of preoperative cessation of smoking and other factors in postoperative pulmonary complications: a blinded prospective study of coronary artery bypass patients. Mayo Clin Proc 1989;64(6):609–16.

[12] Brunelli A, Monteverde M, Al Refai M, et al. Stair climbing test as a predictor of cardiopulmonary complications after pulmonary lobectomy in the elderly. Ann Thorac Surg 2004; 77(1):266–70.

[13] Gerson MC, Hurst JM, Hertzberg VS, et al. Prediction of cardiac and pulmonary complications related to elective abdominal and noncardiac thoracic surgery in geriatric patients. Am J Med 1990;88(2):101–7.

[14] Schwieger I, Gamulin Z, Suter PM. Lung function during anesthesia and respiratory insufficiency in the postoperative period: physiological and clinical implications. Acta Anaesthesiol Scand 1989;33(7):527–34.

[15] Hazzard WR, Blass JP. Nutrition and aging. In: Sullivan DH, Johnson LE, editors. Principles of geriatric medicine and gerontology. 5th ed. New York: McGraw-Hill; 2003. p. 1167.

[16] Souba WW. Nutritional support. N Engl J Med 1997;336(1):41–8.

[17] Daley J, Khuri SF, Henderson W, et al. Risk adjustment of the postoperative morbidity rate for the comparative assessment of the quality of surgical care: results of the National Veterans Affairs surgical risk study. J Am Coll Surg 1997;185(4):328–40.

[18] Persson MD, Brismar KE, Katzarski KS, et al. Nutritional status using mini nutritional assessment and subjective global assessment predict mortality in geriatric patients. J Am Geriatr Soc 2002;50(12):1996–2002.

[19] Sadean MR, Glass PS. Pharmacokinetics in the elderly. Best Pract Res Clin Anaesthesiol 2003;17(2):191–205.

[20] Bailey JM, Mora CT, Shafer SL. Pharmacokinetics of propofol in adult patients undergoing coronary revascularization. The Multicenter Study of Perioperative Ischemia Research Group. Anesthesiology 1996;84(6):1288–97.

[21] Thomson IR, Harding G, Hudson RJ. A comparison of fentanyl and sufentanil in patients undergoing coronary artery bypass graft surgery. J Cardiothorac Vasc Anesth 2000;14(6): 652–6.

[22] Wappler F. Cardiac and thoracic vascular surgery. Best Pract Res Clin Anaesthesiol 2003; 17(2):219–33.

[23] Loick HM, Schmidt C, Van Aken H, et al. High thoracic epidural anesthesia, but not clonidine, attenuates the perioperative stress response via sympatholysis and reduces the release of troponin T in patients undergoing coronary artery bypass grafting. Anesth Analg 1999; 88(4):701–9.

[24] Cook DJ. New frontiers in geriatrics research: an agenda for surgical and related medical specialties. New York: American Geriatrics Society; 2004.

[25] Desbiens NA, Mueller-Rizner N, Connors AF Jr, et al. Pain in the oldest-old during hospitalization and up to one year later. HELP Investigators. Hospitalized Elderly Longitudinal Project. J Am Geriatr Soc 1997;45(10):1167–72.

[26] Aubrun F, Monsel S, Langeron O, et al. Postoperative titration of intravenous morphine in the elderly patient. Anesthesiology 2002;96(1):17–23.

[27] Gagliese L, Jackson M, Ritvo P, et al. Age is not an impediment to effective use of patient-controlled analgesia by surgical patients. Anesthesiology 2000;93(3):601–10.

[28] Mann C, Pouzeratte Y, Boccara G, et al. Comparison of intravenous or epidural patient-controlled analgesia in the elderly after major abdominal surgery. Anesthesiology 2000; 92(2):433–41.

[29] Parikh SS, Chung F. Postoperative delirium in the elderly. Anesth Analg 1995;80(6): 1223–32.

[30] Inouye SK, Charpentier PA. Precipitating factors for delirium in hospitalized elderly persons. Predictive model and interrelationship with baseline vulnerability. JAMA 1996; 275(11):852–7.

[31] Marcantonio ER, Goldman L, Orav EJ, et al. The association of intraoperative factors with the development of postoperative delirium. Am J Med 1998;105(5):380–4.

[32] Moller JT, Cluitmans P, Rasmussen LS, et al. Long-term postoperative cognitive dysfunction in the elderly ISPOCD1 study. ISPOCD investigators. International study of postoperative cognitive dysfunction. Lancet 1998;351(9106):857–61.

[33] Inouye SK, Bogardus ST Jr, Charpentier PA, et al. A multicomponent intervention to prevent delirium in hospitalized older patients. N Engl J Med 1999;340(9):669–76.

[34] Brock MV, Kim MP, Hooker CM, et al. Pulmonary resection in octogenarians with stage I nonsmall cell lung cancer: a 22-year experience. Ann Thorac Surg 2004;77(1):271–7.

SURGICAL
CLINICS OF
NORTH AMERICA

Surg Clin N Am 85 (2005) 1267–1282

Perioperative Management of Special Populations: Immunocompromised Host (Cancer, HIV, Transplantation)

Dev M. Desai, MD, PhD, Paul C. Kuo, MD, MBA*

*Division of General and Transplant Surgery, Department of Surgery,
Duke University School of Medicine, Durham, NC 27710, USA*

Optimal perioperative care of the immunocompromised patient requires an understanding of the consequences of disease-specific pharmacologic therapies. The toxicity profile of these therapies can strongly influence the decision algorithms for delivering care in the perioperative period. In this manuscript, the authors describe the potential effects of drugs commonly used for treatment of patients with cancer, HIV, or transplanted organs, and impact of these drugs on the care of these patients in the perioperative setting.

Cancer

Most antineoplastic drugs are antiproliferative agents and do not differentiate malignant cells from normal cells [1,2]. Tumor selectivity depends on kinetic differences between cancer cells and normal cells. Antineoplastic agents can be divided into three groups: cell-cycle-nonspecific agents, cell-cycle-specific/phase-nonspecific agents, and cell-cycle-specific/phase-specific agents. Cell-cycle-nonspecific agents, such as alkylating agents, are toxic to both dividing and quiescent (cell-cycle phase G0) cells. Cell-cycle-specific/phase-nonspecific agents, such as anthracyclines and mitoxantrone, kill dividing cells regardless of the cells' phase. Cell-cycle-specific/phase-specific agents, such as antimetabolites, epipodophyllotoxins, vinca alkaloids, and bleomycin, kill dividing cells at specific phases of the cell cycle.

* Corresponding author: 110 Bell Building, DUMC, Box 3522, Durham, NC 27710.
E-mail address: kuo00004@mc.duke.edu (P.C. Kuo).

Chemotherapy drugs are most cytotoxic for rapidly proliferating tissues. That is, the drugs will have a greater effect on cell populations with large percentage of cycling cells, as compared to cell populations with a large percentage of cells in the G0 (resting) phase. Most acute side effects of chemotherapy occur in areas of the body where cell turnover is rapid. These include, for example, the gastrointestinal mucosa, the Sertoli cells of the testis, the hair follicles, and the replicating elements in the bone marrow. Drug doses and schedules of administration must be based on the specific mechanism of action and clinical pharmacology of each drug and on the time required for normal tissues to recover from their associated acute toxicities.

Concomitant medical problems or polypharmacy may exacerbate toxicities. Medical conditions that interfere with the metabolism or excretion of chemotherapeutic agents may increase their toxicity greatly. Because the liver may metabolize chemotherapeutic drugs, patients with liver or biliary dysfunction are more likely to experience severe toxic effects. Similarly, drug metabolism that is renal-dependent will induce toxicity in the presence of kidney pathology.

Drug interactions may also play a role. Salicylates displace methotrexate from its binding sites on albumin to increase its toxicity. 6-Mercaptopurine is metabolized by xanthine oxidase and concurrent administration of the xanthine oxidase inhibitor allopurinol can increase its toxicity greatly. Chemotherapeutic agents can synergize with X rays and ultraviolet light. A reaction characterized by skin erythema and inflammation may be seen with doxorubicin or dactinomycin shortly after a course of radiotherapy. Usually, this inflammation is limited to the site of irradiation. Several agents, notably 5-fluorouracil (5-FU) and methotrexate, may act as photosensitizers, increasing susceptibility to inflammation and sunlight-induced damage. Finally, idiosyncratic or allergic reactions may occur with a variety of chemotherapeutic agents. Anaphylaxis has been known to occur in response to the administration of bleomycin, L-asparaginase, and paclitaxel.

Cardiotoxicity

Doxorubicin and daunorubicin are chemotherapeutic agents sometimes associated with cardiac injury. Acute effects on the heart are manifested by electrocardiographic (ECG) abnormalities and are seen in up to 41% of patients receiving the drug. These ECG changes, such as nonspecific ST-T wave changes, sinus tachycardia, premature ventricular and atrial contractions, and low-voltage QRS complexes, are more common in patients who previously have had an abnormal ECG. In the setting of toxicity, mortality is as high as 61%.

The total dose of doxorubicin is the most significant risk factor for cardiomyopathy. Others include the schedule of drug administration, age, preexisting cardiac disease, prior mediastinal or left chest radiotherapy, and concurrent therapy with cytotoxic drugs. Tachycardia may be the first sign of doxorubicin toxicity. Affected patients present with symptoms of congestive heart failure, shortness of breath, or nonproductive cough. Pathologic findings are nonspecific and no morphologic evidence is predictive of doxorubicin-induced heart failure. Cardiomyopathy can be prevented in most affected patients by limiting the dose of doxorubicin.

Pulmonary toxicity

Several chemotherapeutic agents affect the lung, but pulmonary toxicity is most common with bleomycin. The end result is pulmonary fibrosis. Early preclinical studies of bleomycin indicated that it is concentrated preferentially in squamous tissues, particularly the lung and skin. A dry, hacking cough and dyspnea on exertion characterize bleomycin-mediated pulmonary toxicity. Symptoms may develop during the course of drug therapy or 1 to 3 months after the end of treatment. The early findings on physical examination are bibasilar rales, rhonchi, or a pleural friction rub. The radiographic manifestations are fine, reticular, bibasilar infiltrates that may progress to alveolar and interstitial infiltrates, progressive involvement of the lower lobe, and lung consolidation. On blood gas analysis, oxygen and bicarbonate concentrations usually are low. Serial pulmonary function tests should be performed in all patients receiving bleomycin. Bleomycin-induced lung toxicity is dose-related, increasing significantly at doses greater than 500 units. Risk factors include advanced age, preexisting lung disease, and previous radiotherapy. Several other chemotherapeutic agents have been cited as pulmonary toxins, including cyclophosphamide, procarbazine, melphalan, methotrexate, mitomycin C, and carmustine (BCNU).

Hepatotoxicity

Several chemotherapeutic agents may be hepatotoxic. Effects may manifest as a transient elevation in enzymes, while severe damage might result in permanent cirrhosis. The nitrosourea compounds (eg, BCNU, lomustine (CCNU), streptozocin) can cause mild elevations in serum transaminases, alkaline phosphatase, and bilirubin. These levels generally normalize once administration of the offending agent is discontinued. The antimetabolite methotrexate, a dihydrofolate reductase inhibitor, also is associated with liver dysfunction, often causing elevations in aspartate aminotransferase and lactate dehydrogenase. Hepatic fibrosis may resolve once treatment is discontinued. However, cirrhosis will not resolve. Azathioprine and 6-mercaptopurine are associated with intrahepatic cholestasis and parenchymal cell necrosis. Liver enzyme levels can be elevated also by the administration of cytosine arabinoside. The hepatotoxic effects of L-asparaginase, a drug used frequently with acute lymphoblastic leukemia, include fatty changes, decreased serum proteins and coagulation factors, and elevations in liver enzymes. Administration of floxuridine by hepatic artery infusion has been associated with significant hepatotoxicity and biliary injury.

Genitourinary toxicity

Chemotherapeutic agents that cause major renal toxicity include cisplatin, methotrexate, and streptozocin. Toxicity depends on the dose of an agent used and the schedule of administration. Cisplatin toxicity may be potentiated by preexisting renal disease or by the concurrent use of other nephrotoxic agents, such as the aminoglycoside antibiotics. Cisplatin toxicity may be avoided by aggressive hydration with normal saline or mannitol. High-dose methotrexate may cause acute renal failure, although this complication can be avoided through the use of hydration and alkalinization schemes. Cyclophosphamide and ifosfamide have been associated with hemorrhagic cystitis as the result of toxic metabolites in the urine. Hemorrhagic cystitis may be avoided with adequate hydration. Symptoms of cystitis include urgency, frequency, dysuria, and a mild microscopic hematuria. Usually, the cystitis is self-limiting, resolving within 2 to 6 weeks after use of the drug is stopped. Severe hemorrhagic cystitis may require cystoscopy with clot removal, fulguration of discrete bleeding sites, and instillation of such sclerosing agents as formalin. The use of mesna, a synthetic sulfhydryl, reduces the incidence of this complication after the administration of high-dose cyclophosphamide or ifosfamide.

Neurotoxicity

Chemotherapeutic agents have been associated with various neurologic toxicities. Best described is the toxicity related to the vinca alkaloids, particularly vincristine. Vincristine is unique among the antineoplastic agents in that its neurotoxicity is commonly dose-limiting. Early manifestations include distal paresthesias and the loss of deep tendon reflexes. Cranial nerve palsy, autonomic neuropathy, and the syndrome of inappropriate antidiuretic hormone secretion are seen with high cumulative doses of vincristine. Toxicity is usually symmetric, dose-related, and reversible. Peak dose levels correlate best with toxicity. Cisplatin and carboplatin produce a symmetric sensory neuropathy, particularly at high cumulative doses. Other evidence of neurologic toxicity from cisplatin includes tinnitus and hearing loss, especially in the high-frequency range. 5-FU induces cerebellar ataxia, while L-asparaginase is associated with lethargy, confusion, and disorientation. The use of high-dose or intrathecal methotrexate, especially in combination with cranial irradiation, may cause progressive encephalopathy. Paclitaxel induces a symmetric polyneuropathy that is dose-dependent and enhanced by cisplatin.

Emesis is coordinated by receptors in the gastrointestinal tract and the central nervous system. Vagus nerve afferents connect to the "vomiting center" in the medulla. The identification of specific receptor antagonists has allowed more effective drugs to be developed to treat chemotherapy-induced nausea and vomiting. Anticipatory nausea and vomiting is a conditioned response usually found in patients with poor emetic control after initial chemotherapy. Such patients may begin to experience symptoms following triggers, such as entering the hospital. Anticipatory nausea and vomiting may exacerbate postoperative nausea and vomiting. Maximizing the antiemetic regimen during the first course of chemotherapy can prevent this complication. Once established, anticipatory emesis may be treated by desensitization, hypnosis, or relaxation techniques. Delayed emesis, which contributes to morbidity by interfering with nutrition and hydration, is encountered most often following high-dose chemotherapy. Symptoms are noted 48 hours after chemotherapy administration, but may occur up to 5 days later. Effective treatment includes oral dexamethasone plus oral metoclopramide or a phenothiazine.

Myelosuppression

Bone marrow suppression is a toxic effect of many chemotherapeutic agents and typically is the dose-limiting factor. Death occurring after chemotherapy usually results either from infection related to drug-induced leukopenia or from bleeding secondary to thrombocytopenia. The onset of myelosuppression varies among drugs. For example, cell-cycle-specific chemotherapeutic agents affect the rapidly proliferating pool of blood precursors in the marrow (from myeloblasts to promyelocytes). Destruction of this cohort of myeloid precursors leads to a predictable decrease in the peripheral white blood-cell count at approximately 10 to 14 days after the drug is administered, after which the white count rapidly returns to normal. Other chemotherapeutic agents affect stem cells, leading to myelosuppression and a delay in the recovery of normal blood counts. In most cases, myelosuppression is relatively short-lived (3–5 days) and is self-limited.

Infection is a frequent problem associated with leukopenia. As evidence, the most common cause of chemotherapy-related death in neutropenic patients is sepsis. The usual clinical manifestations of infection (eg, erythema, pain, pulmonary infiltrates, pyuria) are absent in patients with neutropenia. The hallmark of infection in neutropenic patients is fever. If the absolute neutrophil count is 500 to 1000/mm^3, indicating neutropenia, broad-spectrum antibiotics should be given emergently. The Infectious Disease Society of America developed guidelines for the use of antimicrobial agents to treat neutropenic patients with cancer, and includes recommendations for monotherapy and combination therapy [3]. On occasion, infection may develop without fever. In such patients, the sudden onset of weakness, hypotension, or confusion may suggest the diagnosis. Initial infections in the neutropenic patient are typically bacterial and involve such gram-positive organisms as *Staphylococcus aureus* and such gram-negative organisms as *Pseudomonas aeruginosa, Escherichia coli, Klebsiella,* and *Serratia* species. Often, the source of the infecting organism is previous colonization. Common sites of infection include the skin, oropharynx, lungs, gastrointestinal and genitourinary tracts, and blood stream. Particular sites may be at higher risk for infection, owing to the specific malignancy or anticancer therapy (eg, an obstructive bronchial lesion, radiation-induced esophagitis).

In febrile neutropenic patients, the routine use of such recombinant colony-stimulating factors as granulocyte colony-stimulating factor (G-CSF) or granulocyte-macrophage colony-stimulating factor (GM-CSF) with antibiotics has not been proven to confer added benefit. Current guidelines suggest using growth factors only in patients at high risk for complications from sepsis. Although bacterial infections may be controlled by prompt administration of antibiotics, treating fungal and viral infections in neutropenic patients is much more difficult. Fungal pathogens may include *Candida, Aspergillus,* and *Mucor* species, among others. Patients who are neutropenic and remain persistently febrile despite adequate antibiotic treatment may benefit from a trial of empiric therapy with the antifungal drugs.

Neutropenia and its subsequent infectious complications represent the most common dose-limiting toxicity of cancer chemotherapy. Febrile neutropenia occurs with common chemotherapy regimens in 25% to 40% of treatment-naïve patients, and may result in subsequent chemotherapy delays or dose reductions.

The American Society of Clinical Oncology (ASCO) guidelines [4] recommend the use of G-CSF as primary prophylaxis (first-cycle use) in patients with ≥40% risk of febrile neutropenia. These patients may include elderly and other high-risk patients. Clinical trials to date have not demonstrated a significant effect on overall survival or disease-free survival, but have demonstrated clinically the benefits of delivering planned chemotherapy doses on schedule, an important clinical goal, especially in curative tumor settings.

In March 2005, the National Comprehensive Cancer Network (NCCN) issued new guidelines advocating the use of CSF to prevent febrile neutropenia in patients with a 20% risk of developing the condition [5]. The panel also recommended that physicians consider CSFs when the risk of febrile neutropenia is between 10% and 20%. The guidelines do not recommend the drugs for patients at a less than 10% risk of febrile neutropenia.

Cutaneous toxicity

A cutaneous complication is the local infiltration of a vesicant drug that may cause severe tissue inflammation and necrosis. The major drugs associated with such reactions include doxorubicin, daunorubicin, dactinomycin, mitomycin C, BCNU, dacarbazine (DTIC), nitrogen mustard, vincristine, vinblastine, and vinorelbine. Managing skin ulceration and inflammation that result from drug extravasation can be extremely difficult. The necrotic process may persist over several months, and excision with skin grafting may be necessary. Specific antidotes have been defined for some of the drugs, and the appropriate agent should be injected promptly into the site. The routine use of steroids in this setting is not recommended. Central venous catheters and subcutaneous infusion ports markedly reduce the risk for extravasation.

HIV

Morbidity and mortality from HIV have been reduced with the introduction of highly active antiretroviral therapy (HAART) [6–11]. More HIV-positive patients require surgical procedures because of their increased survival rate. HAART regimens are comprised of three antiretroviral drugs drawn from four classes: nucleoside or nucleotide reverse transcriptase inhibitors (NRTIs and NtRTIs, respectively), non-nucleoside reverse transcriptase inhibitors (NNRTIs), protease inhibitors, and fusion inhibitors.

Mitochondrial toxicity

Toxicities associated with NRTIs and NtRTIs result from impaired synthesis of mitochondrial enzymes that generate adenosine triphosphate (ATP) [6,7]. This is manifested by elevated plasma lactate with or without acidosis. Risk factors for lactic acidemia include type and duration of RTI therapy, pregnancy (NRTI hepatic steatosis), and concomitant therapy with ribavirin (for hepatitis C) or hydroxyurea. The main mitochondrial toxicities are hepatic steatosis, peripheral neuropathy, peripheral lipoatrophy, pancreatitis, cardiomyopathy, proximal myopathy, renal tubular acidosis, and neonatal encephalopathy. Osteopenia is also possible. Of these toxicities, hepatic steatosis and pancreatitis are the most severe, and are associated with higher lactate levels. Severity of illness correlates with lactate levels. Mortality is about 80% in patients with lactate >10 mM. Lactate levels normalize about three months after NRTI cessation. The clinical illness can take longer to resolve.

Lipodystrophy

Lipodystrophy is characterized by lipoatrophy of the face, limbs, and buttocks with central fat accumulation (within the abdomen and breasts, and over the dorsocervical spine) and is seen in patients being treated with NRTIs and protease inhibitors, particularly when given in combination. Metabolic features include hypertriglyceridemia, hypercholesterolemia, low high-density lipoprotein cholesterol, insulin resistance (elevated C-peptide and insulin), lactic acidemia, and elevated hepatic transaminases. Protease inhibitor therapy has been linked mainly to insulin resistance and hypercholesterolemia. Meanwhile, nucleoside analogs have been linked to lactic acidemia.

Hypersensitivity

Drug hypersensitivity in HIV-infected patients typically manifests as an erythematous, maculopapular, pruritic, and confluent rash after 1 to 3 weeks of therapy and is approximately 100 times more common than in the general population. All NNRTIs, the NRTI abacavir, and the protease inhibitor amprenavir, are common causes.

Liver dysfunction

All antiretroviral drugs are associated with liver dysfunction. Antiretroviral-mediated liver dysfunction does not necessarily require cessation of therapy, as it might be asymptomatic, minimally symptomatic, or transient. Also, nondrug factors, such as opportunistic infections and alcohol abuse, might coexist. Isolated biochemical hepatitis, with or without clinical hepatitis, can occur weeks to more than 6 months after initiation of protease inhibitors or NNRTIs. Risk factors are chronic hepatitis B virus (HBV) infection (specifically, hepatitis B presurface antigen (HbsAg), hepatitis B e antigen (HbeAg) or HBV DNA-positive), hepatitis C infection (HCV), and elevated transaminases pretherapy. Each of these factors is associated with a threefold to eightfold risk. Levels of transaminases are generally substantially higher than those seen in patients with NRTI-associated hepatic steatosis. Most adverse reactions improve despite continuation of the responsible drug. The discontinuation of drug therapy should be reserved for patients with clinically progressive or persistent hepatitis, or for those with hepatic synthetic dysfunction.

Immunological recovery with any antiretroviral therapy can be associated with a clinical flare of a previously latent infection. This recovery stems from better immune recognition of low-level pathogens in which the immune response, rather than the pathogen itself, is partly or entirely the cause of the illness. Pathogens associated with immune restoration illnesses include hepatitis B, *Mycobacterium avium*, cytomegalovirus, cryptococcosis, varicella and HCV.

Miscellaneous

Fusion inhibitors prevent entry of HIV-1 into target cells [6,7]. The major adverse effect is an injection-site reaction, characterized by a mixed neutrophilic and eosinophilic infiltrate. In addition, a higher incidence of bacterial pneumonia of unknown cause has been noted while some patients develop a systemic hypersensitivity reaction. The hypersensitivity manifestations may include fever, constitutional symptoms, glomerulonephritis, pneumonitis, and Guillain-Barre syndrome.

Organ transplant recipients

The field of organ transplantation has undergone tremendous growth with improved outcomes for all solid-organ transplants. The success of organ transplantation stems from improved patient and disease management, surgical techniques, and postoperative care. Also playing an especially important role in that success is the improved and expanded pharmaceutical armamentarium available to physicians to manage immune suppression and complications. A better understanding of the immunologic basis for allograft rejection has fostered the development of more specific agents with improved safety profiles and has led to improvements in the application of drugs already in use.

Corticosteroids

Corticosteroids were the first immunosuppressive medications used in transplant recipients. Steroids have potent anti-inflammatory as well as immunomodulatory properties, and their effects on the immune system are complex. The ubiquitously expressed glucocorticoid receptor, when bound by corticosteroids, translocates from the cytoplasm to the nucleus where it mediates its physiologic effect through modulation of gene transcription. Corticosteroids modulate the immune system by inhibiting the production of T cell cytokines, including interleukin-1 (IL-1), IL-2, IL-3, IL-6, tumor necrosis factor, and gamma interferon. Steroids also exhibit non-specific effects. For example, steroids redistribute lymphocytes back to lymphoid tissues, inhibit monocyte migration, and block the synthesis or release of chemokines, permeability factors, and vasodilatory agents [12].

Complications of steroid therapy are numerous and well documented. Many of these side effects are dose- and chronicity-dependent. In the immediate setting, such as bolus steroid therapy for acute allograft rejection, there is an increased risk for opportunistic infections, avascular necrosis of the femoral heads, altered mental status, and glucose intolerance. Glucose homeostasis can be severely disturbed in brittle type I diabetics, such that the need for continuous insulin infusion is not uncommon.

In the long term, adverse effects of corticosteroid therapy include cosmetic changes, such as Cushingoid facies, acne, and hypertrichosis. Adverse effects can also include medically severe complications, such as impaired wound healing, dermal atrophy, hypertension, proximal muscle wasting, cataracts, glaucoma, growth impairment, and osteoporosis [12].

In the perioperative period, wound healing is of critical concern. Glucocorticoids negatively impact wound healing by altering collagen synthesis, the main structural protein providing tensile strength to wounds. Glucocorticoids inhibit the hydroxylation of proline and lysine residues of the type I collagen protein, which are required for covalent cross-linking of the individual collagen strands to form the final structurally stable collagen triple-helix complex. This effect of glucocorticoids on collagen synthesis can be partially reversed by the use of supplemental zinc, ascorbic acid, and vitamin A [13]. In addition to the effect of glucocorticoids on collagen synthesis, steroids also alter the microenvironment of the wounded site. The early stage of wound healing is characterized by the migration of inflammatory cells, which "clean" the wound site and release chemokines that mediate fibroblast migration to the injured area initiating the repair process. Glucocorticoids impair this wound healing process by inhibiting inflammation, chemokine production, and thus monocyte and macrophage migration to the areas of injury.

In addition to its anti-inflammatory effects, chronic use of glucocorticoids may influence the normal regulatory feedback pathways involved in the production of cortisol. One area of controversy in the management of patients on chronic corticosteroids is the effect of chronic steroids in suppressing the hypothalamic-pituitary-adrenal axis (HPA). In cases of an intact HPA axis, baseline secretion of cortisol increases under situations of stress, such as that of surgery. Fraser, in 1952, described a patient on chronic steroids who died postoperatively of intractable hypotension [14]. Postmortem examination revealed bilateral adrenal atrophy. Thus, it was concluded that adrenal insufficiency from chronic steroid use resulted in the patient's death. This single case report and other evidence have resulted in the general use of stress-dose steroids in the perioperative period in patients on long-term corticosteroids.

In the 50 years since the Fraser report, numerous studies have both supported and refuted evidence that supra-physiologic doses of corticosteroids are required to prevent adrenal insufficiency in the perioperative period. To assess HPA axis function in patients on chronic steroids undergoing surgery, Brown and Buie analyzed 11 related studies that met strict criteria in the assessment of physiologic and biochemical parameters [15]. They concluded that no evidence justifies the use of supra-physiologic doses of steroids in patients undergoing surgery. However, some evidence in case-series reports show a 1% to 2% incidence of hypotensive crisis in patients on chronic steroids. While case reports are generally considered to have poor scientific validity, the investigators suggest that, "because of the risk for mortality from hypotensive crisis, this evidence cannot be ignored". The investigators thus recommend the use of physiologic doses of hydrocortisone (25–100 mg) at the time of surgery as the best way to prevent potential hypotensive crisis while minimizing the deleterious impact of corticosteroids.

Calcineurin inhibitors

The most commonly used and widely known immunosuppressive agents, cyclosporine and tacrolimus comprise the class of drugs known as calcineurin inhibitors (CNIs), as they inhibit the function of calcineurin, a critical T cell serine/threonine phosphatase and a central enzyme in the signal transduction cascade resulting in T cell activation. The introduction of cyclosporine in the early 1980s transformed the field of transplantation, increasing the 1-year patient survival rates from 30% to over 70% [12].

The side-effect profile for both cyclosporine and tacrolimus are similar but do not completely overlap. The therapeutic profile for calcineurin inhibitors is relatively narrow and dosing is based on therapeutic drug monitoring of trough whole blood levels. Target drug levels are predicated by the type of transplanted organ, its level of function and the time since transplant. Calcineurin inhibitors are absorbed throughout the gastrointestinal tract, although the greatest absorption occurs in the stomach, duodenum, and proximal jejunum. CNI absorption in the gastrointestinal tract is highly variable among individual patients and any procedure or disease process that affects gastrointestinal motility and absorption will impact CNI blood levels. Abdominal surgery, which can result in an ileus as well as altered gastrointestinal absorption because of bacterial overgrowth or other factors affecting the mucosal lining of the intestinal tract, will alter calcineurin absorption and drug levels [16]. There are intravenous formulations of CNIs. However, these formulations should be used only as a last resort, as they need to be administered as a continuous infusion and at one tenth the dose of the oral agent. The intravenous formulations can result in severe toxicity and should only be prescribed by physicians who routinely manage transplant recipients. Thus CNIs should be administered enterally under most circumstances; however, regardless of the route of administration in the perioperative period, CNI levels should be monitored on a daily basis and adjusted accordingly.

The metabolism of CNIs is through the microsomal cytochrome P450 system of the liver and intestine. Cyclosporine and tacrolimus are both excreted in the bile with no renal excretion. Thus, no dose adjustments need to be made in the setting of renal dysfunction. However, hepatic dysfunction and drugs that affect the microsomal P450 system have a significant impact on CNI levels (Table 1).

In the perioperative period, CNIs can affect patient recovery as well as result in increased morbidity. Renal toxicity is the most severe and common side effect of CNIs. Both tacrolimus and cyclosporine cause efferent renal artery constriction, which is dose-dependent. Thus, oliguria, renal dysfunction and electrolyte abnormalities can be more pronounced in the postoperative period. Moreover, the renal toxic effects of CNIs can be greatly potentiated through the use of other nephrotoxic agents, such as

Table 1
Drug interaction on calcineurin inhibitor levels

Drug or drug class	Effect on CNI level
Azole antifungals (ketoconazole, fluconazole, itraconazole)	Increase
Dihydropyridine Ca-channel blockers (verapamil, diltiazem)	Increase
Macrolide antibiotics (erythromycin, clarithromycin, azithromycin)	Increase
Grapefruit juice	Increase
HAART protease inhibitors (ritonavir, lopinavir)	Increase
Amiodarone	Increase
Antimycobacterial agents (rifampin, rifabutin)	Decrease
Anticonvulsants (barbiturates, phenytoin, carbamazepine)	Decrease
Saint-John's-wort	Decrease

aminoglycoside antibiotics, amphotericin, nonsteroidal anti-inflammatory agents and angiotensin converting enzyme and receptor antagonists. Chronic calcineurin inhibitor use also can result in renal parenchymal interstitial fibrosis, which is not reversible and results in chronic renal insufficiency.

While the renal side effects of the CNIs are most profound, this class of drugs also produces neurotoxicity, ranging from tremors, insomnia, and headaches, to more severe events that include seizures and coma [16]. The neurologic side effects are dose-dependent. Generally these side effects are seen at higher drug levels and within the first year of drug initiation. However, these adverse events may also be seen with drug levels within the therapeutic window and beyond the first year.

Long term use of cyclosporine and tacrolimus have numerous metabolic and physiologic effects, including promotion and/or exacerbation of hypertension, hypercholesterolemia, hypomagnesemia, and hyperglycemia, which can complicate perioperative patient management and increase the risk for major morbidity and mortality. Moreover, these adverse metabolic and physiologic effects of CNI's can also negatively impact transplant recipients' ability to undergo elective surgery. Take for example, hypertension and hypercholesterolemia, which can result in advanced atherosclerotic disease thus potentially disqualifying patients from undergoing elective surgery or resulting in an increased risk of perioperative stroke or myocardial ischemia.

Hyperglycemia associated with CNI therapy is more pronounced with the use of tacrolimus than cyclosporine. Tacrolimus not only results in increased peripheral insulin resistance, but also results in diminished insulin release from pancreatic islet beta cells. Surgery results in insulin resistance. In the peri-operative period, the additive effects of CNI-mediated alterations in glucose homeostasis and the increase in peripheral insulin resistance due to complex physiologic effects of surgery on glucose metabolism can result in profound hyperglycemia in the peri-operative period. Thus it is not unusual for transplant recipients to require continuous insulin infusions in the peri-operative period following elective surgery [17].

Sirolimus

Sirolimus, a macrolide antibiotic isolated initially from a soil fungus found on the island of Rapa Nui (Easter Island), hence the name rapamycin, is a relatively new maintenance immunosuppressive agent. Thus, sirolimus is known also as rapamycin. While sirolimus is structurally similar to tacrolimus and binds the same cytoplasmic binding protein or immunophilin (FKBP-12), the sirolimus-immunophilin complex does not inhibit calcineurin activity. Instead, the complex binds to target of rapamycin (TOR) proteins. The immunosuppressive effect is mediated through the inhibition of a key regulatory kinase that permits passage of cells from the G1 to S phase of the cell cycle. In T lymphocytes, this kinase is regulated by cytokine receptors, which include interleukin-2, the primary molecule responsible for immune response amplification. Sirolimus dosing, like that of CNIs, is based on therapeutic drug monitoring of trough whole blood concentrations and is adjusted based on the type of transplanted organ, the time since transplant and the current clinical situation [18].

The side effect profile for sirolimus is different from the profile for CNIs because their intracellular targets are different. Serious side effects of sirolimus include thrombocytopenia and leucopenia, which are usually seen when the sirolimus level is maintained at chronically elevated states. The blood counts usually normalize when the use of sirolimus is reduced or discontinued.

Sirolimus is also thought to hinder wound healing by inhibiting fibroblasts and cells of the innate immune system that are critical in the early phases of wound healing. Numerous studies have documented statistically higher rates of wound dehiscence as well as incisional hernia formation [12]. If possible, patients on sirolimus should be converted to a CNI-based regimen 2 to 4 weeks before a major surgical procedure. The administration of sirolimus should not be resumed until postoperative month 2 when approximately 80% of wound tensile strength is restored.

Sirolimus, like the CNIs, does increase levels of serum cholesterol and triglycerides. However, sirolimus does not harm renal function, either acutely or with chronic use. Because of the favorable renal profile of sirolimus, many transplant patients with chronic renal dysfunction are being converted from CNI-based immunosuppressive regimens to those based on sirolimus [12].

Antimetabolites

Azathioprine, a purine analog, interferes with DNA synthesis and consequently exerts its therapeutic effect by suppressing the proliferation of T and B lymphocytes, which undergo rapid cell division during an immune response. The side effects of azathioprine use for immune modulation are the same as those observed when it is used as an antineoplastic agent, as described earlier.

Inosine monophosphate dehydrogenase inhibitors (IMPDH), mycophenolate mofetil and mycophenolic acid, inhibit the de novo purine synthesis pathway, resulting in the S phase arrest of replicating lymphocytes. IMPDH inhibitors preferentially affect T and B lymphocytes because these cells lack the salvage pathway of purine biosynthesis, which many other highly replicative cell types are able to use [19].

The side-effect profile of IMPDH inhibitors is similar to that of other antimetabolites, with a predilection for highly replicative cell types, such as hematopoietic precursors and various cells of the gastrointestinal tract. Gastrointestinal side effects were the most pronounced, with diarrhea, gastroesophageal reflux, gastritis, and vomiting. These side effects are dose-dependent and improve or completely resolve with dose reduction or drug discontinuation. Additionally, IMPDH inhibitors can also cause leukopenia and thrombocytopenia through bone marrow suppression. This side effect is also reversible with drug discontinuation or dose reduction [19].

Biologic and new agents

Numerous antibody preparations are used in the treatment of transplant patients. Most of these agents are administered in the immediate transplant period (induction immunosuppression) or in the treatment of allograft rejection. The biologic agents are directed against single or multiple cell-surface molecules located on the surface of T and B lymphocytes (eg, T cell receptor, interleukin-2 receptor, antithymocyte globulin, CD52, and CD20). In general, these agents are prescribed by physicians involved in the long-term management of transplant recipients. Therefore, these patients are usually undergoing close follow-up with transplant professionals. Thus, these agents will not be reviewed in detail here. Biologic agents are the most potent immunosuppressive medication in the transplant physician's armamentarium, and thus the major side effects of this class of drugs are opportunistic infections, overwhelming systemic infections, and, in the long term, lymphoid-based malignancies [12].

As for pharmaceuticals being developed, some represent new classes of drugs (eg, belatacept, FTY770, leflunomide), while others represent modifications of existing agents (everolimus, SDZ-RAD). The side effect profiles of these agents have not been well established.

Infectious complications

All classes of immunosuppressive drugs used in solid organ transplantation impair the function of the immune system and thus increase the likelihood of opportunistic infections. The risk for infectious complications is proportional to the dose and number of immunosuppressive medications used. In general, most transplant recipients receive the peak doses and number of immunosuppressive medications within the first 1 to 3 months of transplantation, after which the dose and number of medications are reduced, depending on the clinical circumstances. During this period of peak immune suppression, prophylactic antibiotics, such as sulfonamide and trimethoprim combinations for *Pneumocystis carini*, and antiviral medications, such as ganciclovir for cytomegalovirus, are used. Transplant recipients that undergo elective surgery, should be maintained or restarted on their outpatient medications, including prophylactic anti-infective medications as early as possible in the perioperative period.

In terms of perioperative antibiotics for preventing wound infections, the guidelines set forth by various surgical specialty boards for each type of surgery (eg, clean, clean-contaminated, contaminated) should be followed. Perioperative antibiotics should be administered no more than 2 hours before the surgical incision and generally should not be continued for more than 24 hours postprocedure, if at all. As in nonimmunosuppressed patients, excessive use of perioperative antibiotics only results in emergence of drug resistant infections.

Summary

The perioperative management of immunocompromised patients can be successfully undertaken without increased morbidity or mortality through vigilant attention to detail and a basic understanding of the pharmacology and toxic profile of the drugs most commonly used in the management of this patient population. When complications occur, early recognition of these problems and their causes, especially consideration of drug-mediated side effects, are imperative to minimize the potential morbidity.

References

[1] Bland KI, Daly JM, Karakousis CP. Surgical oncology. New York: McGraw-Hill Medical; 2001.

[2] Pazdur R. Cancer management: a multi-disciplinary approach. Melville (NY): PRR; 2000.

[3] Hughes WT, Armstrong D, Bodey GP, et al. 2002 guidelines for the use of antimicrobial agents in neutropenic patients with cancer. Clin Infect Dis 2002;34(6):730–51.

[4] American Society of Clinical Oncology. Recommendations for use of the hematopoietic colony-stimulating factors: evidence-based, clinical practice guidelines. J Clin Oncol 1994; 12(11):2471–508.

[5] McNeil C. NCCN guidelines advocate wider use of colony-stimulating factor. J National Cancer Institute 2005;97(100):710–1.

[6] Carr A, Cooper DA. Adverse effects of antiretroviral therapy. Lancet 2000;356:1423–30.

[7] Carr A. Toxicity of antiretroviral therapy and implications for drug development. Nat Rev Drug Discov 2003;2:624–34.

[8] Lin PH, Bush RL, Yao Q, et al. Abdominal aortic surgery in patients with human immunodeficiency virus infection. Am J Surg 2004;188:690–7.

[9] Grubert TA, Reindell D, Kastner R, et al. Rates of postoperative complications among human immunodeficiency virus-infected women who have undergone obstetric and gynecologic surgical procedures. Clin Infect Dis 2002;34:822–30.

[10] Imanaka K, Takamoto S, Kimura S, et al. Coronary artery bypass grafting in a patient with human immunodeficiency virus: role of perioperative active anti-retroviral therapy. Jpn Circ J 1999;63:423–4.

[11] Albaran RG, Webber J, Steffes CP. CD4 cell counts as a prognostic factor of major abdominal surgery in patients infected with the human immunodeficiency virus. Arch Surg 1998; 133:626–31.

[12] Humar A, Matas AJ. Immunosuppressive drugs. In: Hakim NS, Danovitch GM, editors. Transplantation surgery. London: Springer-Verlag; 2001. p. 373–93.

[13] Hunt TK, Ehrlich HP, Garcia JA, et al. Effects of vitamin A on reversing the inhibitory effects of cortisone on healing of open wounds in animals and man. Ann Surg 1969;170: 633–41.

[14] Fraser CG, Preuss FS, Bigford WD. Adrenal atrophy and irreversible shock associated with cortisone therapy. JAMA 1952;149:1542–3.

[15] Brown CJ, Buie WD. Perioperative stress dose steroids: do they make a difference? J Amer Col Surg 2001;193:678–85.

[16] Plosker GL, Foster RH. Tacrolimus: a further update of its pharmacology and therapeutic use in the management of organ transplantation. Drugs 2001;59:323–89.

[17] Danovitch GM. Immunosuppressant induced metabolic toxicities. Tranpl Rev 2000;14: 65–72.

[18] Kahan B, Camardo J. Rapamycin: clinical results and future opportunities. Transplantation 2001;72:1181–93.

[19] Allison AC, Eugui EM, Sollinger HW. MMF (RS-61443): mechanisms of action and effects in transplantation. Transpl Rev 1993;7:129–33.

ELSEVIER
SAUNDERS

SURGICAL
CLINICS OF
NORTH AMERICA

Surg Clin N Am 85 (2005) 1283–1289

Perioperative Management of Special Populations: Obesity

Eric J. DeMaria, MD*, Brennan J. Carmody, MD

General Surgery Division, Department of Surgery, Medical College of Virginia,
Virginia Commonwealth University, 1200 East Broad Street,
Richmond, VA 23298-0519, USA

Obesity and its complications have reached epidemic proportions. At least two thirds of the adult American population are considered overweight. That is, their body mass index (BMI), calculated as weight in kilograms divided by the square of the height in meters, is ≥25. Half of those overweight people are obese. That is, they have a BMI of ≥30 [1]. By definition, a person has morbid obesity if he or she has a BMI of ≥40. This degree of excess weight is clearly associated with increased morbidity and mortality [2]. Additionally, obesity has become increasingly prevalent in the pediatric population, and 30% of American children have a BMI greater than the 85th percentile for their age [3]. Several obesity-related conditions are underlying causes for earlier mortality associated with obesity, especially morbid obesity. These conditions include coronary artery disease, hypertension, impaired cardiac ventricular function, adult-onset diabetes mellitus, obesity hypoventilation and sleep apnea syndromes, hypercoagulability leading to an increased risk of pulmonary embolism, and development of certain malignancies [4]. As this obesity problem becomes more widespread in the general population, it will become more common for this patient population to seek elective or urgent surgical care. Therefore, surgeons and hospitals alike must be aware of the special considerations involved in treating the obese patient.

Preoperative assessment

Experts disagree about whether obesity itself below the level of morbid obesity is an independent risk factor for increased perioperative morbidity

---

* Corresponding author.
E-mail address: eric.demaria@duke.edu (E.J. DeMaria).

doi:10.1016/j.suc.2005.09.002   *surgical.theclinics.com*

and mortality. Several investigators conclude that while surgical-site infection is more common in this patient population, mortality rates are similar to those of nonobese patients. Besides adding to the complexity of all aspects of care, obesity increases incidence of the aforementioned comorbidities, which raises perioperative risk. Therefore, medical professionals must make thorough evaluations to properly identify and address medical comorbidities in obese patients.

Morbid obesity is often associated with left ventricular enlargement and both systolic and diastolic dysfunction, even in patients without overt cardiac disease [5]. The risk of atrial fibrillation increases 50% in the obese population [6], and factors associated with the development of coronary artery disease, such as hypertension, hyperlipidemias, and diabetes mellitus, are more common in the obese population. Patients should be assessed for risk based on history and physical, planned procedure, and functional capacity [7]. Intermediate- or high-risk patients undergoing major procedures should undergo further noninvasive testing. A reliable clinical predictor for intermediate or high risk is the finding that the patient is unable to perform activities requiring at least four metabolic equivalents. β-Blockade may decrease the risk of perioperative ischemia, infarction, or arrhythmia in patients with coronary artery disease [8]. Cardiac medications should be continued up to the day of surgery.

The prevalence of obstructive sleep apnea (OSA) is higher in the obese population; up to 71% of morbidly obese patients undergoing work-up for bariatric surgery have OSA. No correlation exists between BMI and the presence or severity of OSA [9]. This condition is associated with sudden death during sleep resulting from myocardial infarction or arrhythmia [10]. Characteristics of OSA include apneic periods during sleep, daytime somnolence, loud snoring, morning headaches, and frequent nocturnal awakening. Sleep polysymnography confirms the diagnosis and demonstrates cessation of airflow during sleep associated with persistent respiratory efforts. Preoperative initiation and perioperative use of continuous positive airway pressure (CPAP) can reduce hypercarbia, hypoxemia, and pulmonary artery vasoconstriction and should decrease the incidence of hypoxemic complications. Exertional dyspnea or syncope can indicate pulmonary hypertension; EKG findings include right axis deviation, and an echocardiogram can determine pulmonary vascular resistance [11].

The incidence of perioperative deep venous thrombosis (DVT) and pulmonary embolism (PE) is also higher in the obese population. This relationship between DVT and obesity stems from the increased intra-abdominal pressure and venous stasis most pronounced with central obesity. Both of these effects are accentuated by intraoperative factors, such as pneumoperitoneum and anesthesia-induced paralysis. Obesity is also associated with a hypercoagulable state through increased levels of fibrinogen, factor VIII, and von Willebrand factor. Procedures associated with prolonged immobility, such as those related to orthopedic cases, amplify this risk.

The risk of perioperative thromboembolic events in the obese population has been described in the bariatric surgery literature, which states that the estimated incidence of DVT and PE in patients receiving perioperative prophylaxis ranges from 0.2% to 2.4% [12,13]. Venous stasis ulcers of the lower extremities are relatively common in the morbidly obese. An association between the presence of stasis changes and PE has been described [14]. Prophylactic inferior vena cava filter insertion should be strongly considered in patients with such risk factors. Otherwise, unfractionated or low-molecular-weight heparin should be administered before surgery and continued throughout hospitalization. After the operation, continued short-term outpatient anticoagulation may be necessary for these high-risk patients.

Diabetes mellitus is common in the obese population, and it is likewise an independent risk factor for postoperative morbidity. Additionally, strict perioperative glycemic control reduces morbidity and mortality in cardiothoracic patients [15]. Therefore, care must be taken to ensure that serum glucose is at the appropriate level before proceeding with the intended surgery.

Obesity has been identified as an independent risk factor for surgical-site infection. Possible etiologies include decreased oxygen tension [16], immune impairment [17], and tension and secondary ischemia along long suture lines. Chronic skin infections, such as intertriginous *Candida*, should be treated preoperatively, and preoperative antibiotics should be administered as appropriate for the surgical procedure classification. Laparoscopic techniques offer a significant advantage in reducing surgical site infections and should be considered [18].

Finally, bariatric surgery itself plays a role in improving the medical condition of morbidly obese patients and enhancing the results of a future planned procedure, such as a total knee replacement or renal transplant [19,20]. In fact, satisfactory weight reduction may obviate elective orthopedic surgery because symptoms, such as those asociated with degenerative joint disease, often improve dramatically with weight loss.

Intraoperative management

The operating room table must be able to accommodate the obese patient. The C-Max surgical table (Steris, Mentor, OH), can accommodate patients weighing up to 1100 lb and can be fit with width and length extenders. Bariatric beds such as the Magnum II Bariatric Patient Care System, (Hill-Rom Services, Batesville, IN) can support patients weighing up to 800 pounds and function as chairs and transport vehicles [21]. Obese patients are at risk for slipping off the table during position changes and therefore must be well secured to the table [22]. A bean bag may be used to assist in preventing shifting, especially during position changes. All potential pressure points should be well padded. Reports indicate that rhabdomyolysis of gluteal muscles leading to renal failure has occurred in morbidly obese patients. Also, nerve injuries are more common in obese patients [23]. Sequential compression devices should also be used in combination with subcutaneous heparin for DVT prophylaxis, especially in the setting of laparoscopic access where increases in intra-abdominal pressure are likely to decrease venous return from the lower extremities.

Invasive arterial monitoring should be used for severely obese patients, including so-called "super" obese patients with a BMI ≥ 60. Invasive arterial monitoring is also important for patients with significant cardiopulmonary disease, and in cases where noninvasive blood pressure monitoring devices are unreliable. Blood pressure cuffs should span a minimum of 75% of the patient's upper arm circumference. The ankle or wrist may be used as alternate sites for taking blood pressure [24]. Establishing peripheral intravenous access can be difficult in obese patients. Central venous catheters should be used in cases where peripheral access cannot be obtained or when postoperative access may be difficult.

Endotracheal intubation and airway management in the obese patient can be challenging. These patients as a group are more likely than the general population to have airways difficult to keep open. A large neck circumference appears to be one of the best predictors of a problematic intubation [25]. Towels or a shoulder roll can be used to extend the neck. Other adjuncts include awake flexible fiber-optic intubation and the use of the Bullard Laryngoscope (ACMI, Southborough, MA). Highly lipophilic medications, such as benzodiazepines and barbiturates, must be administered in higher doses to account for increases in volume of distribution (V_D) compared with patients of normal weight. Doses should be calculated according to total body weight [26]. Ventilator strategies include tidal volumes of 10 to 12 mL/kg for limiting volutrauma, respiratory rates up to 14 breaths/minute for maintaining normocapnia, and positive end-expiratory pressure (PEEP) of 5 to 10 cm H_2O for improving oxygenation.

Accurate assessment of volume status can be difficult, and a Foley catheter should be placed at the onset of major procedures. Laparoscopy can confound the issue because pneumoperitoneum itself can decrease renal blood flow and decrease urine output. Hypovolemia can accentuate these effects.

Postoperative management

Obese patients require close postoperative observation. Patients with obstructive sleep apnea, significant cardiac disease, or other significant comorbidity should be admitted to intermediate or intensive care for continuous cardiopulmary monitoring. Obese patients undergoing abdominal or thoracic procedures are at significant risk for pulmonary complications. Atelectasis has been reported in up to 45% of obese patients following upper abdominal surgery and may be worsened by the effects of pneumoperitoneum [27].

Conversely, laparoscopic access has been associated with decreased postoperative pain and a reduction in pulmonary dysfunction [28]. Postoperative ambulation and use of incentive spirometry should be initiated as soon as possible. Ways to reduce pulmonary dysfunction include the use of continuous positive airway pressure (CPAP) [29] or bilevel positive airway pressure (BIPAP) [30].

Adequate analgesia is crucial in allowing early ambulation and restoring the best possible pulmonary function. Patient-controlled narcotics are frequently used following both minimally invasive and open procedures. Potential benefits of nonnarcotic agents include decreased sedation and more rapid return of bowel function. Such agents, including, for example, marcaine and bupivicaine, can be administered via epidural. Recently, agents have been administered adjacent to the surgical site using a marcaine infusion device, such as the On-Q (I-Flow, Lake Forest, CA). Evidence indicates that the administration of agents adjacent to the surgical site reduces both postoperative pain and use narcotics following inguinal hernia repair [31].

The nursing staff plays a crucial role in the postoperative management of the obese patient. Early ambulation may decrease pulmonary dysfunction and increase return to bowel function. Also, early ambulation should reduce the risks of DVT, PE, and the formation of decubitus ulcers. Care providers must be vigilant with regard to the latter and carefully inspect the skin over potential pressure points at frequent intervals. Oscillating beds should be used for patients who cannot shift their own weight, and bariatric beds that can conform into sitting positions are helpful.

Hospitals and health care systems should be prepared to care for the obese patient population. Besides the aforementioned beds and transport devices, doorways and bathrooms should be large enough to accommodate morbidly obese patients. Radiologic equipment, such as CT scanners and interventional radiology tables, should be capable of supporting these patients.

The American College of Surgeons (ACS) has developed the Bariatric Surgery Center Network Accreditation Program to foster high-quality surgical care for patients who undergo bariatric surgery. The program manual (available at http://www.FACS.ORG/CQI/BSCN/index/html) describes the necessary physical resources, human resources, clinical standards, surgeon credentialing standards, data reporting standards and verification and approval processes associated with ACS designation as a bariatric surgery center.

Summary

As obesity becomes more common, more obese patients will require or choose surgical care. A multidisciplinary effort including providers, nursing staff, and health systems must be attuned to the special needs and comorbidities associated with this patient group. Careful preoperative, perioperative, and postoperative care that anticipates issues and complications particular to the obese patient is critical in reducing morbidity and mortality in these patients. All hospitals and surgeons must be prepared to handle surgical issues for this challenging population.

References

[1] National Center for Health Statistics NHANES IV report. Available at: http://www.cdc.gov/nchs/product/pubs/pubd/hestats/obes/obese99.htm2002. Accessed November 29, 2004.

[2] Fontaine KR, Redden DT, Wang C, et al. Years of life lost due to obesity. JAMA 2003;289: 187–93.

[3] Ogden CL, Flegal KM, Carroll MD, et al. Prevalence and trends in overweight among US children and adolescents, 1999–2000. JAMA 2002;288:1728–32.

[4] Health Implications of Obesity. National Institutes of Health Consensus Development Conference Statement. Ann Intern Med 1985;103:147–51.

[5] Wong CY, O'Moore-Sullivan T, et al. Alterations of left ventricular myocardial characteristics associated with obesity. Circulation 2004;110:3081–7.

[6] Wang TJ, Parise H, Levy D, et al. Obesity and the risk of new-onset atrial fibrillation. JAMA 2004;292:2471–7.

[7] Abir F, Bell R. Assessment and management of the obese patient. Crit Care Med 2004; 32(4 Suppl):S87–91.

[8] Eagle KA, Berger PB, Calkins H, et al. ACC/AHA guideline update for perioperative cardiovascular evaluation for noncardiac surgery–executive summary: a report of the American College of Cardiology/American Heart Association Task Force on Practice Guidelines (Committee to Update the 1996 Guidelines on Perioperative Cardiovascular Evaluation for Noncardiac Surgery). J Am Coll Cardiol 2002;39(3):542–53.

[9] Frey WC, Pilcher J. Obstructive sleep-related breathing disorders in patients evaluated for bariatric surgery. Obes Surg 2003;13:676–83.

[10] Shepard JW Jr. Hypertension, cardiac arrhythmias, myocardial infarction, and stroke in relation to obstructive sleep apnea. Clin Chest Med 1992;13(3):437–58.

[11] Abbas AE, Fortuin FD, Schiller NB, et al. A simple method for noninvasive estimation of pulmonary vascular resistance. J Am Coll Cardiol 2003;41(6):1021–7.

[12] Higa KD, Boone KB, Ho T. Complications of the laparoscopic Roux-en-Y gastric bypass: 1,040 patients–what have we learned? Obes Surg 2000;10(6):509–13.

[13] Eriksson S, Backman L, Ljungstrom KG. The incidence of clinical postoperative thrombosis after gastric surgery for obesity during 16 years. Obes Surg 1997;7(4):332–6 [discussion: 336].

[14] Sapala JA, Wood MH, Schuhknecht MP, et al. Fatal pulmonary embolism after bariatric operations for morbid obesity: a 24-year retrospective analysis. Obes Surg 2003;13(6): 819–25.

[15] Goldberg PA, Sakharova OV, Barrett PW, et al. Improving glycemic control in the cardiothoracic intensive care unit: clinical experience in two hospital settings. J Cardiothorac Vasc Anesth 2004;18(6):690–7.

[16] Dindo D, Muller MK, Weber M, et al. Obesity in general elective surgery. Lancet 2003; 361(9374):2032–5.

[17] Tanaka S, Inoue S, Isoda F, et al. Impaired immunity in obesity: suppressed but reversible lymphocyte responsiveness. Int J Obes Relat Metab Disord 1993;17(11):631–6.

[18] Nguyen NT, Goldman C, Rosenquist CJ, et al. Laparoscopic versus open gastric bypass: a randomized study of outcomes, quality of life, and costs. Ann Surg 2001;234(3):279–89.

[19] Parvizi J, Trousdale RT, Sarr MG. Total joint arthroplasty in patients surgically treated for morbid obesity. J Arthroplasty 2000;15(8):1003–8.

[20] Alexander JW, Goodman HR, Gersin K, et al. Gastric bypass in morbidly obese patients with chronic renal failure and kidney transplant. Transplantation 2004;78(3):469–74.

[21] Carbonell AM, Joels CS, Sing RF, et al. Laparoscopic gastric bypass surgery: equipment and necessary tools. J Laparoendosc Adv Surg Tech A 2003;13(4):241–5.

[22] Ogunnaike BO, Jones SB, Jones DB, et al. Anesthetic considerations for bariatric surgery. Anesth Analg 2002;95(6):1793–805.

[23] Bostanjian D, Anthone GJ, Hamoui N, Crookes PF. Rhabdomyolysis of gluteal muscles leading to renal failure: a potentially fatal complication of surgery in the morbidly obese. Obes Surg 2003;13(2):302–5.

[24] Mann GV. The influence of obesity on health. N Engl J Med 1974;291:178–85, 226–32.

[25] Brodsky JB, Lemmens HJ, Brock-Utne JG, et al. Morbid obesity and tracheal intubation. Anesth Analg 2002;94(3):732–6.

[26] Blouin RA, Warren GW. Pharmacokinetic considerations in obesity. J Pharm Sci 1999; 88(1):1–7.

[27] Soderberg M, Thomson D, White T. Respiration, circulation and anaesthetic management in obesity. Investigation before and after jejunoileal bypass. Acta Anaesthesiol Scand 1977; 21(1):55–61.

[28] Nguyen NT, Lee SL, Goldman C, et al. Comparison of pulmonary function and postoperative pain after laparoscopic versus open gastric bypass: a randomized trial. J Am Coll Surg 2001;192(4):469–77 [discussion 476–7].

[29] Oberg B, Poulsen TD. Obesity: an anaesthetic challenge. Acta Anaesthesiol Scand 1996; 40(2):191–200.

[30] Joris JL, Sottiaux TM, Chiche JD, et al. Effect of bi level positive airway pressure (BiPAP) nasal ventilation on the postoperative pulmonary restrictive syndrome in obese patients undergoing gastroplasty. Chest 1997;111(3):665–70.

[31] Sanchez B, Waxman K, Tatevossian R, et al. Local anesthetic infusion pumps improve postoperative pain after inguinal hernia repair: a randomized trial. Am Surg 2004;70(11):1002–6.

ELSEVIER
SAUNDERS

SURGICAL
CLINICS OF
NORTH AMERICA

Surg Clin N Am 85 (2005) 1291–1297

Operating Room Management: Operative Suite Considerations, Infection Control

Maria D. Allo, MD[a,b,*], Maureen Tedesco, MD[c]

[a]Department of Surgery, Santa Clara Valley Medical Center,
751 South Bascom Avenue, San Jose, CA 95128, USA
[b]Division of General Surgery, Stanford University, 300 Pasteur Drive,
Stanford 94305, CA, USA
[c]Stanford University, Old Union, 520 Lasuen Mall, Stanford, CA 94305, USA

For any room, good design not only creates an aesthetically pleasing configuration, it also meets the functional needs of its users. In designing an operating room, this translates into careful attention to traffic patterns; the number and configuration of nearby operating rooms; space required for storage, administration, and staff; provisions for sterile processing; and systems to manage airborne contaminants. This article addresses these issues as they relate to infection control and prevention.

Traffic patterns

Most postoperative surgical infections originate from the patient's own endogenous flora. Thus the integrity of the patient's immune system and other host factors are more important in determining infections than the numbers of bacteria in the operating room environment. Nonetheless, airborne contaminants can cause or aggravate infections. For that reason, as much as possible it is best to create traffic patterns that limit the movement of personnel and materials from outside the surgical suite. This restricts the movement of airborne contaminants, such as organisms carried and shed by people and objects.

* Corresponding author. Department of Surgery, Santa Clara Valley Medical Center, 751 S. Bascom Avenue, San Jose, CA 95128.
E-mail address: mdallo@earthlink.net (M.D. Allo).

There is no perfect traffic plan. However, some guidelines are useful for limiting movement from the outside into the operating suite. First, make sure there are no more people than necessary in the operating room while operations are being performed. Second, limit the amount of movement within the room. Third, keep the doors of each operating room closed during operations. Personnel in an operating room shed squamae from skin and hair, generating most particles and bacteria found in operating room air [1]. Although no one has established a direct relationship between the number of people in an operating room and the development of postoperative infection, the few studies that have been performed suggest that, as the number of people in the operating room increases, so does the incidence of surgical site infection [2]. Whether this has to do with the people per se or the greater amount of traffic into and around the room is not clear. It has been shown that opening the doors to the operating room decreases the effectiveness of the ventilation system to effectively clear potential contaminants from the operating room outward. Laufman [3] argues that a sensible traffic pattern should reflect "the realistic traffic and commerce of patients, personnel and supplies, with careful attention to 'clean' and 'semi-clean' work areas."

Operating rooms

The operating room must be large enough to accommodate the equipment and personnel necessary to perform the operation. As more complex technology has come into use, the recommended size for operating rooms has increased. Current American Institute of Architects (AIA) guidelines recommend that in new construction general operating rooms have "a minimum clear floor area of 400 square feet exclusive of fixed or wall-mounted cabinets and built-in shelves, with a minimum of 20 feet clear dimension between fixed cabinets and built-in shelves." The guidelines also say that rooms "for cardiovascular, neurological, orthopedic and other special procedures that require additional personnel or large equipment" should have "a minimum clear floor area of 600 square feet, with a minimum of 20 feet clear dimension exclusive of fixed or wall-mounted cabinets and built-in shelves" [4]. These standards are also recommended for renovations; however, if that is not possible, the minimum clear floor area for general-purpose rooms and orthopedic rooms should be 360 square feet, and for cardiovascular, neurological and other special purpose rooms, 400 square feet.

If an operating room has windows, those windows should have coved or sloped edges. Designers should make sure that no ledges can collect dust or debris. Windows should be well sealed and function primarily as sources of natural light. They should not be allowed to be opened. The addition of windows is optional. Studies have shown that natural light enhances staff morale. However, for some types of operations, the need to darken the room, control for glare, and other considerations may outweigh any advantages.

Floors should ideally be slip-resistant under wet and dry conditions and should be able to withstand frequent washings and hard cleaning with scrubbing machines. They should also be smooth and able to tolerate rolling loads. Carpeting should not be used in operating rooms because of the frequent spilling of blood and body fluids and the need for efficient, frequent, and thorough cleansing [5].

Walls should be water-impermeable, resistant to cracks and scrubbable. They should also be protected from impact by gurneys and other equipment coming to and from the rooms. There is no evidence that antimicrobial additives to wall surfacing material or paint has any role in infection control.

Monolithic ceilings are recommended for the rooms where operations are actually performed. Ceiling surfaces should be smooth and scrubbable. Ceilings are usually made of plaster; however, moisture-resistant gypsum wallboard systems with special epoxy-based coatings can be a less costly alternative material. Any ceiling-mounted lights or fixtures must be sealed so that dust and contaminants cannot enter through these openings, and so that there is no compromise to the ventilation system. Lay-in ceilings may be used in semirestricted and unrestricted areas, including recovery and holding areas, but are not permitted in operating rooms. Where lay-in ceilings are used, clips must be applied to ensure that dust and other contaminants do not enter the room.

Storage considerations

The task of providing adequate storage is probably one of the most difficult problems in operating room design. In the initial design of an operating room, careful planning must go into determining what equipment, if any, should be stored in the room. In rooms with one purpose, such as a room where only laparoscopic operations are performed, it may be appropriate to provide space to store monitors, insufflators, light sources, and other regularly needed equipment in the room.

However, as a general rule, unless a piece of equipment is almost always and exclusively used in a given operating room, it should be stored elsewhere. Most equipment should be kept in an equipment storage area in the semirestricted area of the operating suite. AIA Guidelines recommend specifying not less than 150 square feet or 50 square feet per operating room, whichever is greater [4]. For specialty rooms, an adjacent space in the restricted area, preferably adjoining the room, should be designated. These would include, but are not limited to a pump room for cardiac surgery, and large equipment storage for the neurological and orthopedic rooms.

There is a strong tendency to opt for more operating room space rather than storage space when putting together a wish list in the design phase of an operating room suite. However, failure to provide adequate space results in cluttered corridors and operating rooms, which can easily become safety hazards. In addition to providing space for storing equipment, designers must also provide space for storing sterile supplies. This is logically placed in the substerile areas between operating rooms. Other storage spaces should be designated for clean supplies and packaged reusable items, and should be in a separate space from the soiled workroom. Carts and gurneys should not be stored where they obstruct corridors.

Sterile processing

All sterile supplies should be transported into operating rooms in closed sterile containers. Inadequate sterilization of surgical instruments has been implicated in outbreaks of surgical site infections [6,7]. For that reason, indicators documenting adequate sterilization should be included in all sterile instrument sets [8,9]. Case carts, when used, should be transported in covered, enclosed units and should not follow a route from the point of assembly to the operating room that traverses public thoroughfares.

Air handling

Proper air handling is the single most important environmental factor in the prevention of surgical site infection. Operating suites should be maintained at positive pressure so that air flows from the cleanest areas to the least clean areas. This means air should flow from the operating rooms toward the corridors and adjacent areas.

Positive pressure should be maintained in corridors and adjacent areas [4,10,11]. At least 15 air changes per minute should be maintained, of which at least three air changes per minute should be made up of fresh air [12,13]. All recirculated air and fresh air should be filtered so as to provide at least 90% efficiency by drop-spot testing [4,13]. Most operating rooms are designed to introduce air at the ceiling with exhaust near the floor (plenum system) [12,13]. This kind of system requires that the opening of doors and other movement be limited to the greatest possible extent because such movements can decrease the efficiency of the system.

Rooms may be engineered for horizontal laminar flow whereby particle-free air is moved over the operative field at a uniform velocity picking up particles in its path and passing them through a high-efficiency particulate air filter. However, it is not clear that this is necessary in any but the highest-risk operations, such as joint replacements where surgical site infections can be devastating. In studies of patients undergoing total hip replacements [12,14], incidence of surgical site infections came to 3.4% when laminar flow systems were employed in combination with antibiotic prophylaxis. This fell to 1.6% when laminar flow systems were employed alone, without antibiotic prophylaxis. The only studies supporting laminar flow rooms were done on patients undergoing orthopedic procedures.

To the extent possible, operating room doors should be kept closed. Entry should be limited to essential equipment and personnel. Every effort should be made to minimize traffic in and out of rooms [15].

Maintenance

Regularly scheduled surveillance and maintenance of the air-handling system is essential. This includes checking for moisture in walls, ceilings, and other potentially porous materials, assuring integrity of the air ducts, and checking fan settings and filters. Temperature and humidity also influence the likelihood of surgical-site infection. Most building codes require stringent humidity control in operating rooms, because water-borne bacteria such as *Legionnella* do not survive at relative humidity below 35%, and many non-bacterial pathogens, such as viruses and fungi, thrive in high humidity.

Conventional cooling systems dehumidify by cooling air to temperatures below its dew point, causing moisture to condense and drip off the coil into a drain pan. The air that leaves the coil is therefore extremely moist, usually close to saturation. When temperatures are kept above about 70°F this poses no problem. However, when the room is cooled significantly below this temperature (eg, to 65°F), the humidity goes up to an unacceptable level, requiring the lowering of the chillers in the heating, ventilating, and air-conditioning (HVAC) system to a low-chilled water temperature, or the use of desiccant dehumidifiers in the cooling system. The latter systems are particularly helpful in places where the climate is very warm and humid. The systems work by removing the moisture from the outside air before it reaches the chilled-water coil, allowing the chilled-water temperature to be raised in the cooling system with less moisture condensing into the drain pains and ductwork. Most modern systems can maintain adequate temperature, humidity, and pressure relationships; however, any disruption of the ductwork can change internal pressure relationships and cause airborne particles to migrate into the system.

Room "turnover"

Although no data support routine disinfecting of operating rooms and equipment between operations in the absence of visible soiling or contamination, standard practice is to routinely clean rooms after each operation to provide a clean environment for the next one [8,9,11,15,16]. CDC guidelines specify that hospitals use a one-step process and a hospital detergent registered with the Environmental Protection Agency (EPA) and designed for general housekeeping purposes where there may be blood or body fluid contamination on surfaces [12]. Similarly, the Occupational Safety and Health Administration (OSHA) requires that any equipment or surfaces contaminated with blood or potentially infectious agents be cleaned and decontaminated [17]. If single-use, disposable mops and cloths are not used, mop heads and cloths should be cleaned after each use and allowed to dry before reuse [17,18]. Following the last surgical procedure of the day or night, operating room floors should be wet-mopped with a single-use mop and an EPA-registered hospital disinfectant [19]. Tacky surfaces and mats should not be used at the entrances of operating rooms, [19] nor should ultraviolet lights. Despite the common practice of closing operating rooms or having special procedures to clean rooms after contaminated or dirty operations, no data support such practices [12].

Repairs and renovations

Nosocomial infections ranging from *Aspergillus* and mold in ceilings to *Legionella* in wet areas have prompted support of mandatory proactive infection control risk assessments (ICRAs) by the Joint Commission for the Accreditation of Hospitals, the American Society of Hospital Epidemiologists, and the AIA. Major renovations, particularly those involving air-handling systems or ventilation, require an ICRA before beginning any remodeling or new construction. A multidisciplinary team should conduct ICRAs. This team might include infection control personnel, risk managers, contractors, facility designers, HVAC specialists, structural engineers, safety officers, and hospital epidemiologists. ICRAs should be initiated in the earliest stages of the design or development phase of a project to identify potential infectious risks to the patient population, any risks associated with the mechanical systems of the building, and the areas that will be affected by the project. Its goals include defining necessary containment measures (such as traffic diversion, waste removal, and work disruption) during construction and anticipating any safety hazards that can result from the construction.

References

[1] Laufman H. Design, devices, and discipline in operating room infection control. Med Instrum 1978;12(3):158–60.
[2] Pryor F, Messmer PR. The effect of traffic patterns in the OR on surgical site infections. AORN Online 1998;68(4):649–60.
[3] Laufman H. What's wrong with our operating rooms. Am J Surg 1971;122:332–42.
[4] The American Institute of Architects and the Facilities Guidelines Institute. Guidelines for design and construction of hospital and health care facilities. Washington (DC): American Institute of Architects Press; 2001. 7.7. A; p. 35.
[5] Suzuki A, Naba Y, Matsuura M, Horisawa A. Bacterial contamination of floors and other surfaces in operating rooms: a five-year survey. J Hyg (Lond) 1984;93:559–66.
[6] Soto LE, Bobadilla M, Villalobos Y, Sifuentes J, Avelar J, Arrieta M, et al. Post surgical nasal celulitis outbreak due to *Mycobacterium chelonae*. J Hosp Inf 1991;19(2):99–106.
[7] Center for Disease Control. Postsurgical infections associated with nonsterile implantable devices. MMWR Morb Mortal Wkly Rep 1992;41(15):63.
[8] Association of Operating Room Nurses. Standards, recommended practices guidelines. Denver (CO): Association of Operating Room Nurses; 2004.

[9] Committee on Control of Surgical Infections of the Committee on Pre- and Postoperative Care. American College of Surgeons manual on control of infection in surgical patients. Philadelphia: JB Lippincott Co.; 1984.

[10] Lidwell OM. Clean air at operation and subsequent sepsis in the joint. Clin Orthop 1986;211: 91–102.

[11] Nichols RL. The operating room. In: Bennett JV, Brachman PS, editors. Hospital infections. 3rd edition. Boston: Little, Brown and Co; 1992. p. 61–73.

[12] Mangram AJ, Horan TC, Pearson ML, Silver LC, Jarvis WR. Guideline for prevention of surgical site infection. Infect Control Hosp Epidemiol 1999;20:247–80.

[13] Babb JR, Lynam P, Ayliffe GA. Risk of airborne transmission in an operating theater containing four ultraclean air units. J Hosp Infect 1995;31:159–68.

[14] Lidwell OM, Elson RA, Lowbury EJ, et al. Ultraclean air and antibiotics for prevention of postoperative infection. A multicenter study of 8,052 joint replacement operations. Acta Orthop Scand 1987;58:4–13.

[15] Ayliffe GA. Role of the environment of the operating suite in surgical wound infection. Rev Infect Dis 1991;13(Suppl 10):S800–4.

[16] Hambraeus A. Aerobiology in the operating room—a review. J Hosp Infect 1988;11(Suppl A):68–76.

[17] US Department of Labor, Occupational Health and Safety Administration. Occupational exposure to bloodborne pathogens; final rule (29 CFR Part 1910.1030). Fed Regist 1991; 56:64175–82.

[18] Ayliffe GA, Collins BJ, Lowbury EJ, et al. Ward floors and other surfaces as reservoirs of hospital infection. J Hyg (Lond) 1967;65:515–37.

[19] Scott E, Bloomfield SF. The survival and transfer of microbial contamination via cloths, hands and utensils. J Appl Bacteriol 1990;68:271–8.

ELSEVIER
SAUNDERS

SURGICAL
CLINICS OF
NORTH AMERICA

Surg Clin N Am 85 (2005) 1299–1305

Strategies for Preventing Sharps Injuries in the Operating Room

Ramon Berguer, MD[a],*, Paul J. Heller, MD[b]

[a]Contra Costa Regional Medical Center, Department of Surgery,
2500 Alhambra Avenue, Martinez, CA 94553, USA
[b]VA Connecticut Healthcare System, Anesthesia Service, 950 Campbell Avenue,
West Haven, CT 06516, USA

With the discovery AIDS and HIV, the medical community began to recognize widely the dangers of serious illnesses spreading through contact with contaminated blood and body fluids. Responding to this growing awareness, the Centers for Disease Control (CDC) in 1987 came out with Universal Precautions [1], guidelines for contamination issues involving blood and body fluid for all patients. In 1991, with the enactment of the Blood Borne Pathogen Standard [2], the Occupational Safety and Health Administration began requiring the use of Universal Precautions. Although this standard has been revised and updated several times (most recently in 2001 [3]), the published literature indicates that surgeons continue to demonstrate poor compliance with Universal Precautions [4]. Equally unfortunate is the failure of Universal Precautions and the Blood Borne Pathogen Standard to fully address the needs of the high-risk operating room environment. Thus, sharps injuries to surgeons and scrub personnel continue to occur.

The operating room

Ensuring a safe operating room environment is challenging because surgeons, scrub nurses, and operating room technicians work closely together handling the same instruments in a confined space. Consequently, surgeons and scrub personnel are injured in similar ways with similar equipment and often by each other. To reduce injury rates in the operating room, a team

---

* Corresponding Author.
E-mail address: rberguer@yahoo.com (R. Berguer).

0039-6109/05/$ - see front matter © 2005 Elsevier Inc. All rights reserved.
doi:10.1016/j.suc.2005.09.012
surgical.theclinics.com

approach to safety is critical for examining the patterns of injuries typical of the operating room.

According to reports, the skin or mucous membranes of operating room personnel may have contact with patient blood in as many as 50% of operations, and cuts or needle sticks may occur in as many as 15% of operations [5,6]. Not surprisingly, the risk of sharps injury increases with longer, more invasive, and higher blood-loss procedures [5–9]. Most injuries are self-inflicted, but a significant number, perhaps as many as 24%, are inflicted by co-workers [6,10,11,13]. The most common body part injured is the non-dominant hand [10,11,13].

Surgeons and first assistants are at highest risk for injury [10], suffering as many as 59.1% of injuries in the operating room [10]. Scrub nurses and scrub technicians in the operating room sustain the second highest frequency of injuries (19.1%), followed by anesthesiologists (6.2%) and circulating nurses (6%) [10]. Although the risk of injury and exposure is different for various personnel, the risk in the operating room is never zero (Table 1).

Suture needles are the most frequent source of injury and are involved in as many as 77% of injuries [11]. Interestingly, while the largest number of injuries occurs with curved suture needles, the rate of injuries involving straight suture needles is higher considering the number of needles used [12]. Many suture needle injuries occur while suturing muscle and fascia during wound closure, often as the fingers manipulate needles and tissue [10,11]. Up to 16% of injuries occur while passing sharp instruments hand to hand (range 6%–16%). As many as one third of devices that cause injuries come in contact with the patient after the injury to the health care worker. That means that in addition to the risk of disease transmission from patient to health care worker, there is also a risk of disease transmission from health care worker to patient [9,11]. Fortunately, only about 0.5% of injuries to surgeons are "high risk," which are defined as injuries from hollow bore vascular access needles [10]. Unfortunately, surgeons fail to report as many as

Table 1
Risk of needle injuries in the operating room

Job category	Percent of total needlestick exposures
Surgeons	59.1%
Scrub nurses	19.1%
Anesthesiologists	6.2%
Circulating nurses	6.0%
Medical students	3.1%
Attendants	0.8%
Other	5.7%

Data from Jagger J, et al. A study of patterns and prevention of blood exposures in OR personnel. Aorn J 1998;67(5):979–96.

70% of their injuries, and therefore rarely participate in recommended post-exposure strategies [4].

Double gloving

Surgeons and scrub personnel realize that glove barrier failure is common. In fact, the Food and Drug Administration (FDA) accepts a failure rate of 2.5% for new unused sterile gloves in standardized quality-control tests [14]. Perforation rates as high as 61% for thoracic surgeons and 40% for scrub nurses have been reported [15]. Initial intraoperative glove perforation occurs an average of 40 minutes [15,16] into a procedure and is not detected by the surgeon in as many as 83% of cases [17].

Therefore, the practice of wearing two pairs of gloves offers a higher degree of protection from this common event. Double gloving reduces the risk of exposure to patient blood by as much as 87% when the outer glove is punctured [18–22]. While puncture of the outer glove remains common, corresponding punctures of both the inner and outer gloves are rare. Additionally, the volume of blood on a solid suture needle is reduced as much as 95% when passing through two glove layers, thereby reducing the viral load in the event of a contaminated percutaneous injury [23]. Because of the occult nature of intraoperative glove failures, double gloving may prevent prolonged occult hand contact with patient blood. Using electronic detection of glove barrier failure, one study estimated that surgeons wearing a single pair of gloves would have contact with patient blood for 42 hours for every 100 hours of operating time [19]. Several reports indicate that better barrier protection might protect the patient from exposure to blood-borne pathogens from members of the operating team [24–28].

Surgeons have been reluctant to adopt this safety measure largely because of the widespread perception that double gloving reduces hand sensitivity and dexterity. One study compared knot-tying ability and moving two-point discrimination tests (under non-surgical conditions) between single- and double-gloved surgeons and found no difference [29]. A more recent study demonstrated that double-gloved surgeons experienced decreased hand sensibility during evaluations of pressure sensitivity and moving two-point discrimination. However, static two-point discrimination for those surgeons was not impaired [30]. Subjective evaluations comparing surgeons' comfort, sensitivity, and dexterity with single and double gloves indicated subjective impairment of all parameters [31], and surgeons involved in clinical studies with double gloving remove the outer glove before the end of surgery in about 26% of cases [32]. Nevertheless, surgeons who always or usually double glove report that a period of 1 to 120 days (2 days in most cases) is required to fully adapt to double gloving. Also, surgeons who routinely double glove report decreased hand sensation much less frequently than those who do not [4]. It appears that a period of adaptation and "retraining" is required for practitioners to feel comfortable with the technique.

Use blunt suture needles

Curved suture needles used during fascial closure cause as many as 59% of suture needle injuries in the operating room [12] (Table 2).

To decrease this risk of needle-stick injury to the surgeon, the use of blunt suture needles has been proposed and studied. To date, four prospective randomized trials have demonstrated that the use of blunt suture needles leads to a significant reduction in, and in some cases the elimination of, needle injuries to operating room staff. Wright et al. [37] reported that the use of blunt needles during hip arthroplasty significantly decreased glove perforations. Mingoli [38] reported that blunt needles reduce sharp injuries sevenfold in emergency abdominal procedures. Rice [39] reported no glove perforations or needle sticks using blunt suture needles in 68 total hip replacements. By comparison, rates using sharp needles are 16 percent for perforations and 6 percent for needle sticks. Hartley [40] reported a significant decrease in glove puncture rates (38% versus 6.5%) with the use of blunt suture needles. In a 1994 report, the CDC indicated that the use of blunt suture needles reduced percutaneous injuries from 1.9/1000 for curved suture needles to 0/1000 for blunt needles [12].

Several case series also support the safety and usability of blunt suture needles. Dauleh [41] reported that blunt suture needles eliminated needle-prick injury to surgeons' hands and were technically satisfactory in abdominal wall closure, hernia repair, and even in colonic anastomosis. Monz [42] reported ease of use and no percutaneous injuries with the use of blunt needles in 50 cases of abdominal wound closure.

Therefore, compelling published evidence supports the routine use of blunt suture needles for the closure of fascia and muscle. With further experience, these needles may be found to be safe and useful for suturing tissues other than fascia.

Use a neutral zone for passing sharps

The neutral zone has been defined as "a previously agreed upon location on the field where sharps are placed from which the surgeon or scrub can retrieve them. Therefore, hand-to-hand passing of sharps is limited" [33].

Table 2
Needle injuries relative to needle type

Type of needle	Injuries per 1000 needles used
Blunt suture needle	0
Straight suture needle	14.2
Curved suture needle	1.9

Data from Evaluation of blunt suture needles in preventing percutaneous injuries among health-care workers during gynecologic surgical procedures—New York City, March 1993–June 1994. MMWR Morb Mort Wkly Rep 1997;46(2):25–9.

The use of the neutral zone to transfer sharps (otherwise known as the hands-free technique (HFT)) has been proposed as a method to reduce exposure of operating room personnel to blood during surgery and is recommended by the American College of Surgeons and the Association of PeriOperative Registered Nurses. The American College of Surgeons offers the following guidelines:

> Avoid accidents and self-wounding with sharp instruments by following these measures: Do not recap needles, Use needle-less systems when possible, Use cautery and stapling devices when possible, and *pass sharp instruments in metal trays during operative procedures* [34].

Meanwhile, the Association of PeriOperative Registered Nurses offers the following precautions:

> Surgical team members should use hands-free techniques whenever possible and practical instead of passing needles and other sharp items hand to hand...Changes in surgical practice to minimize manual manipulation of sharps (ie, no touch techniques) can have a major impact on these injuries...Creation of a neutral zone (ie, where instruments are put down and picked up, rather than passed hand to hand) may decrease injuries from sharp instruments [35].

A study of 3765 operations [33] reported that, when HFT was judged by the scrub nurse to have been used 75% of the time or more often during the operation, the number of "incidents" fell by 59% in operations with a blood loss of 100 mL or greater. Incidents were defined as sharps injuries, cutaneous blood exposure, or glove tears. In contrast, one smaller randomized prospective study of the use of HFT compared with control during 156 cesarean sections demonstrated no reduction of the incidence of glove perforations with HFT compared with control [36].

While data regarding the efficacy of the HFT remains inconclusive, the technique is recommended by several leading professional organizations and its use is mandated in many hospitals as a safety measure to reduce sharps injuries during surgery.

Summary

Sharps injuries remain a significant health risk for surgeons and nurses in the operating room. health care workers must be made aware of this important issue. A number of related resources are available. These include:

1. International Sharps Injury Prevention Society. Education, information and product knowledge to help reduce the number of sharps injuries. Available at: http://www.isips.org.
2. International Health Care Worker Safety Center EPInet.. Exposure prevention information network. Available at http://www.med.virginia.edu/medcntr/centers/epinet/.

3. Joint Commission for Accreditation of Health Care Organizations. Sentinel alert: preventing needle stick and sharps injuries. August 2001. Available at: http://www.jcaho.org/about+us/news+letters/sentinel+event+alert/sea_22.htm.
4. Davis, MS. Advanced precautions for today's O.R. In: The operating room professional's handbook for the prevention of sharps injuries and bloodborne pathogen exposures. Atlanta (GA): Sweinbinder Publications; 2001.

References

[1] Recommendations for prevention of HIV transmission in health-care settings. MMWR Morb Mortal Wkly Rep 1987;36(Suppl 2):1S–18S.
[2] Bloodborne pathogens. Toxic and hazardous substances. Occupational safety and health standards. Washington, DC; 1991. Department of Labor, Occupational Safety and Health Administration. Standard Number 1910.1030.
[3] Occupational exposure to bloodborne pathogens; needlestick and other sharps injuries; final rule. Washington, DC: Occupational Safety and Health Administration, Department of Labor. Fed Regist 2001;66(12):5318–25.
[4] Patterson JM, Novak CB, Mackinnon SE, et al. Surgeons' concern and practices of protection against bloodborne pathogens. Ann Surg 1998;228(2):266–72.
[5] Gerberding JL, Littell C, Tarkington A, et al. Risk of exposure of surgical personnel to patients' blood during surgery at San Francisco General Hospital. N Engl J Med 1990;322(25): 1788–93.
[6] Quebbeman EJ, Telford GL, Hubbard S, et al. Risk of blood contamination and injury to operating room personnel. Ann Surg 1991;214(5):614–20.
[7] Panlilio AL, Foy DR, Edwards JR, et al. Blood contacts during surgical procedures. JAMA 1991;265(12):1533–7.
[8] Popejoy SL, Fry DE. Blood contact and exposure in the operating room. Surg Gynecol Obstet 1991;172(6):480–3.
[9] White MC, Lynch P. Blood contact and exposures among operating room personnel: a multicenter study. Am J Infect Control 1993;21(5):243–8.
[10] Jagger J, Bentley M, Tereskerz P. A study of patterns and prevention of blood exposures in OR personnel. AORN J 1998;67(5):979–81, 983–4, 986–7 passim.
[11] Tokars JI, Bell DM, Culver DH, et al. Percutaneous injuries during surgical procedures. JAMA 1992;267(21):2899–904.
[12] Evaluation of blunt suture needles in preventing percutaneous injuries among health-care workers during gynecologic surgical procedures—New York City, March 1993–June 1994. MMWR Morb Mortal Wkly Rep 1997;46(2):25–9.
[13] Wright JG, McGeer AJ, Chyatte D, et al. Mechanisms of glove tears and sharp injuries among surgical personnel. JAMA 1991;266(12):1668–71.
[14] Patient examination gloves and surgeons' gloves; sample plans and test method for leakage defect; adulteration. Washington, DC. Code of Federal Regulations: 2005. US Printing Office, 21CFR800.20.
[15] Hollaus PH, Lax F, Janakiev D, et al. Glove perforation rate in open lung surgery. Eur J Cardiothorac Surg 1999;15(4):461–4.
[16] Hentz VR, Stephanides M, Boraldi A, et al. Surgeon-patient barrier efficiency monitored with an electronic device in three surgical settings. World J Surg 2001;25(9):1101–8.
[17] Thomas S, Agarwal M, Mehta G. Intraoperative glove perforation—single versus double gloving in protection against skin contamination. Postgrad Med J 2001;77(909):458–60.

[18] Aarnio P, Laine T. Glove perforation rate in vascular surgery—a comparison between single and double gloving. Vasa 2001;30(2):122–4.

[19] Caillot JL, Cote C, Abidi H, et al. Electronic evaluation of the value of double gloving. Br J Surg 1999;86(11):1387–90.

[20] Jensen SL. Double gloving—electrical resistance and surgeons' resistance. Lancet 2000; 355(9203):514–5.

[21] Laine T, Aarnio P. How often does glove perforation occur in surgery? Comparison between single gloves and a double-gloving system. Am J Surg 2001;181(6):564–6.

[22] Naver LP, Gottrup F. Incidence of glove perforations in gastrointestinal surgery and the protective effect of double gloves: a prospective, randomised controlled study. Eur J Surg 2000;166(4):293–5.

[23] Bennett NT, Howard RJ. Quantity of blood inoculated in a needlestick injury from suture needles. J Am Coll Surg 1994;178(2):107–10.

[24] Esteban JI, Gomez J, Martell M, et al. Transmission of hepatitis C virus by a cardiac surgeon. N Engl J Med 1996;334(9):555–60.

[25] Harpaz R, Von Seidlein L, Averhoff FM, et al. Transmission of hepatitis B virus to multiple patients from a surgeon without evidence of inadequate infection control. N Engl J Med 1996;334(9):549–54.

[26] McNeil SA, Nordstrom-Lerner L, Malani PN, et al. Outbreak of sternal surgical site infections due to Pseudomonas aeruginosa traced to a scrub nurse with onychomycosis. Clin Infect Dis 2001;33(3):317–23.

[27] van den Broek PJ, Lampe AS, Berbee GA, et al. Epidemic of prosthetic valve endocarditis caused by Staphylococcus epidermidis. Br Med J (Clin Res Ed) 1985;291(6500):949–50.

[28] Wooster DL, Louch RE, Krajden S. Intraoperative bacterial contamination of vascular grafts: a prospective study. Can J Surg 1985;28(5):407–9.

[29] Webb JM, Pentlow BD. Double gloving and surgical technique. Ann R Coll Surg Engl 1993; 75(4):291–2.

[30] Novak CB, Patterson JM, Mackinnon SE. Evaluation of hand sensibility with single and double latex gloves. Plast Reconstr Surg 1999;103(1):128–31.

[31] Wilson SJ, Sellu D, Uy A, et al. Subjective effects of double gloves on surgical performance. Ann R Coll Surg Engl 1996;78(1):20–2.

[32] Matta H, Thompson AM, Rainey JB. Does wearing two pairs of gloves protect operating theatre staff from skin contamination? BMJ 1988;297(6648):597–8.

[33] Stringer B, Infante-Rivard C, Hanley JA. Effectiveness of the hands-free technique in reducing operating theatre injuries. Occup Environ Med 2002;59(10):703–7.

[34] American College of Surgeons. ACS surgery: principles and practice. New York: Web MD; 2002.

[35] AORN Recommended Practices Committee, Association of PeriOperative Registered Nurses. Recommended practices for sponge, sharp, and instrument counts. AORN J 1999;70(6):1083–9.

[36] Eggleston MK Jr, Wax JR, Philput C, et al. Use of surgical pass trays to reduce intraoperative glove perforations. J Matern Fetal Med 1997;6(4):245–7.

[37] Wright KU, Moran CG, Briggs PJ. Glove perforation during hip arthroplasty. A randomised prospective study of a new taperpoint needle. J Bone Joint Surg Br 1993;75(6):918–20.

[38] Mingoli A, Sapienza P, Sgarzini G, et al. Influence of blunt needles on surgical glove perforation and safety for the surgeon. Am J Surg 1996;172(5):512–6 [discussion 516–7].

[39] Rice JJ, McCabe JP, McManus F. Needle stick injury. Reducing the risk. Int Orthop 1996; 20(3):132–3.

[40] Hartley JE, Ahmed S, Milkins R, et al. Randomized trial of blunt-tipped versus cutting needles to reduce glove puncture during mass closure of the abdomen. Br J Surg 1996;83(8):1156–7.

[41] Dauleh MI, Irving AD, Townell NH. Needle prick injury to the surgeon—do we need sharp needles? J R Coll Surg Edinb 1994;39(5):310–1.

[42] Montz FJ, Fowler JM, Farias-Eisner R, et al. Blunt needles in fascial closure. Surg Gynecol Obstet 1991;173(2):147–8.

ELSEVIER
SAUNDERS

Surg Clin N Am 85 (2005) 1307–1319

SURGICAL
CLINICS OF
NORTH AMERICA

Patient Safety Practices in the Operating Room: Correct-Site Surgery and NoThing Left Behind

Verna C. Gibbs, MD[a,b,*]

[a]*Department of Surgery QI Program, University of California at San Francisco,*
533 Parnassus Avenue U-157, Box 0617, San Francisco, CA 94143-0617, USA
[b]*San Francisco Veterans Affairs Medical Center, 4150 Clement Street (112),*
San Francisco, CA 94121, USA

Workplace safety standards for the operating room have existed for decades. These standards have traditionally focused on equipment, fire prevention and environmental controls with the primary aim of protecting the people who work in the room. That is, surgeons, perioperative care nurses and anesthesiologists. Not until the late 1990s, after the publication of the National Academy of Medicine's treatise "To Err Is Human," did safety standards specifically for patients begin to be considered [1] in operating room practices. Attention turned to developing ways to ensure that patients would be free from injuries caused by mistakes in the operating room.

Patient safety practices in the operating room are based on strategies for reducing error. Such strategies may require systems in which perioperative care providers work is redesigned. Newly redesigned systems may include standards for processes of care, the use of protocols and checklists to reduce reliance on memory, and simplification of all processes as much as possible. Furthermore such systems should eliminate or minimize conditions that lead to human error (eg, interruptions, fear, anger, time pressure, anxiety), include devices designed to be error-proof and incorporate frequent training in the use of those devices [2]. Additional practices include the creation by senior management of an environment of "no fault" reporting of errors and "near misses," feedback on performance improvement in employee and staff reviews, and evaluation of safety practices in institutional performance measures.

---

* Department of Surgery QI Program, University of California at San Francisco, 533 Parnassus Avenue U-157, Box 0617, San Francisco, CA 94143-0617.
 E-mail address: gibbsv@surgery.ucsf.edu

0039-6109/05/$ - see front matter. Published by Elsevier Inc.
doi:10.1016/j.suc.2005.09.007

Safety practices generally cover broad structural elements within a health care system. Such measures include steps for creating appropriate environments for safe delivery of care and practices for proper patient identification. In medicine, patient safety efforts have focused on prevention of medication errors and improvement in the transmission of medical orders through computerized entry systems [2]. In surgery, the first patient safety initiative was directed against the problem of wrong-site surgery.

Correct-site surgery

In 1998, the Joint Commission on Accreditation of Health Care (JCAHO) issued a sentinel event alert on the problem of wrong-site surgery. This alert was based on a review of 15 cases reported to the organization [3]. Wrong-site surgery is the performance of an operation or surgical procedure on the wrong part of the body. This can include the wrong side of the body in cases involving laterality or it can be the wrong level of the spine in cases involving spine surgery. Wrong-procedure surgery is the performance of a procedure other than that intended or indicated. Wrong-person surgery is the performance of an operation or procedure on a person other than the one for whom the procedure was intended. All of these events are errors of commission and are the result of mistakes in applying identification procedures. Although these errors happened before with astonishing regularity in the most modern health care environments, the initial impetus to systematically address this problem came only after the JCAHO review.

By 2000, the JCAHO sentinel event database contained 150 reported cases of wrong-site, wrong-person or wrong-procedure surgery, and 126 of these cases had root-cause analysis information available for them [4]. Root-cause analysis is an investigative technique for drilling down to underlying organizational causes or factors that contribute to an event, and for identifying corrective opportunities that could reduce the likelihood of a similar error recurring [2]. The JCAHO has promoted this detailed and time-consuming technique in the investigation of all reported sentinel events. Institutions are expected to report sentinel events and root-cause analysis findings to the JCAHO to discover trends, learn lessons and develop better patient safety practices.

Of the 126 cases that involved wrong-site surgery, 41% involved orthopedic surgery, 20% involved general surgery, 14% neurosurgery, 11% urology and the remaining cases involved other surgical disciplines [4]. The high percentage of wrong-site orthopedic cases is related to the likelihood that orthopedic surgeons operate on bilaterally symmetric or paired structures involving multiple digits or toes and levels. Operations of this nature present more opportunities for error. Fifty-eight percent of the cases occurred in hospital-based ambulatory surgery units, 29% occurred in inpatient operating rooms, and 13% at other inpatient clinical care settings, such as the emergency department or the ICU. Seventy-six percent involved surgery on the wrong body part or site, 13% involved surgery on the wrong patient, and 11% involved the wrong surgical procedure.

After reviewing the cases, hospitals identified many factors as root causes for the errors. However, the most noteworthy factor shared by all the cases was poor communication between members of the clinical care team and the patient. Poor communication stemmed from factors related to both the health care provider and the patient. Provider-related factors included unclear determination of the operative site, deficient verification checklists of patient status or procedure in the operating room, incomplete patient perioperative assessments, and inadequate policies and practices related to patient identification. Patient-related factors included the patient's physical characteristics, the patient's lack of knowledge of procedures to be performed, and communication difficulties among physicians, patients, and families [5].

In 1997, the American Academy of Orthopedic Surgeons issued recommendations and promulgated methods for eliminating wrong-site surgery. However, a survey in 2000 showed that only 30% of orthopedic surgeons actually followed these recommendations [6]. The most important directive was to mark the operative site in the preoperative area with the surgeon's initials, the so-called "sign your site" initiative. This marking procedure was to be done whenever possible with the active involvement of the patient and after the completion of adequate patient identification procedures. By 2001, reports showed continuing occurrences of cases involving wrong-site surgery. A survey of hand surgeons revealed that 20% of the respondents had operated on the wrong site at least once in their career. An additional 16% had almost operated on the wrong site but their errors were caught and the cases became near misses [7]. These events illustrated the difficulties inherent in a system where people under operating-room conditions were making decisions involving symmetrical organs, multiple digits and spinal levels that often depended on radiographs. Responding to this problem, the American College of Surgeons, in 2002, issued its "Statement on Ensuring Correct Patient, Correct Site and Correct Procedure Surgery" [8].

The problem persisted. The JCAHO received reports of 60 cases of wrong-site surgery in 2002 and 50 in 2003, leading the JCAHO to develop and implement on July 1, 2004, the Universal Protocol for Preventing Wrong Site, Wrong Procedure, and Wrong Person Surgery [9] (Fig. 1). The primary components of the protocol address the primary issues of patient identification, unambiguous communication and perioperative environmental confusion. The universality of the protocol lies in its application in all health care settings where invasive procedures that expose patients to harm are performed.

The universal protocol mandates that medical professionals must follow a preoperative verification process, mark the operative site, and take a "time out" immediately before starting the procedure [9]. The goal of the

Universal Protocol For Preventing Wrong Site, Wrong Procedure, Wrong Person Surgery™

Wrong site, wrong procedure, wrong person surgery can be prevented. This universal protocol is intended to achieve that goal. It is based on the consensus of experts from the relevant clinical specialties and professional disciplines and is endorsed by more than 40 professional medical associations and organizations.

In developing this protocol, consensus was reached on the following principles:

❑ Wrong site, wrong procedure, wrong person surgery can and must be prevented.

❑ A robust approach—using multiple, complementary strategies—is necessary to achieve the goal of eliminating wrong site, wrong procedure, wrong person surgery.

❑ Active involvement and effective communication among all members of the surgical team is important for success.

❑ To the extent possible, the patient (or legally designated representative) should be involved in the process.

❑ Consistent implementation of a standardized approach using a universal, consensus-based protocol will be most effective.

❑ The protocol should be flexible enough to allow for implementation with appropriate adaptation when required to meet specific patient needs.

❑ A requirement for site marking should focus on cases involving right/left distinction, multiple structures (fingers, toes), or levels (spine).

❑ The universal protocol should be applicable or adaptable to all operative and other invasive procedures that expose patients to harm, including procedures done in settings other than the operating room.

In concert with these principles, the following steps, taken together, comprise the Universal Protocol for eliminating wrong site, wrong procedure, wrong person surgery:

❑ Pre-operative verification process
  o Purpose: To ensure that all of the relevant documents and studies are available prior to the start of the procedure and that they have been reviewed and are consistent with each other and with the patient's expectations and with the team's understanding of the intended patient, procedure, site and, as applicable, any implants. Missing information or discrepancies must be addressed before starting the procedure.
  o Process: An ongoing process of information gathering and verification, beginning with the determination to do the procedure, continuing through all settings and interventions involved in the preoperative preparation of the patient, up to and including the "time out" just before the start of the procedure.

❑ Marking the operative site
  o Purpose: To identify unambiguously the intended site of incision or insertion.
  o Process: For procedures involving right/left distinction, multiple structures (such as fingers and toes), or multiple levels (as in spinal procedures), the intended site must be marked such that the mark will be visible after the patient has been prepped and draped.

❑ "Time out" immediately before starting the procedure
  o Purpose: To conduct a final verification of the correct patient, procedure, site and, as applicable, implants.
  o Process: Active communication among all members of the surgical/procedure team, consistently initiated by a designated member of the team, conducted in a "fail-safe" mode, i.e., the procedure is not started until any questions or concerns are resolved.

© Copyright 2003

Fig. 1. Universal protocol for preventing wrong site, wrong procedure and wrong person surgery. Reprinted with permission of the Joint Commission on Accreditation of Healthcare Organizations.

preoperative verification process is to ensure that all relevant documents and studies are available before the procedure is performed and that the studies have been reviewed. Furthermore, the process should confirm that all team members agree that the intended procedure is being performed on the correct patient at the correct site. Many health care entities have developed preoperative checklists that are completed before every procedure to document compliance with the universal protocol.

The marking of the operative site identifies unambiguously the intended incision or insertion. The site marking is especially important in cases involving right/left distinction and in cases with multiple structures or levels. The marking should take place before the patient has been prepped and draped. Nonoperative sites are not to be marked and the marking should be done by a person who will be performing the procedure. The marking should preferably be with indelible ink that won't be removed by the surgical prep.

The institution of a final "time-out" to bring everyone on the team to the same place provides the opportunity for a final verification of the correct patient, procedure and site. During the time-out, members of the operating team should employ active communication techniques. All questions and concerns are to be addressed before the incision is made. The performance of the time-out must be documented in the medical record. Active communication requires that a member of the operative team gathers the attention of the team and states the patient's name, procedure and site, and ensures the verbal acknowledgment of the team that the information is correct. Many health care entities have developed standardized scripts that are followed by the team members to ensure that the proper information is covered.

Not enough time has passed since the introduction of this universal protocol to determine its effectiveness in decreasing the incidence of wrong-site surgery. The universal protocol has brought about changes in the way invasive procedures are planned and started, and has influenced the way team members communicate with each other. What effect these changes have had is still unknown. New technology, such as the SurgiChip, is under development for prevention of wrong-site, wrong-procedure, and wrong-person surgery. The SurgiChip uses radio frequency identification (RFID) technology that generates adhesive labels containing a computer chip with detailed patient identification information. The chip can be read by a handheld scanner. The US Food and Drug Administration approved the SurgiChip for this application in 2004 [10].

NoThing left behind

A less tragic but probably more common surgical error is that of retained foreign bodies [11]. One estimate says that one case of a retained item occurs at least once a year in a major hospital where 8,000 to 18,000 major cases are performed per year [12]. Data from a retrospective case-control study of medical records associated with claims filed between 1985 and 2001 found that the likelihood of retained-foreign-body cases was higher for patients who had emergency surgery, an unexpected change in surgical procedure, and a higher mean body-mass index. Incidents were less likely if sponge counts were performed at the time of operation. This estimate was based on claims data and thus did not include data about many cases that are settled quietly outside of the legal system. Nor did it include the many near misses that have occurred. Near misses involve, for example, incorrect sponge and needle counts that are resolved before a procedure is concluded. The JCAHO in June 2005 made cases of retained surgical items a sentinel event which will require reporting and root cause analysis. Changing this requirement may help identify how frequently these events actually occur nationwide. Recognizing the problem of retained foreign bodies, the American College of Surgeons in June 2005 approved the "Statement on Prevention of Retained Foreign Bodies after Surgery" (www.facs.org/fellows_info/statements/st-51.html) (Box 1).

A retained foreign body occurs when a surgical tool, usually a sponge, needle or instrument, is unintentionally left behind in a patient. In 2001, after the institution of heightened airport security measures, surgical retractors, scissors and clamps were being discovered in unsuspecting former patients as they went through processes for boarding flights. Retained objects can be left behind in any part of the body, but most frequently are reported lost in the abdominal cavity, chest, pelvis and vagina [13]. The surgical tools can be discovered weeks, months or years after the original operation, usually because of the development of patient symptoms [14]. The foreign body can cause an acute injury leading to early discovery, or it can induce a reaction with local or systemic signs. Fistulization may occur leading to spontaneous extrusion, or a fibrinous response can be elicited, which leads to encapsulation of the foreign body, causing a mass effect or a bowel obstruction. Any of these findings can lead providers to investigate possible causes and obtain a CT scan [15]. Most retained objects require an operation for removal. While cases of retention of surgical instruments garner the biggest headlines, cases of retained sponges probably occur more frequently.

No experimental evidence directly addresses the problem of retained foreign bodies. However, anecdotal and experiential evidence, such as quality improvement reviews, risk management reports, and closed claims studies, show that these events occur, just like wrong-site surgery cases, because of poor communication among perioperative care personnel and faulty processes of care in the operating room. Examples of poor communication include instances where surgeons and nurses fail to work together cooperatively to rectify an incorrect count, where surgeons dismiss requests to look for missing objects, and where personnel are changed multiple times during a procedure without accurate cross-informational reporting. Faulty processes of care include inadequate or incomplete wound explorations, poorly performed

Box 1. Statement on the Prevention of Retained Foreign Bodies after Surgery

The American College of Surgeons (ACS) recognizes patient safety as being an item of the highest priority and strongly urges individual hospitals and healthcare organizations to take all reasonable measures to prevent the retention of foreign bodies in the surgical wound. The ACS offers the following guidelines that can be adapted to various practice settings, including traditional operating rooms, ambulatory surgery centers, surgeons' offices, and other areas where operative and invasive procedures are performed:

- Surgical procedures take place within a system of perioperative care composed of surgeons, perioperative registered nurses, surgical technologists and anesthesia professionals. These individuals share a common ethical, legal and moral responsibility to promote an optimal patient outcome.
- Prevention of foreign body retention requires good communication among perioperative personnel and the consistent application of reliable and standardized processes of care.
- Recommendations to prevent the retention of sponges, sharps, instruments and other designated miscellaneous items include:
  - consistent application and adherence to standardized counting procedures
  - performance of a methodical wound exploration before closure of the surgical site
  - use of X-ray detectable items in the surgical wound
  - maintenance of an optimal OR environment to allow focused performance of operative tasks
  - employment of Xray or other technology (e.g. radiofrequency detection, bar coding) as indicated, to ensure there is no unintended item remaining in the operative field
  - suspension of these measures as required in life-threatening situations
- Documentation should include, but not be limited to: results of surgical item counts, notification of the surgical team members, instruments or items intentionally left as packing, and actions taken if count discrepancies occur.

- Surgical facilities must provide resources to ensure that necessary equipment and personnel are available to support these perioperative surgical safety measures.
- Policies and procedures for the prevention of retained foreign bodies should be developed, reviewed periodically, revised as necessary, and available in the practice setting.

Notes:

Gibbs VC and Auerbach, AD "The Retained Surgical Sponge" in "Making Health Care Safer: A Critical Analysis of Patient Safety Practices." Shojania KG, Duncan BW, McDonald KM, Wachter RM, editors. *Evidence Report/Technology Assessment No. 43, AHRQ Publication No. 01-E058*; July 2001. Report available at http://www.ahrq.gov/clinic/ptsafety/chap22.htm

Gwande AA, Srudert DM, Orav TA, et al. "Patient Safety: Risk Factors for Retained Instruments and Sponges after Surgery", *New England Journal of Medicine* 2003;348:229–35.

"Recommended Practices for Sponge, Sharp, and Instrument Counts," in *AORN Standards, Recommended Practices & Guidelines* (Denver, AORN, Inc., 2004), 229–34.

From the Bulletin of the American College of Surgeons 2005;90(10):15, with permission.

sponge and instrument counts, and incomplete, inadequate or misread intra-operative radiographs. Most evidence suggests that the existing system of prevention fails because of human-related communication factors [16].

The airline industry has a good model for dealing with communication between persons with diverse skills and roles. The airline safety program has addressed communication issues by developing team communication and performance standards, training to these standards, reviewing performance in simulated learning environments, and enforcing standards equally among all team members. Developing team training and enhanced communication skills and behaviors among perioperative care professionals would likely go a long way toward preventing miscounts and errors in the management of surgical paraphernalia.

Standardized processes of care are important. One widely used operating room practice is the manual counting of sponges, sharps, and instruments [17]. While no good evidence of the effectiveness of this procedure has been published, it is the only available safety modality currently in use to track surgical tools. While the practice of counting is standard procedure for operating room personnel, the process by which counts are performed is not standardized and components of the processes are subject to individual hospital policy.

Counting procedures can be supplemented with assistive devices, such as the widely used plastic hanging pocket counting device. Counting procedures are often omitted or abbreviated in emergency cases or in cases where a significant risk for leaving instruments in the surgical site does not exist. The adjunctive procedure to the count is the performance of a radiograph examination to identify any objects that may remain in a body cavity. This practice is not universally used and can only identify objects, such as metal objects, that a radiograph can reveal. When a confirmatory radiograph is requested, hospital personnel must be available and expeditiously dispatched. Expert radiological review when available is recommended. In trauma settings, or when the patient is in a critical life-threatening situation in the operating room, the usual procedures for counting may be suspended and replaced with a mandatory radiological evaluation in an alternative care setting once the patient has been stabilized.

Counting alone does not prevent foreign body retention. All members of the operating team have a responsibility to adopt safe surgical practices and help account for surgical tools and objects. Sponges, towels, gauze and cotton pads placed in the operative field should contain a radio-opaque marker. A strongly recommended safety practice for surgeons is to use in the surgical wound only items detectable on a radiograph. Surgeons should execute a careful and thoughtful exploration of the operative site before the closure of the wound. This methodical exploration, especially important in the chest, abdomen, and pelvis, should be performed every time and before the final sponge and needle count (Box 2).

Following an incorrect count and the determination that an item is missing, the wound should be reopened and carefully re-explored. Anesthesiologists often use non–radio-opaque gauze sponges in their work area and they should be mindful and cooperative in working with fellow members of the operating room team in keeping unmarked items out of the wound and in disposing of them in separate containers from those used to track the radiograph-detectable sponges. Many companies are developing devices to facilitate the detection of surgical tools. New technology that will help with accounting should be evaluated and considered for adoption as they become available [18]. These technologies include the use of bar codes on instruments, detection systems for sponges (eg, radio-frequency identification), and electronic surveillance systems.

As a general principal, the maintenance of an optimal operating room environment allows everyone to mindfully accomplish their work. Allowing time for the focused performance of operative tasks is likely to enhance accuracy and reduce errors. Distractions, interruptions, personnel changes, noise, conversation and traffic should be limited and kept to a minimum. Process review and improvement should be performed regularly and routinely after any near-miss or retained-foreign-body event. A focused review or analysis of contributing factors can often identify areas within established processes of care that need revision. The incidence of retained foreign

Box 2. Methodical exploration of operative site(s)

Process:

A methodical exploration of the operative wound should be
conducted prior to closure. Carefully examine the space to be
closed, and especially prior to closure of a cavity within a cavity
(i.e. stomach, bladder, uterus, vagina). Reliance on only one
element of sensory perception is discouraged, strive to **SEE
AND TOUCH** during the exploration whenever possible. All
items placed in the operative site should contain a radiopaque
marker whenever possible to ease in xray detection should the
item be lost. These instructions are based upon experiential
and published case reports of where missing objects were
found.

Wound/operative site(s)

1. Place retractors in the incision to provide adequate exposure
   to perform visual and manual exploration of the operative
   site. Do not be deceived by the size of the wound or the
   nature of the operation.
2. Look and feel in the recesses of the wound and under fatty
   protuberances and soft-tissue appendages.

Abdomen/pelvis

1. Place retractors in the incision to provide adequate exposure
   to perform visual and manual exploration of the peritoneal
   and retroperitoneal spaces if these areas were entered.
2. Examine all four quadrants of the abdomen with attention to:
   i.   Lift the transverse colon
   ii. Check above/around the liver and above/around the spleen
   iii. Examine within and between loops of bowel
   iv. Look where there was a retractor or retractor blades were
        placed
3. Examine the pelvis
   i. Look behind the bladder, uterus (if present) and around the
      upper rectum
4. If the vagina was entered, explored or part of the procedure it
   should be examined.

Mediastinum/thorax

1. In the mediastinum, reflect the heart and examine the
   retrocardiac space.
2. Elevate the apex of the heart to look behind it and look in
   the transverse sinus to the right and left of the aorta
   and pulmonary artery.

3. Examine the thoracic cavity with attention to the thoracic apex and base of the lungs. Place a hand or finger behind the lung and palpate from apex to base.

When there is an incorrect count:
When the surgeon(s) is informed by nursing professionals that there is an incorrect count, while all perioperative care personnel are looking for the missing object, the surgeon(s) should participate in this endeavor by repeating the methodical wound examination.
1. STOP CLOSING THE WOUND
2. Remove enough fascial suture to replace a retractor and obtain adequate visual AND tactile information to locate the surgical item. Examine the full length and depth of the wound
3. Repeat the methodical operative site examination as described above
4. Obtain a radiograph and strong consideration should be given to not having the patient leave the OR until the xray is reviewed by a radiologist.

bodies can be brought to zero. With effective perioperative care systems in place, the surgical patient can be assured that there will be "NoThing Left Behind."

Summary

Attention has turned to issues of surgical patient safety. Essential patient safety practices in the operating room include the application of standard processes of care, the use of protocols and checklists to reduce reliance on memory, the employment of simpler processes as much as possible, the alleviation of conditions that predispose to human error (eg, interruptions, fear, anger, time pressure, anxiety), and the design and use of error-proof devices coupled with frequent training in the use of these devices. These practices can be applied to two issues in surgical patient safety: assurance of correct site surgery and prevention of incidents involving retained foreign bodies. Both of these safety problems involve poor communication between perioperative care personnel and faulty processes of care. Recommendations to ensure that the correct procedure is performed on the correct patient at the correct site have been mandated by the JACHO Universal Protocol. The protocol mandates using a preoperative verification process, marking the operative site, and taking a "time out" immediately before starting the procedure. All health care facilities where invasive procedures that expose patients to harm are performed are required to comply with this protocol. Recommendations to prevent the retention of sponges, sharps, instruments, and other miscellaneous items include consistent application and adherence to standardized counting procedures, performance of a methodical wound exploration before closure of the surgical site, use of radiograph-detectable items in the surgical wound, maintenance of an optimal operating room environment to allow focused performance of operative tasks, and application of radiographs or other technology as indicated to ensure there is no item left by mistake in the operative field. All perioperative care personnel can work together to ensure that these events never happen. Getting to zero is possible.

References

[1] Kohn LT, Corrigan JM, Donaldson MS, editors. To err is human: building a safer health system. Washington (DC): National Academy Press; 2000.

[2] Wachter RM, Shojania K. Internal bleeding: the truth behind America's terrifying epidemic of medical mistakes. New York: Rugged Land; 2004.

[3] Joint Commission on Accreditation of Healthcare Organization. Lessons learned: wrong-site surgery. Sentinel event alert. Issue 6. 1998. Available at: http://www.jcaho.org/about+us/news+letters/sentinel+event+alert/sea_6.htm. Accessed September 28, 2005.

[4] Joint Commission on Accreditation of Healthcare Organizations. A follow-up review of wrong-site surgery. Sentinel Event Alert 2001; 24.

[5] DiGiovanni CW, Kang L, Manuel J. Patient compliance in avoiding wrong-site surgery. J Bone Joint Surg [Am] 2003;85-A:815–9.

[6] OK plan to end wrong-site surgeries. AAOS Bulletin. Available at: http://www.aaos.org/wordhtml/bulletin/oct97/wrong.htm. Accessed September 28, 2005.

[7] Meinberg EG, Stern PJ. Incidence of wrong-site surgery among hand surgeons. J Bone Joint Surg [Am] 2003;85-A:193–7.

[8] American College of Surgeons. [ST-41] Statement on ensuring correct patient, correct site, and correct procedure surgery. Available at http://www.facs.org/fellows_info/statements/st-41.html. Accessed September 27, 2005.

[9] Joint Commission on Accreditation of Healthcare Organizations. Universal protocol for prevention of wrong site, wrong procedure, wrong person surgery. Available at www.jcaho.org/accredited+organizations/patient+safety/universal+protocol/. Accessed September 27, 2005.

[10] Sandlin D. SurgiChip—new technology for prevention of wrong site, wrong procedure, wrong person surgery. J Perianesth Nurs 2005;20(2):144–6.

[11] Gibbs VC, Auerbach AD. The retained surgical sponge. In: Shojania KG, Duncan BW, McDonald KM, Wachter RM, editors. Making health care safer: a critical analysis of patient safety practices. Rockville (MD): Agency for Healthcare Research and Quality; 2001. p. 255–7.

[12] Gawande AA, Studdert DM, Orav EJ, et al. Risk factors for retained instruments and sponges after surgery. N Engl J Med 2003;348:229–35.

[13] Kaiser CW, Friedman S, Spurling KP, et al. The retained surgical sponge. Ann Surg 1996; 224:79–84.

[14] Gibbs VC. Retained surgical sponge; cases and commentaries: surgery-anesthesia. September 2003. AHRQ WebM&M cases. Available at: http://webmm.ahrq.gov/case.aspx?caseID=27. Accessed September 28, 2005.

[15] O'Connor AR, Coakley FV, Meng MV, et al. Imaging of retained surgical sponges in the abdomen and pelvis. Am J Roentgenol 2003;180:481–9.

[16] Thomas EJ, Moore FA, The missing suction tip. Spotlight case, November 2003. AHRQ WebM&M cases. Available at http://webmm.ahrq.gov/case.aspx?caseID=37. Accessed September 28, 2005.

[17] Association of PeriOperative Registered Nurses. Recommended practices for sponge, sharp and instrument counts in AORN standards, recommended practices and guidelines. Denver (CO): AORN, Inc.; 2004.

[18] Fabian C. Electronic tagging of surgical sponges to prevent their accidental retention. Surgery 2005;137:298–301.

SURGICAL
CLINICS OF
NORTH AMERICA

Surg Clin N Am 85 (2005) 1321–1327

Standardization of Perioperative Management: Clinical Pathways

Lena M. Napolitano, MD[a,b,*]

[a]*University of Michigan School of Medicine, Ann Arbor, MI, USA*
[b]*Department of Surgery, University of Michigan Medical Center,*
1500 East Medical Center Drive, 1C340 University Hospital, Box 0033,
Ann Arbor, MI 48109-0033, USA

Many initiatives have been introduced in the past decades to standardize and improve clinical perioperative care and thereby improve patient care. Clinical pathways (also known as integrated care pathways, critical pathways, critical paths, care paths) are structured multidisciplinary care plans that detail essential steps in the care of patients with a specific clinical problem [1]. They are designed to support the implementation and translation of national guidelines into local protocols and their subsequent application to clinical practice. In surgery, clinical pathways are standardized protocols for the management of patients who have common conditions undergoing common surgical procedures.

Clinical pathways were introduced in the early 1990s in the United Kingdom and the United States and are being increasingly used throughout the developed world. They provide detailed guidance for each stage in the management (eg, treatments, interventions) of a patient who has a specific condition over a given time period and include progress and outcomes details. In particular, clinical pathways aim to improve the continuity and coordination of care across different disciplines and sectors within the hospital setting.

Clinical pathways can be viewed as algorithms in that they offer a flow chart format of the decisions to be made and the care to be provided for a given patient or patient group for a given condition in a step-wise sequence. Clinical pathways have four main components: a timeline, the categories of care or activities and their interventions, intermediate and

* Correspondence. Department of Surgery, University of Michigan Health System, Room 1C340, University Hospital, 1500 East Medical Center Drive, Ann Arbor, MI 48109.
E-mail address: lenan@umich.edu

doi:10.1016/j.suc.2005.10.011   *surgical.theclinics.com*

long-term outcome criteria, and the variance record (to allow deviations to be documented and analyzed).

Clinical pathways differ from practice guidelines, protocols, and algorithms because they are used by a multidisciplinary team and focus on the quality and coordination of care. Clinical pathways should be the quality-assessed and evidence-based way of consistently delivering high-quality care for a particular circumstance. The goals of clinical pathways [2] are

- Selecting the best practice when practice varies unnecessarily
- Defining the standards for the expected duration of hospital stay and for the use of tests and treatments
- Examining the interrelations among the different steps in the care process to find ways to coordinate or decrease the time in the rate-limiting step
- Giving all hospital staff a common plan from which to view and understand their various roles in the overall care process
- Providing a framework for collecting data on the care process so that providers can learn how often and why patients do not follow an expected course during their hospitalization
- Decreasing documentation burdens
- Improving patient satisfaction with care by educating patients and their families about the plan of care

The American Heart Association [3] recently reviewed critical pathways in the context of cardiovascular medicine and concluded that

- Critical pathways are being implemented in a broad range of patients who have cardiovascular disease
- Although cost savings can and should be evaluated with the critical pathway, the goal of improving guideline compliance and overall quality of care should be the primary focus
- Additional rigorous research into the cost of pathway development and implementation, as well as the outcomes of critical pathway use, is essential before further dissemination of this tool.
- Clinical protocols can and should be used to decrease variation in care, improve guideline compliance, and potentially improve overall quality of care in patients who have cardiovascular disease.

Practitioners and administrators should work together to incorporate similar and compatible features of clinical protocols and critical pathways. This process may result in improved quality of care and reduced costs.

Clinical pathways: common features

Clinical pathways, in medicine and in other areas, have a number of consistent features. Clinical pathways

- Examine the external evidence for individual technologies

- Combine this evidence with local knowledge and experience and conditions
- Involve a number of persons from different disciplines in a team decision, creating ownership of the product
- Measure the results of the actions
- Have information systems feeding back to the team on a timely basis
- Amend the pathway in the light of results

They also have in common perhaps the single most important result: they deliver a better quality of care and almost always manage to do so at lower cost.

Clinical pathways traditionally have been developed by a multidisciplinary team familiar with the care of specific patients who have specific diseases or who are undergoing specific procedures. The goal of these clinical pathways has been to make health care delivery more efficient, more standardized, more effective, and less error-prone. Newer technologic computer-based approaches for the development of clinical pathways have been developed and are undergoing critical evaluation to assess future potential [4].

The benefits and potential problems associated with clinical pathways are listed in Box 1. These issues must be addressed for each individual clinical pathway. If numerous potential problems are associated with a particular pathway, implementation of the clinical pathway will be problematic. Continual reevaluation and update of clinical pathways is necessary.

Clinical pathways in surgery

Standardized clinical pathways have been established for a number of common surgical procedures, including laparoscopic cholecystectomy [5,6], colon surgery [7,8], minimally invasive surgery [9,10], and more complex adult surgery such as pulmonary and esophageal resections [11], pancreaticoduodenectomy [12], and revision of total hip replacement [13]. Critical pathway methodology has also been established as an effective strategy in complex pediatric and neonatal surgical procedures such as congenital heart surgery [14]. Implementation of these clinical pathways in pediatric heart surgery has also been associated with a significant reduction in length of stay and resource use [15].

With the recent advent and expansion of bariatric surgery, the use and subsequent modification of clinical pathways for bariatric surgery has been shown to achieve superior outcomes, including reduced length of stay, reduced complication rates, and decreased duration of nasogastric tube decompression [16]. Once implemented, an established clinical pathway can be used to modify patient care to achieve specific goals, in this circumstance the specific goal of reducing the duration of nasogastric tube decompression.

Similarly, comprehensive clinical pathways have been associated with improved outcome and reduced length of hospital stay in patients undergoing

Box 1. Benefits and potential problems of clinical pathways

Benefits
Support the introduction of evidence-based medicine and use of
    clinical guidelines
Support clinical effectiveness, risk management, and clinical auditing
Improve multidisciplinary communication, teamwork, and care
    planning
Can support continuity and coordination of care across different
    clinical disciplines and sectors
Provide explicit and well-defined standards for care
Help reduce variations in patient care (by promoting standardization)
Help improve clinical outcomes
Help improve and even reduce patient documentation
Support training
Optimize the management of resources
Help ensure quality of care and provide a means of continuous
    quality improvement
Support the implementation of continuous clinical auditing in
    clinical practice
Support the use of guidelines in clinical practice
Help empower patients
Help manage clinical risk
Help improve communications between different care sectors
Disseminate accepted standards of care
Provide a baseline for future initiatives
Are not prescriptive: do not override clinical judgment
Are expected to help reduce risk
Are expected to help reduce costs by shortening hospital stays

Potential problems and barriers
May seem to discourage personalized care
Risk increasing litigation
Do not respond well to unexpected changes in a patient's condition
Are better suited to standard conditions than to unusual or
    unpredictable ones
Require commitment from staff and establishment of an adequate
    organizational structure
May create problems in introducing new technology
May take time to be accepted in the workplace
Need provisions to ensure variance and outcomes are properly
    recorded, audited, and acted upon

_____

Adapted from http://www.openclinical.org/clinicalpathways.html, with permission.

radical cystectomy [17]. The clinical pathway included improvements in preoperative, intraoperative, and postoperative care. The preoperative care included limited outpatient standardized bowel preparation and patient education. Operative modifications included reduced incision length, initial preperitoneal dissection, and the use of internal surgical stapling devices. The postoperative care included the use of prokinetic agents, early nasogastric tube removal, the use of non-narcotic analgesics, and the early institution of an oral diet. These advances resulted in improved morbidity and recovery and earlier hospital discharge.

The fast-track approach

Cardiac surgery has led the clinical pathway initiative with the fast-track approach, defined as a perioperative process involving rapid progress from preoperative preparation through surgery and discharge from the hospital [18]. Although highly individualized among the various cardiac surgery centers and dependent on local surgeon preferences and local practices, the fast-track process is a team activity. The necessary elements of the fast-track program are the use of short-acting anesthetic drugs, standardized surgical procedures, early extubation, rewarming and sustained postoperative normothermia, optimal postoperative pain control, early ambulation, alimentation, and discharge, and follow-up after discharge.

This approach has been carefully studied and was not associated with higher 60-day rates of death or readmission in 83,347 Medicare patients who underwent coronary artery bypass grafting in the United States. In fact, risk-adjusted rates of death or cardiovascular readmission were lower among patients discharged earlier [19]. Subsequent studies have confirmed similar findings in Europe [20] and Canada [21].

Fast-tracking has now been applied to other surgical procedures, including pulmonary resections [22,23] and colorectal surgery [24]. Fast-track abdominal aortic aneurysm repair has also been described [25]. This approach requires a cooperative team of motivated individuals, including nurses, anesthesiologists, surgeons, respiratory therapists, and others involved in the perioperative care of patients, and a commitment to continuous reevaluation and improvement of the processes involved. Most importantly, increased efforts in educating patients and providing information about the procedure, the expected time course, and outcome are of great importance, emphasizing the active role of the patient. The implementation of this approach in colorectal surgery was again associated with a shorter hospital stay, reduced morbidity, and no increase in postoperative complications after discharge.

Summary

Clinical pathways are promoted for standardizing patient care, reducing length of stay, and decreasing resource utilization without compromising outcome. Development and improvement of multimodal interventions within the context of fast-track surgery programs represent the major challenge for all medical professionals working to achieve an optimal perioperative course [26]. New approaches in pain control, introduction of techniques that reduce the perioperative stress response, and the more frequent use of minimally invasive surgical techniques will continue to be introduced into clinical pathways in an effort to optimize surgical patient outcomes. Electronic clinical care pathways will be utilized in the future as part of the electronic medical record and may further simplify and standardize patient care to achieve optimal surgical patient outcomes [27].

References

[1] Campbell H, Hotchkiss R, Bradshaw N, et al. Integrated care pathways. BMJ 1998;316: 133–7.

[2] Pearson SD, Goulart-Fisher D, Lee TH. Critical pathways as a strategy for improving care: problems and potential. Ann Intern Med 1995;123:941–8.

[3] Every NR, Hochman J, Becker R, et al, for the Committee on Acute Cardiac Care, Council on Clinical Cardiology, American Heart Association. Critical pathways: a review. AHA Scientific Statement. Circulation 2000;101:461.

[4] Kopec D, Shagas G, Reinharth D, et al. Development of a clinical pathways analysis system with adaptive Bayesian nets and data mining techniques. Stud Health Technol Inform 2004; 103:70–80.

[5] Calland JF, Tanaka K, Foley E, et al. Outpatient laparoscopic cholecystectomy: patient outcomes after implementation of a clinical pathway. Ann Surg 2001;233(5):704–15.

[6] Soria V, Pellicer E, Flores B, et al. Evaluation of the clinical pathway for laparoscopic cholecystectomy. Am Surg 2005;71(1):40–5.

[7] Bradshaw BG, Liu SS, Thirlby RC. Standardized perioperative care protocols and reduced length of stay after colon surgery. J Am Coll Surg 1998;186(5):501–6.

[8] Stephen AE, Berger DL. Shortened length of stay and hospital cost reduction with implementation of an accelerated clinical care pathway after elective colon resection. Surgery 2003;133(3):277–82.

[9] Webster TM, Baumgartner R, Sprunger JK, et al. A clinical pathway for laparoscopic pyeloplasty decreases length of stay. J Urol 2005;173(6):2081–4.

[10] Uchiyama K, Takifuji K, Tani M, et al. Effectiveness of the clinical pathway to decrease length of stay and cost for laparoscopic surgery. Surg Endosc 2002;16(11):1594–7.

[11] Zehr KJ, Dawson PB, Yang SC, et al. Standardized clinical care pathways for major thoracic cases reduce hospital costs. Ann Thorac Surg 1998;66:914–9.

[12] Porter GA, Pisters PW, Mansyur C, et al. Cost and utilization impact of a clinical pathway for patients undergoing pancreaticoduodenectomy. Ann Surg Oncol 2000;7(7):484–9.

[13] Dracass M, Sharland C. Southampton University Hospitals NHS Trust integrated care pathway for revision of total hip replacement. Journal of Integrated Care Pathways 2002; 6:26–51.

[14] Turley K, Tyndall M, Roge C. Critical pathway methodology: effectiveness in congenital heart surgery. Ann Thorac Surg 1994;58:57–65.

[15] DeSomma M, Divekar A, Galloway AC, et al. Impact of a clinical pathway on the postoperative care of children undergoing surgical closure of atrial septal defects. Appl Nurs Res 2002;15(4):243–8.

[16] Yeats M, Wedergren S, Fox N, et al. The use and modification of clinical pathways to achieve specific outcomes in bariatric surgery. Am Surg 2005;71(2):152–4.

[17] Pruthi RS, Chun J, Richman M. Reducing time to oral diet and hospital discharge in patients undergoing radical cystectomy using a perioperative care plan. Urology 2003;62(4):661–5 [discussion: 665–6].

[18] Pande RU, Nader ND, Donias HW, et al. Fast-tracking cardiac surgery: review. Heart Surg Forum 2003;6(4):244–8.

[19] Cowper PA, Peterson ED, DeLong ER, et al. Impact of early discharge after coronary artery bypass graft surgery on rates of hospital readmission and death. The Ischemic Heart Disease (IHD) Patient Outcomes Research Team (PORT) Investigators. J Am Coll Cardiol 1997; 30(4):908–13.

[20] Loubani M, Mediratta N, Hickey MS, et al. Early discharge following coronary bypass surgery: Is it safe? Eur J cardiothoracic Surg 2000;18(1):22–6.

[21] Moon MC, Abdoh A, Hamilton GA, et al. Safety and efficacy of fast track in patients undergoing coronary artery bypass surgery. J Card Surg 2001;16(4):319–26.

[22] Cerfolio RJ, Pickens A, Bass C, et al. Fast-tracking pulmonary resections. J Thorac Cardiovasc Surg 2001;122(2):318–24.

[23] Lin J, Iannettoni MD. Fast-tracking: eliminating roadblocks to successful early discharge. Thorac Surg Clin 2005;15(2):221–8.

[24] Kremer M, Ulrich A, Buchler MW, et al. Fast-track surgery: the Heidelberg experience. Recent Results Cancer Res 2005;165:14–20.

[25] Mukherjee D. Fast-track abdominal aortic aneurysm repair. Vasc Endovasc Surg 2003; 37(5):329 34.

[26] Kehlet H, Wilmore DW. Multimodal strategies to improve surgical outcome. Am J Surg 2002;183(6):630–41.

[27] Clarke A. Implementing electronic integrated care pathways: learning from experience. Nurse Manag 2005;12(2):28–31.

ELSEVIER
SAUNDERS

SURGICAL
CLINICS OF
NORTH AMERICA

Surg Clin N Am 85 (2005) 1329–1340

Patient Safety: Latex Allergy

H. David Reines, MD[a],*, Patricia C. Seifert, RN, MSN[b]

[a]*Department of Surgery, Inova Fairfax Hospital, 3300 Gallows Road,
Falls Church, VA 22042-3300, USA*
[b]*Inova Heart and Vascular Institute, 3300 Gallows Road, Falls Church, VA 22042-3300, USA*

Allergic reaction to the natural material latex rubber is a growing problem. The implications for hospital staff, physicians, and patients make this potentially fatal reaction a serious safety issue for all health practitioners. This article will give the historical background and the scientific basis for the reactions and summarize the various evidenced-based and practical recommendations for balancing requirements related to patient safety with the realities of the current health-care milieu.

History

Indigenous people of Central and South America, as well as Southeastern Asia, have for centuries used rubber, the milky sap of the rubber tree, *Hevea brasiliensis*. Richard Cook first used india rubber for surgical gloves in 1834 [1]. Not until Charles Goodyear developed the process of vulcanization to stabilize rubber and prevent it from easily melting or freezing, did the rubber industry become important. Although J.C. Bloodgood used gloves with his surgical team in 1893 [1], it was William Halsted in 1894 who popularized the use of gloves in surgery. Caroline Hampton, who was Halsted's scrub nurse and later his wife, developed a dermatitis from mercuric chloride used to disinfect instruments. Because of this dermatitis, Halsted required her to use rubber gloves to protect her hands [2]. Other members of his team then began to protect themselves similarly with gloves.

Not until 1928 was a process developed to dip gloves into latex, thereby producing a glove that was both stronger and thinner [1]. These gloves finally gave surgeons enough tactile sensation to become practical. Because of cost, most rubber gloves were washed, spun with powder to prevent

---

* Corresponding author.
E-mail address: h.david.reines@inova.com (H.D. Reines).

doi:10.1016/j.suc.2005.09.014
surgical.theclinics.com

sticking, and then sterilized for reuse. This practice persisted until the 1960s, when disposable gloves came into common use.

Although no randomized prospective studies have proven the efficacy of gloves, conventional wisdom requires sterile gloves for two purposes: 1) to protect the patient from microorganisms of the hands (after a cleaning solution is applied) of the team members, and 2) to protect the team from the transmission of microorganisms and viruses from the patient's blood and fluids. Because of the incidence of perforation of latex gloves (13%) the Occupational Safety and Health Administration recommends double gloving and sterile gloves for all members of the scrubbed surgical team as a Category 1B recommendation [3] after donning a sterile gown.

Latex is used in the operating room not only in the form of gloves, but in many other ways, which makes the elimination of latex problematic. Latex is found in multiple medical products, including blood-pressure cuffs, stethoscopes, oral and nasal airways, tourniquets, Penrose drains, syringes, and electrode pads, as well as in gloves, urinary drainage catheters, esophageal dilators, and ventilator connections. Even intravenous connectors are frequently latex-based. It is estimated that latex is used in 40,000 medical and nonmedical products [1], and therefore exposure to latex is almost unavoidable in everyday life.

The first scientific paper describing dermatitis from rubber gloves was published in 1933 [4]. From 1979 to 1988, multiple reports of localized reactions to gloves appeared in Europe and America. Several reports of anaphylaxis began appearing in the anesthesia literature in the late 1980s [5,6]. However, the problem of latex as an allergen was still not widely recognized. As universal precautions (now termed "standard precautions") became the norm following the recognition that AIDS and other viruses were transmitted through human fluids, the use of latex gloves accelerated. Still, knowledge and concern about latex sensitivity was minimal and the allergic reaction was frequently attributed to other sources. It has been estimated that in 1987, 1 billion gloves were imported for medical use. This grew to 20.8 billion gloves imported in 1996 [7]. In the United States, about 5.6 million health-care workers and other persons now use latex gloves daily [8].

One group identified early on as high risk for latex allergy was spina bifida patients, who frequently undergo numerous operative procedures for multiple reasons [9]. It was thought that the rise in latex-related allergies was related to the deterioration in the latex that occurred with low-quality gloves.

Latex—what is it?

Natural rubber latex is a milky fluid that is a mixture of proteins, phospholipids, and polyisoprene. Natural latex is combined with other chemicals, primarily ammonia, to enhance the natural qualities and yield commercial latex. It is postulated that the latex proteins are the major cause of the

IgE-mediated allergic reaction [10]. Added accelerators and antioxidants may also be significant mediators of the type IV (allergic contact dermatitis) allergic reaction [11].

Latex gloves, balloons, and condoms are made either by molds or by a dipping process. The softest rubber products appear to have the highest allergenic potential. The addition of cornstarch powder to gloves in 1947 to prevent sticking and give a smoother fit has been shown to increase the leaching of latex proteins and exposure of latex proteins on the surface. Cornstarch also promotes aerosolization of the latex proteins when gloves are removed. Low-protein, powder-free gloves decrease the sensitization potential of the latex and avoid some of the granuloma formation associated with powder [11].

Incidence of later allergy

Although data is difficult to obtain, estimates now indicate that 1% to 6% of the general population has some sensitivity or allergy to latex, and about 8% to 12% of health-care workers regularly exposed to latex develop sensitivity. Meanwhile, as many as 20% of operating room personnel may have developed sensitivity [12]. European studies found a 0.9% to 10% incidence of positivity to pin prick, while a Brazilian study found a 6% allergic sensitization rate [13]. Other estimates of latex sensitivity are as high as 17% [14]. Because of the explosion in the incidence of later allergy and the worldwide potential for problems, a better understanding of the problem is required for all health-care providers (Appendix 1).

Latex is ubiquitous in our society and is especially prevalent in the health professions. Exposure occurs frequently through cutaneous contact, although mucous membranes, intravenous routes, and inhalation pathways are all portals of entry. Mucous membranes, especially in the mouth, vagina, and rectum are common areas of exposure. The release of latex particles in the air is particularly dangerous to individuals who are already sensitized. Such release can lead to bronchospasm and laryngeal edema. As noted, the addition of powder to the particles makes them particularly dangerous. Outside the operating room, latex is found in elastic bands, erasers, automobile tires, bicycle handgrips, shoe soles, and pacifiers. Therefore, the incidence of latex sensitivities and allergies will likely grow.

Differentiating later allergic reactions

Reactions to natural rubber latex range from mild irritation to anaphylactic latex allergy (Box 1). Irritant contact dermatitis is the most common reaction and is evidenced by sore, red, dry, and chapped hands. This is a nonallergic reaction that is localized to the skin. Thorough washing and drying of hands, the use of powder-free gloves, and the practice of changing

---

Box 1. Types of latex and other glove-associated reactions

A) Irritation: nonallergic irritation caused by hand washing, insufficient rinsing, and glove powder. Clinical signs: dry, crusty, hard bumps; sore and horizontal cracks on skin, which may itch. Treatment: avoid or remove the irritant and use nonpetroleum-based moisturizing creams.

B) Allergic contact dermatitis: chemical allergy from exposure to chemicals in latex manufacture. Clinical signs: red, raised bumps; sore and horizontal cracks, which may extend up forearm. Signs usually appear slowly after exposure and may persist for days. Treatment: use of moisturizing creams and avoidance of petroleum-based products, which may be latex incompatible. Avoidance of latex especially important if there are breaks in the skin.

C) Latex allergy: type I hypersensitivity from exposure to proteins in latex or suspended in air. Clinical signs: wheal and flare response within minutes of exposure under glove. May mimic irritant and allergic contact dermatitis. Severe forms include facial swelling, generalized urticaria, respiratory distress, and anaphylaxis. Treatment: immediate removal from the latex-containing environment and anaphylaxis therapy if needed.

---

gloves frequently to minimize sweating under the gloves can reduce skin irritation.

Allergic contact dermatitis, which may result from the chemical additives used in the glove manufacturing process, is usually localized to the area of contact. This form of dermatitis is not caused by the latex itself. Repeated exposure to the allergens can lead to increased sensitization and an increasingly severe reaction.

True latex allergy occurs when repeated sensitization to latex produces anti-latex IgE antibodies that stimulate mast cells, basophils, and histamine release. Local and systemic reactions can occur. The allergic reaction is immediate, with symptoms occurring in minutes [15]. The patient may display symptoms of urticaria, laryngeal edema, bronchospasm, and asthma. Anaphylaxis and death can occur. Basic life support should be instituted promptly to maintain the airway, breathing, and circulation. Latex-containing products should be removed promptly.

Latex-induced anaphylaxis has been reported to account for up to 17% of cases of intraoperative anaphylaxis [16]. The diagnosis and management of latex-induced anaphylaxis is reviewed in detail in a national practice parameter on anaphylaxis and summary statements are listed in Box 2 [17]. It's

---

Box 2. Summary of parameters for managing latex-induced anaphylaxis

- Latex (rubber) hypersensitivity is a significant medical problem and three groups are at a higher risk of reaction: health-care workers, children with spina bifida and genitourinary abnormalities, and workers with occupational exposure to latex.
- To identify IgE-mediated sensitivity, skin-prick tests with latex extracts should be considered for patients who are members of high-risk groups or who have a clinical history of possible latex allergy. Although a standardized commercial skin test reagent for latex is not available in the United States, many allergy centers have prepared latex extracts from gloves to be used for clinical testing. Such extracts, prepared from gloves, demonstrate tremendous variability in the content of latex antigen. In vitro assays for IgE are generally less sensitive than skin tests.
- Patients with spina bifida (regardless of a history of latex allergy) and other patients with a positive history of latex allergy ideally should have all medical, surgical, and dental procedures performed in a latex-safe environment and as the first case of the day.
- A latex-free environment is an environment in which no latex gloves are used in the room or surgical suite and no latex accessories (eg, catheters, adhesives, tourniquets, and anesthesia equipment) come into contact with the patient.
- In health-care settings, general use of latex gloves with negligible allergen content, powder-free latex gloves, and non-latex gloves and medical articles should be considered to minimize exposure to latex allergen. Such a combined approach might reduce latex sensitization of health-care workers and patients and should lower the risk of inadvertent reactions to latex in previously sensitized individuals.

From Joint Task Force on Practice Parameters for Allergy & Immunology. The diagnosis and management of anaphylasis: an updated practice parameter. J Allergy Clin Immunol 2005;115:S483–523; with permission.

---

important to convert a latex-free environment during the resuscitation of patients with sudden intraoperative cardiovascular collapse of unknown cause. Latex must always be considered as a potential culprit, even in patients without obvious risk factors [18].

Evidenced-based information

There is no level I evidence-based data about latex-induced anaphylaxis because there is no way to design a study to look at a potentially lethal complication. On the other hand, the goal of zero tolerance is also impractical at this point. Therefore, most findings and recommendations are based on case reports and immunological findings. The recommendations are mostly class C. However, the implications of missing a possible latex allergic patient are significant. Obviously, there are important financial and practical obstacles to becoming latex-free, and each institution and surgeon needs to examine the cost/benefit ratio. However, the following recommendations have emerged from the realization that the problem is spreading and has worldwide implications.

Recommendations

The most certain way to prevent latex allergy is to eliminate latex, a solution that is nearly impossible. The goal should be education and lowering of risk to health-care practitioners and patients. Industry is rapidly responding to the problem with the introduction of latex-free gloves, intravenous needles, tubing, and other medical supplies. Eventually, the marketplace will provide solutions. In the meantime, to reduce the exposure to latex and risk of developing latex allergies in health-related fields, health-care institutions should adopt practical recommendations that protect personnel.

Preoperative screening

Screening patients is the first step for minimizing the risk of a latex allergic reaction. Practice guidelines for determining latex sensitivity are imperative to ensure that all patients are identified. Patients first should be asked if they have a confirmed latex sensitivity or allergy. Patients at special risk even without documented latex allergy are those individuals with frequent or prolonged exposure to latex products. This group can include health-care workers who have worn gloves for long periods and patients who have undergone multiple surgeries or procedures. Three groups are at higher risk of later allergic reaction: health-care workers, patients with spina bifida or genitourinary abnormalities, and workers with occupational exposure to latex. These individuals may display irritant or contact dermatitis. Allergic patients may show signs of skin rash, hives, itching, flushing, rhinitis, and shock.

Patients with a history of allergy (eg, asthma, environmental or drug allergens) or a history of unexplained anaphylaxis during surgical, dental, or interventional procedures may also be at risk. When a history of latex sensitivity is suspected, a patient questionnaire, such as the questionnaire in Box 3, can be administered.

Box 3. Patient questionnaire for detecting latex sensitivity

1. Have you ever had allergies, asthma, hay fever, eczema, or problems with rashes?
2. Have you ever had anaphylaxis or an unexpected reaction during a medical procedure?
3. Have you ever had swelling, itching, or hives on your lips or around your mouth after blowing up a balloon?
4. Have you ever had swelling, itching, or hives on your lips or around your mouth during or after a dental examination or procedure?
5. Have you ever had swelling, itching, or hives following a vaginal or rectal examination or after contact with a diaphragm or condom?
6. Have you ever had swelling, itching, or hives on your hands during or within 1 hour after wearing rubber gloves?
7. Have you ever had a rash on your hands that lasted longer than 1 week?
8. Have you ever had swelling, itching, or hives after being examined by someone wearing rubber or latex gloves?
9. Have you ever had swelling, itching, hives, running nose, eye irritation, wheezing, or asthma after contact with any latex or rubber product?
10. Has a physician told you that you have rubber or latex allergy?
11. Are you allergic to bananas, avocados, chestnuts, pears, figs, papayas, or passion fruit?
12. Are you presently on beta-blockers?

Data from Association of periOperative Registered Nurses. AORN latex guidelines. In AORN: 2004 standards, recommended practices and guidelines. Denver (CO): AORN, 2004. Latex sensitivity: current issues. Healthc Hazard Mater Manage 1999;16:103–118. Catalano K. Risk management and latex allergies. Surgical Services Management 1997;42:44–6.

The National Institute for Occupational Safety and Health (NIOSH) [19] recommends steps that employers, workers, and patients can take to reduce latex exposure and to protect patients with possible allergies from undue risk. Those steps are listed in Box 4:

Setting up a latex-safe operating room

Setting up a latex-safe operating room begins with educating staff about the incidence, risk factors, identification, and management of latex sensitivity.

Box 4. NIOSH steps for reducing latex exposure

Steps for employers
1. Provide workers with non-latex gloves to use when there is little potential for contact with infectious materials (eg, food industry workers).
2. Appropriate barrier protection is necessary when handling infectious material [20]. If latex gloves are chosen, provide reduced-protein, powder-free gloves to protect workers from infectious materials.
3. Ensure that workers use good housekeeping practices to remove latex-containing dust from the workplace.
4. Provide workers with education programs and training materials about latex allergy. Post signs and materials in visible places.
5. Periodically screen workers for latex allergy symptoms.

Steps for all workers
1. Use non-latex gloves when possible, especially when not dealing with infectious materials
2. If latex barrier protection is used, choose powder-free gloves with reduced protein content [21].
3. Wash hands after removing latex-containing gloves.
4. Learn to recognize the signs and symptoms of latex allergy and report them promptly

Steps for workers dealing directly with patients
1. Urge patients to notify health-care workers of latex sensitivity.
2. Assess all patients for latex sensitivity.
3. Administer patient questionnaire (Box 3) to patients with suspected or known sensitivity.
4. Apply latex allergy band or medic alert bracelet to patients with suspected or known sensitivity.
5. Perform latex sensitivity testing on patient as indicated.
6. Advise patients that latex is present in many surgical supplies.
7. Institute basic life support to patients with allergic reaction to latex.
8. Use latex-free products for patients with suspected or known sensitivity.
9. Follow institutional latex-safe policy for patients with suspected or known sensitivity.

Adapted from the National Institute of Occupational Safety and Health (NIOSH). Latex allergy: a prevention guide. Available at: www.cdc.gov/niosh/98-113.html. US Department of Health and Human Services, 1999.

Protocols, policies, and procedures related to latex safety should be developed and implemented. Collaborating and communicating with pharmacy, dietary, and other departments can help to avoid latex exposure on, for example, drug vials and food trays. Mock latex allergy situations should be performed at least annually to maintain staff competency.

Health-care workers should identify and avoid (when possible) latex products in the operating room. Identifying alternative products and storing them away from latex products provides latex-free resources for patients suspected or known to have sensitivity. Institutions should consider purchasing latex-free procedure modules for anesthesia and surgical specialties. Developing a mobile cart containing latex-free supplies for sensitive patients facilitates a rapid response.

When a patient is identified as being latex sensitive, the latex-free case should be scheduled as the first of the day. The operating room should be cleaned (with non-latex gloves) before the patient enters the surgical suite. The operating room itself should be closed for 30 minutes after cleaning. Frequent cleaning of areas and equipment contaminated with latex-containing dust can reduce the number of ambient latex particles [21].

Staff should use latex-free gloves and thoroughly wash their hands with soap and dry after removing gloves. Nitrile (eg, polymer of butadiene, acrylonitrile, and carboxylic acid) and neoprene (chloroprene) are acceptable for prolonged exposure to blood and body fluids. Vinyl (polyvinyl chloride) does not provide sufficient barrier protection against blood and body fluids. The management of cardiac surgery patients with latex allergy can be particularly challenging, and an integrated multidisciplinary approach is necessary [22].

Cost considerations

Computing the cost of latex allergy requires a review of morbidity, mortality, and financial factors. Studies have demonstrated cost savings (One institution realized savings of $200,000.) when converting to low-powder or powder-free gloves [23,24]. Removing latex gloves (and other latex products) altogether from a supply inventory is an option undergoing increasing scrutiny.

In a cost analysis of health-care worker disability from latex allergy and asthma, Phillips and colleagues [25] found that health-care facilities can save money by creating a latex-safe environment. In their study, they focused on the cost of replacing latex gloves with non-latex gloves. The investigators compared those costs to the payments for workers' compensation. The study calculated the value of total disability wage replacement for one employee with latex allergy at $108,917. The cost of partial disability for one employee was $61,988. When only the cost of gloves was considered, the latex-free approach was more expensive than the continued use of latex

---

Box 5. Latex-related cost considerations

Sick leave of latex-sensitive staff
Diagnostic tests to determine sensitivity
Latex-related medical care
Decreased staff productivity
Lost staff work time
Employee turnover
Workers' compensation
Cancelled or delayed surgery for latex-sensitive patients
Latex supply replacement
In-service training for staff
Time for developing policies and procedures
Regulatory accommodation (eg, compliance with Americans with
    Disabilities Act)

---

gloves. When other factors were considered (Box 5), the latex-safe approach was more cost-effective, even when latex disability levels were very low.

Summary

As the use of latex has increased, so has the concern over latex reactions among health-care providers. To reduce the risk to health-care personnel and patients, surgeons need to insist on powder-free gloves and be willing to use latex-free products when possible [26]. Converting operating rooms to latex-free environments may be necessary in the future. For now, however, the goals are to lessen exposure to latex-containing products and create a latex-safe environment [23]. Screening for latex allergy, educating health-care providers to the problem, and alerting patients to be aware of the possible risks are all necessary for ensuring the safety and effectiveness of the health-care system. A team approach to eliminate the problem is necessary, and surgeon buy-in is a key element of the solution. The recommendations given above can help establish a framework to minimize or prevent serious latex-related reactions.

Appendix 1. Definitions related to latex sensitivity

> **Allergen**. A substance that can induce an allergic or specific hypersensitivity reaction; an antigen.
> **Allergy**. An immune response to an antigen producing a symptomatic reaction in a susceptible individual.
> **Dermatitis**. Inflammation of the skin.

Allergic contact dermatitis. (Type IV, delayed hypersensitivity) A delayed, T-cell—mediated, hypersensitivity reaction attributed to antigenic chemicals added during the harvesting, processing, or manufacturing of latex products.

Irritant contact dermatitis. Nonallergic, localized cutaneous response to a substance contacting the skin.

Latex. Viscid, milky juice secreted by the rubber tree *Hevea brasiliensis*; contains lipids, phospholipids, proteins, carbohydrates, and cis-1, 4-polyisoprene; also known as natural rubber latex.

Latex allergy. (Type I, type IgE-mediated, immediate hypersensitivity) Localized or systemic allergic response to one or more latex proteins (antigens) to which the individual has been sensitized and developed antibodies; true latex allergy.

Latex-free environment. An environment in which all latex-containing products have been removed.

Latex-safe environment. An environment in which every reasonable effort has been made to remove high-allergen and airborne latex sources from coming into direct contact with affected individuals.

Sensitization. Immunological memory in response to exposure to an antigen.

Sensitivity. Clinical expression of symptoms developing after sensitization.

Data from Association of periOperative Registered Nurses. AORN latex guidelines. In: AORN: 2004 standards, recommended practices and guidelines. Denver (CO): AORN; 2004. p. 103–18. Janeway CA, et al. The induction, measurement, and manipulation of the immune response. In: Immuno biology: the immune system in health and disease, 4th edition. New York: Elsevier; 1999, p. 33–75. American Society of Anesthesiologists Natural rubber latex allergy: considerations for anesthesiologists. Available at: http://www.asahq.org/publicationsAndServices/latexallergy.html. Accessed October 19, 2003. National Institute for Occupational Safety and Health (NIOSH). Preventing allergic reactions to natural rubber latex in the workplace. Available at: http://www.cdc.gov/niosh/latexalthtml. Accessed February 26, 2005.

Further reading

American Latex Allergy Association, www.latexallergyresources.org.

References

[1] Dyck RJ. Historical development of latex allergy. AORN J 2000;72(1):27–40.
[2] Miller JM. William Stewart Halsted and the use of the surgical rubber glove. Surgery 1982; 92:541–3.
[3] Occupational Safety & Health Administration (OSHA). Safety and health topics: latex allergy. Available at: www.osha.gov/SLTC/latexallergy/index.html. Accessed October 17, 2005.

[4] Downing J. Dermatitis from rubber gloves. N Engl J Med 1933;208:196–8.

[5] Hancock DL. Latex allergy: prevention and treatment. Anesthesiol Rev 1994;21:153–63.

[6] Leynadier F, Pecquet C, Dry J. Anaphylaxis to latex during surgery. Anaesthesia 1989;44:547–50.

[7] US Food and Drug Administration. Center for Devices and Radiological Health. Medical glove powder report. Available at www.fda.gov/cdrh/glvpwd.html. Accessed April 24, 2005.

[8] Muller BA. Minimizing latex exposure and allergy. Postgrad Med 2003;113(4):91–7.

[9] Sussman GL. Latex allergy: an overview. Canadian Journal of Allergy and Clinical Immunology 2000;5:317–22.

[10] Reddy S. Latex allergy. American Family Physician 1988:57(1). Available at http://www.aafp.org/afp/98101/reddy.html. Accessed April 11, 2005.

[11] Kwittken P, Sweinberg S. Childhood latex allergy: an overview. American Journal of Asthma and Allergies in Pediatrics 1992;6:27–33.

[12] Porri F, et al. Prevalence of latex sensitization in subjects attending health screening: implications for a perioperative screening. Clin Exp Allergy 1997;27(April):413–7.

[13] Lopes RAM, Benatti MCC, Zollner RL. A review of latex sensitivity related to the use of latex gloves in hospitals. AORN J 2004;80(1):64–71.

[14] Reed D. Update on latex allergy among health care personnel. AORN J 2003;78(3):409–26.

[15] Latex sensitivity: current issues. Healthc Hazard Mater Manage 1999;16:1–12.

[16] Alenius H, Kurup V, Kelly K, et al. Latex allergy: frequent occurrence of IgE antibodies to a cluster of 11 latex proteins in patients with spina bifida and histories of anaphylaxis. J Lab Clin Med 1994;123:712–20.

[17] Joint Task Force on Practice Parameters. The diagnosis and management of anaphylaxis: an updated practice parameter. J Allergy Clin Immunol 2005;115:S483–523.

[18] Hebl JR, Hall BA, Sprung J. Prolonged cardiovascular collapse due to unrecognized latex anaphylaxis. Anesth Analg 2004;98:1124–6.

[19] National Institute of Occupational Safety & Health (NIOSH). Latex allergy: a prevention guide. Available at: www.cdc.gov/niosh/98-113.html. Accessed October 17, 2005.

[20] Fogg DM. Infection prevention and control. In: Rothrock JC, editor. Alexander's care of the patient in surgery. 12th edition. St Louis (MO): Mosby; 2003. p. 97–158.

[21] Association of periOperative Registered Nurses. AORN latex guidelines. In: AORN: 2004 Standards, Recommended Practices and Guidelines. Denver (CO): AORN, 2005. p. 103–18.

[22] Rossi M, De Paulis S, Gaudino M, et al. Managing latex-free mitral valve replacement. Ann Thoracic Surgery 2005;79(2):703–5.

[23] Yip ES. Accommodating latex allergy concerns. AORN J 2003;78(4):595–603.

[24] Hunt LW, et al. Management of occupational allergy to natural rubber latex in a medical center: the importance of quantitative latex allergen measurement and objective follow-up. J Allergy Clin Immunol 2002;110(2)(Suppl):S96–106.

[25] Phillips VL, Goodrich MA, Sullivan TJ. Health care worker disability due to latex allergy and asthma: a cost analysis. Am J Public Health 1999;89:1024–8.

[26] Meyer KK, Beezhold DH. Latex allergy: how safe are your gloves? Bulletin of the American College of Surgeons 1997;82(7). Available at www.latexallergylinks.org/ACSBulletin.html. Accessed February 26, 2005.

ELSEVIER
SAUNDERS

Surg Clin N Am 85 (2005) 1341–1346

SURGICAL
CLINICS OF
NORTH AMERICA

Risk-adjusted Outcomes and Perioperative Care

Lena M. Napolitano, MD[a,b,*], Barbara L. Bass, MD[c]

[a]University of Michigan School of Medicine, Ann Arbor, MI, USA
[b]Department of Surgery, University of Michigan Medical Center,
1500 East Medical Center Drive, Ann Arbor, MI 48109, USA
[c]Carolyn and John F. Bookout Chair, Department of Surgery,
The Methodist Hospital, 6550 Fannin, Ste 1661A, Houston, TX 77030, USA

The ultimate measure of whether perioperative care has been optimal is the determination of patient outcome. Outcome-based comparative measures of the quality of surgical care among surgical services and surgical subspecialties have been elusive in the past. During the past decade there has been a great interest in surgical outcomes research focused on adequate risk adjustment of surgical patients. This initiative has been led by the National Surgery Quality Improvement Program (NSQIP) of the Department of Veterans Affairs (VA).

National Surgery Quality Improvement Program

During the mid- to late-1980s, the VA came under a great deal of public scrutiny over the quality of surgical care in their 133 VA hospitals. At issue were the operative mortality rates in the VA hospitals and the perception in Congress that these rates were significantly higher than the national (private sector) norm. To address the gap, Congress passed law 99-166, which mandated the VA to report its surgical outcomes annually, on a risk-adjusted basis to factor in a patient's severity of illness, and to compare these outcomes with national averages.

VA surgeons recognized that there were no national averages or risk-adjustment models for the various surgical specialties. Prompted by the 1986 congressional mandate, the VA conducted the National VA Surgical

* Corresponding author. Department of Surgery, University of Michigan Health System, Room 1C421, University Hospital, 1500 East Medical Center Drive, Ann Arbor, MI 48109.
E-mail address: lenan@umich.edu (L.M. Napolitano).

0039-6109/05/$ - see front matter © 2005 Elsevier Inc. All rights reserved.
doi:10.1016/j.suc.2005.10.014
surgical.theclinics.com

Risk Study (NVASRS) in 44 VA medical centers between October 1,1991, and December 31,1993 [1]. The aim was to develop and validate risk-adjustment models for the prediction of surgical outcome and the comparative assessment of the quality of surgical care among multiple facilities.

A dedicated clinical nurse reviewer in each medical center collected preoperative, intraoperative, and 30-day outcome variables (Box 1) on a total of more than 117,000 major operations. Using these data, the NVASRS was able to develop risk models for 30-day mortality and morbidity in nine surgical specialties. Additionally, they found that the risk-adjusted outcomes produced by the models matched the quality of systems and processes in the hospitals. Their work allowed, for the first time, a comparative measurement of the quality of surgical care in the nine specialties.

The NVASRS also demonstrated that significant differences in several dimensions of process and structure of the delivery of surgical care were associated with differences in risk-adjusted surgical morbidity and mortality among the 44 VA medical centers [2].

A subsequent publication reported NSQIP data including major surgical procedures (n = 417,944) performed between October 1, 1991, and September 30, 1997 [3]. This study established that, since 1994, the 30-day mortality and morbidity rates for major surgery had fallen 9% and 30%, respectively, in the VA hospitals. This study also established that reliable, valid information on patient presurgical risk factors, process of care during surgery, and 30-day morbidity and mortality rates could be captured for all major surgical procedures in the 123 VA hospitals performing surgery. The VA established the first prospective outcome-based program for comparative assessment and enhancement of the quality of surgical care among multiple institutions for several surgical subspecialties.

The success of the NVASRS study encouraged the VA to establish an ongoing program for monitoring and improving the quality of surgical care across all VA medical centers, and the NSQIP was initiated. The NSQIP

Box 1. Data capture elements for the National Surgery Quality Improvement Program

The following variables are collected on each surgical case:
  Demographics: 9 variables
  Surgical profile: 9 variables
  Preoperative data: 40 clinical variables and 13 laboratory
    variables
  Intraoperative data: 18 clinical variables and 3 occurrence
    variables
  Postoperative data: 20 occurrence variables, 12 laboratory
    variables, and 9 discharge variables

determined the most predictive preoperative risk factors for mortality in noncardiac surgery (Table 1) [3], with the top five risk factors confirmed as (1) admission serum albumin level, (2) American Society of Anesthesiology class, (3) disseminated cancer, (4) emergency operation, and (5) increased age. Careful tracking of postoperative complications and occurrences (Box 2) was also an important component of NSQIP.

Since the inception of the NSQIP data collection process, the 30-day postoperative mortality after major surgery in the VA has decreased by 27%, and the 30-day morbidity has decreased by 45%; median postoperative length of hospital stay has been reduced from 9 to 4 days, and patient satisfaction has improved [4]. In October 2002, the Institute of Medicine named the NSQIP the "best in the nation" for measuring and reporting surgical quality and outcomes.

The National Surgery Quality Improvement Program and perioperative care

The importance of the use of risk-adjusted outcomes in surgery as related to perioperative care has been clearly documented. Specific risk factors (including general anesthesia and blood transfusion) are associated with increased risk for pneumonia [5]. Additional studies have documented that anemia and blood transfusion are associated with increased risk for

Table 1
Most predictive preoperative risk factors for mortality in noncardiac surgery patients

Risk Factor	Order of Entry into Logistic Regression Model for All Operations				
	Phase 1	Phase 2	FY 96	FY 97	Average Rank
Serum albumin (G/dl)	1	1	1	1	1
ASA class	2	2	2	2	2
Disseminated cancer	4	3	3	3	3.3
Emergency operation	3	4	5	5	4.3
Age	5	5	4	6	5
BUN > 40 mg/dl	6	7	6	9	7
DNR	7	10	8	4	7.3
Operation complexity score	12	9	10	13	11
SGOT > 40 IU/ml	11	8	9	17	11.3
Weight Loss > 10% in 6 months	9	13	14	10	11.5
Functional status	24	6	11	8	12.3
WBC > 11,000/mm^3	16	14	15	11	14

Abbreviations: ASA, American Society of Anesthesiology; BUN, blood urea nitrogen; DNR, do nor resuscitate; SGOT, serum giutarnic; WBC, white blood cell count.

From Khuri SF, Daley J, Henderson W, et al. The Department of Veterans Affairs' NSQIP: the first national, validated, outcome-based, risk-adjusted, and peer-controlled program for the measurement and enhancement of the quality of surgical care. National VA Surgical Quality Improvement Program. Ann Surg 1998;228(4):501; with permission.

Box 2. Postoperative occurrences collected by the National Surgery Quality Improvement Program

Wound occurrences
Superficial incisional surgical site infection
Deep incisional surgical site infection
Organ/space surgical site infection
Wound disruption

Respiratory occurrences
Ventilator support needed for longer than 48 hours
Pneumonia
Pulmonary embolism
Unplanned intubation

Urinary tract occurrences
Acute renal failure
Progressive renal insufficiency
Urinary tract infection

Cardiac occurrences
Cardiac arrest requiring cardiopulmonary resuscitation
Myocardial infarction

Central nervous system occurrences
Coma for more than 24 hours
Peripheral nerve injury
Stroke/cerebrovascular accident

Other surgical occurrences
Bleeding/transfusions
Deep vein thrombosis/thrombophlebitis
Graft/prosthesis/flap failure
Sepsis
Septic shock
Systemic inflammatory response syndrome

---

perioperative infection and mortality [6]. Future studies in perioperative care will require the use of risk-adjusted outcome measures.

The National Surgery Quality Improvement Program private sector initiative

In 1999, the private sector became interested in the NSQIP. It was unclear whether the NSQIP methodology was applicable outside the VA and if the risk-adjustment models would hold true for private sector patient populations, which are more heterogeneous than the predominantly male population in the VA system.

A pilot study initiated in 1999 determined the feasibility of implementing the NSQIP in non-VA hospitals. Surgeons at three academic nonfederal hospitals (Emory University, the University of Michigan, and University of Kentucky) volunteered to participate in the pilot study and to donate the time of a nurse coordinator to collect data. The pilot study included only general and vascular surgery. The three centers found that after the first complete year of analysis both the data collection/transmission methods and the predictive and risk-adjustment models of the NSQIP were applicable to their non-VA environments [7].

Administrative databases

Administrative databases that rely primarily on information collected for billing purposes increasingly have been used as tools for public reporting of outcomes quality. Comparative studies assessing correlation between administration data and clinical data collected for quality assurance purposes (eg, NSQIP and the Society of Thoracic Surgeons database) document significant variance between the two, with greater error identified in the administrative databases. A recent study of cardiac surgery found that mortality in administrative data exceeded that reported in clinical data by 21% [8].

The American College of Surgeons National Surgery Quality Improvement Program

In 2001, the American College of Surgeons (ACS) began to take an active interest in the NSQIP and its results in reducing surgical mortality and morbidity rates. The development of a national system to collect and report risk-adjusted event data for surgical services was of great importance to the ACS.

Based on the success of the pilot program, and in collaboration with the VA, the ACS applied for an Agency for Health care Research and Quality grant to expand the program further into the private sector. Funding was awarded to the ACS to expand the pilot program to an additional 14 medical centers including Massachusetts General Hospital, the University of Virginia Medical Center, and New York's Columbia Presbyterian Hospital. Later, data were included from four affiliated community hospitals. The NSQIP functioned well in the 18 private-sector hospitals. Three years of private-sector experience have demonstrated the effectiveness of the NSQIP as a quality improvement tool and as a source of new clinical knowledge for hospitals outside the VA system.

The ACS has announced the expansion of the ACS National Surgical Quality Improvement Program (ACS NSQIP) to all private-sector hospitals that meet the minimum participation requirements. The ACS believes that

NSQIP is one of the best ways to benchmark and improve surgical care. The program includes continuously updated and available Web-based benchmark reporting, ongoing nurse training and data audits, and annual clinical performance reports and evaluations. The VA program will continue its parallel system (the VA NSQIP) and will continue to compare its results against the ACS NSQIP private-sector data.

Summary

Risk-adjusted patient outcomes are developing as accurate measures of adequacy of perioperative care. NSQIP has become the standard tool for assessment of risk-adjusted mortality and morbidity in surgical patients in the United States.

References

[1] Khuri SF, Daley J, Henderson W, et al. The National Veterans Administration Surgical Risk Study: risk adjustment for the comparative assessment of the quality of surgical care. J Am Coll Surg 1995;180(5):519–31.

[2] Daley J, Forbes MG, Young GJ, et al. Validating risk-adjusted surgical outcomes: site visit assessment of process and structure. National VA Surgical Risk Study. J Am Coll Surg 1997;185(4):341–51.

[3] Khuri SF, Daley J, Henderson W, et al. The Department of Veterans Affairs' NSQIP: the first national, validated, outcome-based, risk-adjusted, and peer-controlled program for the measurement and enhancement of the quality of surgical care. National VA Surgical Quality Improvement Program. Ann Surg 1998;228(4):491–507.

[4] Khuri SF, Daley J, Henderson WG. The comparative assessment and improvement of quality of surgical care in the Department of Veterans Affairs. Arch Surg 2002;137(1):20–7.

[5] Arozullah AM, Khuri SF, Henderson WG, et al, for the participants in the National Veterans Affairs Surgical Quality Improvement Program. Development and validation of a multifactorial risk index for predicting postoperative pneumonia after major noncardiac surgery. Ann Intern Med 2001;135(10):847–57.

[6] Dunne JR, Malone D, Tracy JK, et al. Perioperative anemia: an independent risk factor for infection, mortality, and resource utilization in surgery. J Surg Res 2002;102(2):237–44.

[7] Fink AS, Campbell DA Jr, Mentzer RJ Jr, et al. The National Surgical Quality Improvement Program in non-Veterans Administration hospitals: initial demonstration of feasibility. Ann Surg 2002;236(3):344–53 [discussion: 353–4].

[8] Mack MJ, Herbert M, Prince S, et al. Does reporting of coronary artery bypass grafting from administrative databases accurately reflect actual clinical outcome? J Thorac Cardiovasc Surg 2005;129(6):1309–17.

ELSEVIER
SAUNDERS

Surg Clin N Am 85 (2005) 1347–1380

SURGICAL
CLINICS OF
NORTH AMERICA

Cumulative Index 2005

Note: Page numbers of article titles are in **boldface** type.

Changing Your Address?

Make sure your subscription changes too! When you notify us of your new address, you can help make our job easier by including an exact copy of your Clinics label number with your old address (see illustration below.) This number identifies you to our computer system and will speed the processing of your address change. Please be sure this label number accompanies your old address and your corrected address—you can send an old Clinics label with your number on it or just copy it exactly and send it to the address listed below.

We appreciate your help in our attempt to give you continuous coverage. Thank you.

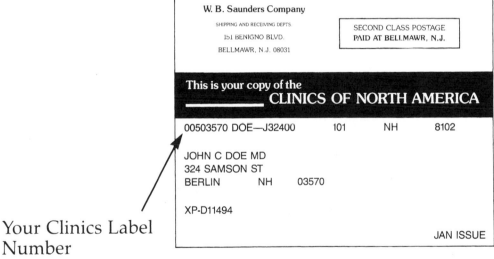

W. B. Saunders Company

SHIPPING AND RECEIVING DEPTS.
151 BENIGNO BLVD.
BELLMAWR, N.J. 08031

SECOND CLASS POSTAGE
PAID AT BELLMAWR, N.J.

This is your copy of the
CLINICS OF NORTH AMERICA

00503570 DOE—J32400   101   NH   8102

JOHN C DOE MD
324 SAMSON ST
BERLIN   NH   03570

XP-D11494

JAN ISSUE

Your Clinics Label Number
Copy it exactly or send your label
along with your address to:
W.B. Saunders Company, Customer Service
Orlando, FL 32887-4800
Call Toll Free 1-800-654-2452

Please allow four to six weeks for delivery of new subscriptions and for processing address changes.

United States Postal Service
Statement of Ownership, Management, and Circulation

1. Publication Title	2. Publication Number										3. Filing Date
Surgical Clinics of North America	0	0	3	9	-	6	1	0	0	9	9/15/05

4. Issue Frequency	5. Number of Issues Published Annually	6. Annual Subscription Price
Feb, Apr, Jun, Aug, Oct, Dec	6	$190.00

7. Complete Mailing Address of Known Office of Publication (Not printer) (Street, city, county, state, and ZIP+4)

Elsevier Inc.
6277 Sea Harbor Drive
Orlando, FL 32887-4800

Contact Person
Gwen C. Campbell

Telephone
215-239-3685

8. Complete Mailing Address of Headquarters or General Business Office of Publisher (Not printer)

Elsevier Inc, 360 Park Avenue South, New York, NY 10010-1710

9. Full Names and Complete Mailing Addresses of Publisher, Editor, and Managing Editor (Do not leave blank)

Publisher (Name and complete mailing address)

Tim Griswold, Elsevier Inc., 1600 John F. Kennedy Blvd., Suite 1800, Philadelphia, PA 19103-2899

Editor (Name and complete mailing address)

Catherine Bewick, Elsevier Inc., 1600 John F. Kennedy Blvd., Suite 1800, Philadelphia, PA 19103-2899

Managing Editor (Name and complete mailing address)

Heather Cullen, Elsevier Inc., 1600 John F. Kennedy Blvd., Suite 1800, Philadelphia, PA 19103-2899

10. Owner (Do not leave blank. If the publication is owned by a corporation, give the name and address of the corporation immediately followed by the names and addresses of all stockholders owning or holding 1 percent or more of the total amount of stock. If not owned by a corporation, give the names and addresses of the individual owners. If owned by a partnership or other unincorporated firm, give its name and address as well as those of each individual owner. If the publication is published by a nonprofit organization, give its name and address.)

Full Name	Complete Mailing Address
Wholly owned subsidiary of	4520 East-West Highway
Reed/Elsevier Inc. US holdings	Bethesda, MD 20814

11. Known Bondholders, Mortgagees, and Other Security Holders Owning or Holding 1 Percent or More of Total Amount of Bonds, Mortgages, or Other Securities. If none, check box ☐ None

Full Name	Complete Mailing Address
N/A	

12. Tax Status (For completion by nonprofit organizations authorized to mail at nonprofit rates) (Check one)
The purpose, function, and nonprofit status of this organization and the exempt status for federal income tax purposes:
☐ Has Not Changed During Preceding 12 Months
☐ Has Changed During Preceding 12 Months (Publisher must submit explanation of change with this statement)

(See Instructions on Reverse)

PS Form 3526, October 1999

13. Publication Title			14. Issue Date for Circulation Data Below
Surgical Clinics of North America			August 2005

15.	Extent and Nature of Circulation		Average No. Copies Each Issue During Preceding 12 Months	No. Copies of Single Issue Published Nearest to Filing Date
a.	Total Number of Copies (Net press run)		7067	6700
b. Paid and/or Requested Circulation	(1)	Paid/Requested Outside-County Mail Subscriptions Stated on Form 3541. (Include advertiser's proof and exchange copies)	3625	3449
	(2)	Paid In-County Subscriptions Stated on Form 3541 (Include advertiser's proof and exchange copies)		
	(3)	Sales Through Dealers and Carriers, Street Vendors, Counter Sales, and Other Non-USPS Paid Distribution	1966	1947
	(4)	Other Classes Mailed Through the USPS		
c.	Total Paid and/or Requested Circulation [Sum of 15b. (1), (2), (3), and (4)]	▲	5591	5396
d. Free Distribution by Mail (Samples, complimentary, and other free)	(1)	Outside-County as Stated on Form 3541	131	182
	(2)	In-County as Stated on Form 3541		
	(3)	Other Classes Mailed Through the USPS		
e.	Free Distribution Outside the Mail (Carriers or other means)			
f.	Total Free Distribution (Sum of 15d. and 15e.)	▲	131	182
g.	Total Distribution (Sum of 15c. and 15f.)	▲	5722	5578
h.	Copies not Distributed		1345	1122
i.	Total (Sum of 15g. and h.)	▲	7067	6700
j.	Percent Paid and/or Requested Circulation (15c. divided by 15g. times 100)		98%	97%

16. Publication of Statement of Ownership
☐ Publication required. Will be printed in the December 2005 issue of this publication.   ☐ Publication not required

17. Signature and Title of Editor, Publisher, Business Manager, or Owner

[signature]

Tim Fanucci – Executive Director of Subscription Services

Date 9/15/05

I certify that all information furnished on this form is true and complete. I understand that anyone who furnishes false or misleading information on this form or who omits material or information requested on the form may be subject to criminal sanctions (including fines and imprisonment) and/or civil sanctions (including civil penalties).

Instructions to Publishers

1. Complete and file one copy of this form with your postmaster annually on or before October 1. Keep a copy of the completed form for your records.

2. In cases where the stockholder or security holder is a trustee, include in items 10 and 11 the name of the person or corporation for whom the trustee is acting. Also include the names and addresses of individuals who are stockholders who own or hold 1 percent or more of the total amount of bonds, mortgages, or other securities of the publishing corporation. In item 11, if none, check the box. Use blank sheets if more space is required.

3. Be sure to furnish all circulation information called for in item 15. Free circulation must be shown in items 15d, e, and f.

4. Item 15h., Copies not Distributed, must include (1) newsstand copies originally stated on Form 3541, and returned to the publisher, (2) estimated returns from news agents, and (3), copies for office use, leftovers, spoiled, and all other copies not distributed.

5. If the publication had Periodicals authorization as a general or requester publication, this Statement of Ownership, Management, and Circulation must be published; it must be printed in any issue in October or, if the publication is not published during October, the first issue printed after October.

6. In item 16, indicate the date of the issue in which this Statement of Ownership will be published.

7. Item 17 must be signed.

Failure to file or publish a statement of ownership may lead to suspension of Periodicals authorization.

PS Form 3526, October 1999 (Reverse)